**Practical
Diabetes Care**

D1158980

Cover illustration: Continuous glucose monitoring study (FreeStyle Navigator(R), Abbott) of a type 1 male one year after a combined pancreas-pre-emptive kidney transplant. Diagnosed age 10, duration 30 years; advanced neuropathic complications, stage 4 CKD. Near-constant glucose levels 5 mmol/L overnight, with post-meal levels rarely above 10 mmol/L. Blood glucose oscillations during the day in part may be caused by glucose intake in response to perceived hypoglycaemia, not documented during this study. Almost non-diabetic HbA$_{1c}$ 5.8% (40 mmol/mol).

Practical Diabetes Care

THIRD EDITION

David Levy MD FRCP

Consultant Physician, Gillian Hanson Centre
Whipps Cross University Hospital;
Honorary Senior Lecturer
Queen Mary University of London
London, UK

WILEY-BLACKWELL

A John Wiley & Sons, Ltd., Publication

This edition first published 2011, © 2011 by David Levy.
1st edition 1998 (Greenwich Medical Media/Cambridge University Press)
2nd edition 2006 (Altman Publications)

Blackwell Publishing was acquired by John Wiley & Sons in February 2007. Blackwell's publishing program has been merged with Wiley's global Scientific, Technical and Medical business to form Wiley-Blackwell.

Registered office: John Wiley & Sons Ltd, The Atrium, Southern Gate, Chichester, West Sussex, PO19 8SQ, UK

Editorial offices: 9600 Garsington Road, Oxford, OX4 2DQ, UK
The Atrium, Southern Gate, Chichester, West Sussex, PO19 8SQ, UK
111 River Street, Hoboken, NJ 07030-5774, USA

For details of our global editorial offices, for customer services and for information about how to apply for permission to reuse the copyright material in this book please see our website at www.wiley.com/wiley-blackwell

Library of Congress Cataloging-in-Publication Data:

Levy, David, 1954- author.
Practical diabetes care / David Levy, MD, FRCP, Consultant Physician, Gillian Hanson Centre, Whipps Cross University Hospital; Honorary Senior Lecturer, Queen Mary University of London, London, UK.—Third Edition.
       p. ; cm.
   Includes bibliographical references and index.
   ISBN 978-1-4443-3385-5 (pbk. : alk. paper)—ISBN 978-1-4443-9113-8 (ePDF)—ISBN 978-1-4443-9115-2 (Wiley online library)—ISBN 978-1-4443-9114-5 (ePub)
   1. Diabetes—Treatment. 2. Primary care (Medicine) I. Title.
   [DNLM: 1. Diabetes Mellitus—therapy. 2. Diabetes Mellitus—diagnosis.
WK 815]
      RC660.H553 2011
      616.4′62—dc22   2010047258

ISBN: 978-1-4443-3385-5

A catalogue record for this book is available from the British Library.

This book is published in the following electronic formats: ePDF 9781444391138; Wiley Online Library 9781444391152; ePub 9781444391145

Set in 9/12pt Palatino by MPS Limited, a Macmillan Company, Chennai, India
Printed in Singapore by Ho Printing Singapore Pte Ltd

1 2011

Contents

Preface

It was rash and naive to say in the preface to the second edition (2006) that we were entering a post-millennial phase of stability in the practical management of diabetes. No sooner had it gone to press than the results of megatrials started appearing in pairs and sometimes trios. Insulin studies in type 2 diabetes began to invade almost every imaginable (and a few almost unimaginable) regimen, and after a quiet phase in the early 2000s, new and alluring medications began to arrive (though a few others fell spectacularly by the wayside).

In the midst of this rapid expansion, a cohort of massive studies, quietly brewing since the beginning of the millennium, finally exploded. The seismic activity was due to the publication of four important randomised trials – VADT, ACCORD and ADVANCE in the latter part of 2007 and early 2008, BARI 2D in mid-2009 – and the complementary findings of the long-term UKPDS follow-up. Accordingly, guideline production and revision accelerated to near-maniacal levels, to the point at which practitioners are now challenged over the choice of second-, never mind third- or fourth-line glycaemic treatments. The uniform, and for some uncomfortable, conclusion from VADT, ACCORD and ADVANCE is that after 10 years or more of diagnosed type 2 diabetes, especially in the presence of macrovascular complications, undue efforts at glycaemic control confer no macrovascular and only slight microvascular benefit, and may even increase mortality; this should have been wise practice in elderly patients even without this evidence. BARI 2D tells us unequivocally that insulin treatment confers no advantage over insulin-sensitizing treatment in diabetic people with symptomatic coronary artery disease. The statistical navel-gazing resulting from the troubling conclusions of the ACCORD glycaemic study is still in full swing as I write this introduction, and it may be that these critical points will never adequately be explained, though it certainly won't be for want of trying. Perhaps of all the ACCORD substudies, ACCORD Eye, published just before the book went for copy-editing, represents the apogee of intricacy in diabetes RCTs and, while I would not wish nightmares on anyone, should give hard-headed mechanistic evidence-based practitioners at least pause for thought that the more 'definitive' a trial is touted to be, the more complex and subtle its conclusions are likely to be. I date this phenomenon to the early 2000s when even the huge, but conceptually simple, ALLHAT hypertension trial failed to land the knockout blow of determining once and for all the 'right' first-line treatment for high blood pressure, but we should have taken the hint from the University Group Diabetes Project decades before. Quite simply, there is probably not a right first-line treatment for any long-term condition.

I have rewritten much of the material on type 2 diabetes to try to reflect these trials, though the results of VADT and Steno-2 do not in any way let us off the hook over blood pressure, lipids, albuminuria and lifestyle intervention, especially smoking cessation. Barely recovering from this onslaught, we felt the aftershocks in 2009 and 2010: the proposal that HbA_{1c} measurements really could be used to diagnose diabetes (and, more contentiously, pre-diabetes as well), and the ACCORD lipid and blood pressure substudies, which showed that people with unremarkable lipid profiles gain unremarkable benefits from statin–fibrate combination treatment, and I think more significantly hinted that 'lower is better' might not even apply to blood pressure.

Still, the UKPDS follow-up permits us to be 'aggressive' (the only use I will permit myself of this pervasive and self-serving word) over glucose treatment in 'early' type 2 diabetes, whatever that means. All these results now sit uncomfortably with protocol-driven strategies for type 2 diabetes management that fail to take into account the extraordinary variety of this condition; we can take this as a liberating opportunity, as I would prefer, or we can try to emulate the artificial intelligence consensus that all we need is more and more comprehensive and prescriptive procotols, guidelines and guidance. However, there was a refreshing and radically different approach in the 2009 reappraisal of the 2007 European Society for Hypertension Guidelines, well worth a complete read-through (don't be put off by the formidable bureaucratic title), and an eminently sensible and patient-orientated approach [1].

On the plus side, bariatric surgery is finally established in the UK, albeit in an unsystematic way, and the advent of the incretin-related therapies means that in some we can achieve the elusive combination of avoiding weight gain while improving glycaemic control and reducing the risk of hypoglycaemia; but we have seen the false dawn of safety and durability of treatments many times over the years, and we need due caution and humility. Insulin pump treatment finally looks as if it is beginning to take hold, though troubling differences in local availability persist in the UK, despite its endorsement by the National Institute for Health and Clinical Excellence (NICE), a requirement, so far as I am aware, not thought to be necessary in most other countries for such an obviously useful treatment.

I have updated and rewritten most of the material of the second edition, de-emphasizing some areas such as retinopathy that are more the province of the UK screening service than the individual practitioner (who shortly is not going to know one end of an ophthalmoscope from the other), and the metabolic syndrome, to which I previously devoted a brief chapter: a combination of impenetrable existential philosophy and the threat of world war persuaded me within a few seconds to abandon the risk of further increasing readers' anxiety on this tendentious entity [2].

Nearly as many medications have been withdrawn since the last edition as have been introduced, some after commercial launch (inhaled insulin, rimonabant, sibutramine), some after unsuccessful late-stage trials (torcetrapib, dual PPAR-α/γ agonists). The glitazones, especially rosiglitazone, wobbled badly from 2007 onwards as a result of a widely discussed meta-analysis, and though the outcomes were not confirmed in major RCTs, the controversy rumbles do, and as the book went to press, the licence for rosiglitazone was withdrawn in Europe and its use still further restricted in the USA. One of the several lessons learned from this unfortunate episode – the FDA requirement to establish cardiovascular safety of new glycaemic agents at launch rather than many years later – was timely and welcome, and should discourage the widespread practice of hinting at clinical advantage on the basis of animal and laboratory studies and of surrogate clinical measurements.

Over the past few years, the management of diabetes in hospitalized patients has rightly come to the fore, but again the trial results swerve from the certainties of tight glycaemic control in Van den Berghe's studies in the early 2000s to the cautions of NICE-SUGAR (2008), and although the UK campaign for better management of diabetes in hospital ('Think Glucose', 2009 onwards) is also timely and welcome, the emphatic message from the assembled trials in glycaemic control, both acute and chronic, is that hypoglycaemia is a very serious consequence of type 2 diabetes and must be avoided as zealously as in type 1. Despite being nearly two decades old, the DIGAMI study, unlike UKPDS and DCCT, is universally recognized by trainees, though not remembered in any detail that could usefully contribute to patient care, but cult memory is long – they still use 'BM' as a measurement of glucose, rather than capillary blood glucose (CBG) – although the demise of the colour BM (Boehringer-Mannheim) strips predated their conception by a good decade or more.

We are still ineffective in educating our patients on sustained lifestyle interventions and I have further emphasized them, with a brief personal viewpoint (I am not a dietitian) on dietary management of type 2 diabetes, based on limited but important clinical trial results that, like the glycaemic trials, challenge conventional thinking. I have also cautiously entered the fascinating area of psychiatry and diabetes (Chapter 13); some material in this chapter, and scattered among other chapters as well, is taken from *Type 1 Diabetes* (Oxford Diabetes Library, Oxford University Press, 2010).

Beyond the glycaemia trials, other studies persist in yielding surprising and counter-intuitive results. Unexpectedly, CHOIR and CREATE (2006) did not support full correction of renal anaemia in patients with chronic kidney disease (CKD), and TREAT (darbepoetin in type 2 CKD patients, 2009) confirmed this. Haemoglobin, like HbA_{1c}, carries very different significance according to the clinical situation.

Added to this disequilibrating melange, we have to prepare for a major change in the practicalities of managing diabetes. Rumours about the unacceptability of HbA_{1c} reported in percentages had been occasionally transmitted over the past few years, but our quarter-century relationship with DCCT-aligned HbA_{1c} percentages was disrupted by the International Federation of Clinical Chemistry's (IFCC) demand that, pending a wholesale downward shift of the measurement when the 'absolute' measurement of HbA_{1c} with mass spectrometry becomes a reality, we must change the units of measurement, and educate the whole diabetes world and our patients in these changes by mid-2011. The chemical pathologists have also been slow to recognize that *changes* in HbA_{1c} are as important to our patients as absolute values. The educational hurdle is daunting, and the likely real advantage rather limited. Sadly, it appears that the heroic ADAG study correlating estimated average glucose values with DCCT-aligned HbA_{1c} measurements – and these *would* be of enormous value to our patients – has, unintentionally I am sure, been supplanted by the rush to global conformity in HbA_{1c} reporting; all these suggestions surfaced around the same time. I have reluctantly quoted IFCC measurements with the traditional DCCT values; less reluctantly, there are traditional biochemical values together with their SI equivalents, and I hope this helps transatlantic and European readers alike.

Fortunately, clinical research and insight are not quite dead – yet. Morris Brown's sophisticated but simple approach to difficult hypertension means that despite the introduction of only one new drug class in the past 12 years or so, the careful use of older and sometimes almost forgotten antihypertensive drugs should have a renaissance in resistant hypertension in diabetes, a very common clinical problem, not addressed in the standard guidelines. The management of hyperglycaemic emergencies is still problematic (a glaring example of an evidence black hole), and I have included some personal views gathered from my experience and that of other, cleverer, colleagues, over the years.

As the book has grown, it was high time for some references. They are quoted in PubMed format, including their unique PMID numbers; type the 7- or 8-digit number into the pubmed.gov search line and it will bring up the abstract. This may be useful for guidelines and other publications that do not have consistent referencing. I hope the suggestions for further reading and internet sources move occasionally beyond the humdrum.

As usual, my colleagues have continued to enthuse me during these difficult times for hospital diabetes practice in the UK. Laura Liew kept me to schedule, helped with illustrations, tables, and changes in insulins, pens, CGMs and other critical paraphernalia. Only she knows how deeply grateful I am to her. Angela Edwards scoured PubMed for the correct citations and punctuation and Timo Pilgram (Medical Education Centre Library) cheerfully and determinedly sourced reprints within days, sometimes hours. Clency Payaneeandee continues to educate me about diabetic feet. Oliver Walter and Jennifer Seward at Wiley-Blackwell enthusiastically took on this new edition, with its slightly altered title; their invigorating light-touch management style would go down a storm in the NHS at present.

Attempting in the same single-author book to cover both type 1 and 2 diabetes (and all the interesting intervening varieties), and acute and ambulatory care while targeting everyone who is practising advanced diabetes care almost guarantees that some will feel short-changed, patronized, lectured at or just plain confused. I can plead no extenuation other than areas of diabetes care that were once the province of the hospital specialist will now be managed by others in many different settings. There is no specialty in which it is more important than ever to balance numbers and the desirability of achieving targets against the primacy of outcomes that are relevant and meaningful to our patients, most importantly of course their long-term well-being. But most important in achieving the equilibrium is – and I will use this as justification for the proliferation of data and trial results in the book – knowing the literature intimately, which is not quite the same as familiarity with the the evidence, or even performing a systematic review and meta-analysis. If we are successful in this most difficult aspect of our art, then our patients and our sanity will be fine. Let me know if I don't manage to achieve it, and I will put it right (and change the title) if I ever make it to the fourth edition.

David Levy
London

1. Mancia G, Laurent S, Agabiti-Rosei E *et al*. Reappraisal of European guidelines on hypertension management: a European Society of Hypertension Task Force document. *J Hypertens* 2009;27:2121–58. PMID 19838131.
2. Alberti KG, Eckel RH, Grundy SM *et al*. Harmonizing the metabolic syndrome. A joint interim statement of the International Diabetes Federation Task Force on Epidemiology and Prevention; National Heart, Lung, and Blood

Institute; American Heart Association; World Heart Federation; International Atherosclerosis Society; and International Association for the Study of Obesity. *Circulation* 2009;120:1640–5. PMID: 19805654. And the devastating WHO riposte: Simmons RK, Alberti KG, Gale EA *et al.* The metabolic syndrome: useful concept or clinical tool? Report of a WHO Expert Consultation. *Diabetologia* 2010;53:600–5. PMID 20012011.

Numbers, conversions and tables

Conversions from SI to traditional units

Cholesterol	×39 (mmol/L to mg/dL)
Creatinine	÷88.4 (μmol/L to mg/dL)
Glucose	×18 (mmol/L to mg/dL)
β-Hydroxybutyric acid (ketone body)	÷10 (mmol/L to mg/dL)
Insulin	×9 (pmol/L to μunit/mL)
Testosterone	×29 (nmol/L to ng/dL)
Triglycerides	×89 (mmol/L to mg/dL)
Urinary albumin/creatinine ratio	×8.8 (mg/mmol to mg/mg)

Glucose-related values

HbA_{1c} (DCCT and IFCC) and estimated average glucose (eAG)

% (DCCT)	mmol/mol (IFCC)	eAG (mmol/L)	95% confidence interval (mmol/L)	eAG (mg/dL)	95% confidence interval (mg/dL)
5	31	5.4	4.2–6.7	97	76–120
5.5	37	6.2		111	
6	42	7.0	5.5–8.5	126	100–152
6.5	48	7.7		140	
7	53	8.6	6.8–10.3	154	123–185
7.5	58	9.3		169	
8	64	10.2	8.1–12.1	183	147–217

(*Continued*)

% (DCCT)	mmol/mol (IFCC)	eAG (mmol/L)	95% confidence interval (mmol/L)	eAG (mg/dL)	95% confidence interval (mg/dL)
8.5	69	10.9		197	
9	75	11.8	9.4–13.9	212	170–249
9.5	80	12.5		226	
10	86	13.4	10.7–15.7	240	193–282
10.5	91	14.1		255	
11	97	14.9	12.0–17.5	269	217–314
11.5	102	15.6		283	
12	108	16.5	13.3–19.3	298	240–347
12.5	113	17.2		312	
13	119	18.0		326	
14	130	19.6		355	

The regression equations for eAG are:
$1.59 \times HbA_{1c} - 2.59$ (mmol/L)
$28.7 \times HbA_{1c} - 46.7$ (mg/dL)
From Nathan DM, Kuenen J, Borg R, Zheng H, Schoenfeld D, Heine RJ. Translating the A1C assay into estimated average glucose values. A1c-Derived Average Glucose Study Group. *Diabetes Care* 2008;31:1473–8. PMID 18540046.

Online calculator relating HbA_{1c} (DCCT) to eAG (mg/dL or mmol/L)
http://professional.diabetes.org/eAG

Online calculator converting DCCT HbA_{1c} values to IFCC values
www.diabetes.org.uk/Professionals/Publications-reports-and-resources/Tools/Changes-to-HbA1c-values/

Diabetic emergencies
Plasma osmolality
$2[Na^+] + 2[K^+] + [urea] + [glucose]$ (normal value 280–300 mosmol/L)

Anion gap
$[Na^+ + K^+] - [HCO_3^-] + [Cl^-]$ (normal anion gap is 7–9 mmol/L; in anion gap acidosis > 10–12 mmol/L)

Hypertension
Classification of stages of hypertension and their predicted ambulatory blood pressures (BP, mmHg).

	Seated clinic BP threshold	Predicted day-time ambulatory equivalent	Predicted 24-hour ambulatory equivalent
Normal BP	120/80	120/78	117/76
Target BP with proteinuria	125/75	124/74	121/71
Target BP plus one condition	130/80	128/78	125/76
Grade 1 (mild) hypertension	140/90	136/87	133/84
Grade 2 (moderate) hypertension	160/100	152/96	148/93
Grade 3 (severe) hypertension	180/110	168/105	163/101

From Head GA, Mihallidou AS, Duggan KA *et al*. Definition of ambulatory blood pressure targets for diagnosis and treatment of hypertension in relation to clinic blood pressure: a prospective cohort study. Ambulatory Blood Pressure Working Group of the High Blood Pressure Research Council of Australia. *Br Med J* 2010;340;c1104.

Selected blood pressures in young people by height centiles, age and gender

Boys

Age	BP percentile	Height percentile	
		50th	75th
13	90th	122/77	124/78
	95th	126/81	128/82
14	90th	125/78	126/79
	95th	128/82	130/83
15	90th	127/79	129/80
	95th	131/83	133/84
16	90th	130/80	131/81
	95th	134/84	135/85
17	90th	132/82	134/83
	95th	136/87	138/87

Girls

Age	BP percentile	Height percentile	
		50th	75th
13	90th	121/77	122/78
	95th	124/81	126/82
14	90th	122/78	124/79
	95th	126/82	127/83
15	90th	123/79	125/80
	95th	127/83	129/84
16	90th	124/80	126/81
	95th	128/84	130/85
17	90th	125/80	130/85
	95th	129/84	137/92

From www.nhlbi.nih.gov/guidelines/hypertension/child_tbl.htm, where the full tables are available (age 1–17, 5th to 95th height percentiles, 50th to 99th BP percentiles).

Estimate of waist circumference from BMI (from VA-HIT study)

Waist (cm) = $2.096 \times$ BMI (kg/m^2) + 40.355 ($r = 0.84$)

From Vittone F, Chait A, Morse JS, Fish B, Brown BG, Zhao X-Q. Niacin plus simvastatin reduces coronary stenosis progression among patients with metabolic syndrome despite a modest increase in insulin resistance: a subgroup analysis of the HDL-Atherosclerosis Treatment Study (HATS). *J Clin Lipidol* 2007;1:203–10. PMID 18591993.

Online cardiovascular risk prediction tools

UKPDS Risk Engine (SI units). Available at www.dtu.ox.ac.uk/riskengine/index.php

ARIC (Atherosclerosis Risk in Communities) (traditional units). Available at www.aricnews.net/riskcalc/html/RC1/html

University of Edinburgh Cardiovascular Risk Calculator (SI units). Patient-friendly online presentation of the Joint British Societies (JBS) Cardiovascular Disease Risk Prediction Charts, developed by the University of Manchester, and published in the *British National Formulary* (BNF). ASSIGN and Framingham risk calculations are also obtainable. Available at www.cvrisk.mvm.ed.ac.uk/calculator/calc.asp

Classification and diagnosis

CHAPTER 1

Key points

- The four major diagnostic categories of diabetes (type 1, type 2, gestational diabetes mellitus and other specific categories) have been blurred by the recognition of clinically important syndromes, for example latent autoimmune diabetes of adults and type 2 diabetes presenting with clear diabetic ketoacidosis.
- The diagnosis of diabetes in adolescents and young adults can be particularly difficult. Tests for antibodies, for example those to glutamic acid decarboxylase, may be of value in individual cases.
- In type 1 patients, be vigilant for associated and emerging autoimmune conditions especially hypothyroidism, coeliac disease and Addison's disease.
- Suggested diagnostic criteria for gestational diabetes mellitus, and for diabetes and pre-diabetes using HbA_{1c} measurements, will probably be widely adopted.
- Screen opportunistically for diabetes in high-risk groups and their offspring; intensive lifestyle intervention and some drugs have been shown to prevent or at least delay the onset of type 2 diabetes by up to 4 years.
- Trials continue into preserving β-cell function in subjects at high risk of developing type 1 diabetes and those with recently diagnosed clinical diabetes.

Introduction

The history of the classification and biochemical diagnosis of diabetes is long and involved, with incomplete agreement between America

Practical Diabetes Care, 3rd edition. © David Levy.
Published 2011 by Blackwell Publishing Ltd.

1

(American Diabetes Association, ADA) and the world (World Health Organization, WHO and the International Diabetes Federation, IDF). The revised ADA classification (1997) was generally agreed in the WHO report of 1999, as was the major change to lower the diagnostic criterion for diabetes from a fasting venous plasma glucose (FPG) of ≥ 7.8 mmol/ L (140 mg/dL) to ≥ 7.0 mmol/L (126 mg/dL). Epidemiological evidence for the lower value was solid. The prevalence of retinopathy (and probably other microvascular complications [1]) is stable and low (but not zero, perhaps around 5%) at FPG below 7.0 mmol/L, but rises rapidly above this value. Normal (non-diabetic) FPG was until quite recently considered to be 6.0 mmol/L (110 mg/dL) or less but there was a feeling that this was too high, and the most recent definition of normal glucose (ADA 2003) is 5.5 mmol/L (100 mg/dL) or less. Values intermediate between normality and overt diabetes (5.6 or 6.1 to 6.9 mmol/L, 100 or 110 to 125 mg/dL), designated 'impaired fasting glucose' (IFG), were intended to define a group of people with a higher prevalence of impaired glucose tolerance (IGT), without the need for the cumbersome and time-consuming oral glucose tolerance test (OGTT), but this potentially efficient move was thwarted by the continued recognition that elevated post-load, rather than fasting, glucose levels appear, at least epidemiologically, to define a group at higher cardiovascular risk. In addition, there is poor agreement between IFG and IGT on OGTT, and diabetes is more reliably identified in some groups (e.g. the elderly, the non-obese, and Southeast Asians) by post-load glucose levels.

There is still uncertainty about the IFG criterion level, and WHO (2006) recommends that the value should remain 6.1 mmol/L (110 mg/dL). The true cardiovascular risk associated with isolated IFG using the lower current cut-off is not known, but is probably not high. Since there is continuing controversy about the cardiovascular benefit of treating isolated near-normal glucose levels, the best clinical approach is to globally assess all cardiovascular risk factors in individual people.

The OGTT is still recommended when there is diagnostic doubt, i.e. persistent FPG in the IFG range (5.6–6.9 mmol/L). The scheme is complex and difficult for the non-specialist to use, but it is nevertheless valuable. All subjects can be classified using FPG together with the OGTT in a well-defined group; more than ever there is no justification for terms such as 'borderline', 'potential', 'slightly elevated', etc. However, the limitations of the OGTT must be recognized: it is poorly reproducible, especially the 2-hour values, even when retesting after only 2 weeks [2]. Relatively small changes in weight, exercise, diet, medication, and no doubt many other factors, including time, may result in changes in apparent glucose tolerance status, especially where values hover around threshold. Nevertheless, because of the adverse cardiovascular impact of

IGT and perhaps more importantly its strong associations with the metabolic syndrome, this particular diagnosis should be carefully sought and acted on.

Classification

The 1997 ADA scheme laudably attempted to classify diabetes by pathophysiology rather than treatment modality. This is particularly important now that markers of islet-cell autoimmunity (see below) are widely available. The terms 'insulin-dependent' and 'non-insulin-dependent' are obsolete, and the non-synonymous terms type 1 and type 2 should now be used (a point of detail, still overlooked, is the use of Arabic, not Roman, numerals – so type 2, not type II diabetes). In practice, however, hybrid terminology still persists, for example 'insulin-treated type 2 diabetes', since treatment modality remains important to clinicians and patients alike. One old term, ketosis-prone diabetes, is becoming more widely used again, and a tentative but promising classification of people presenting with ketosis based on the presence or absence of autoimmune markers and presence or absence of β-cell reserve (Aβ) may become more widely adopted (see below) [3]. Other obsolete terms are shown in Table 1.1.

Type 1 diabetes (β-cell destruction, usually leading to complete insulin deficiency)

Type 1 diabetes is relatively uncommon, occurring in about 1 in 300 of a northern white population, and comprises only 5–10% of all diagnosed cases. Incidence increases with geographical latitude. Formally, it is

Table 1.1 Obsolete terms for type 1 and type 2 diabetes

Type 1	Type 2
Type I	Type II
Insulin-dependent	Non-insulin-dependent
Juvenile-onset	Adult-onset, maturity-onset
IDDM	NIDDM
Ketosis-prone (now less obsolete)	Non-ketosis-prone

classified as type 1A diabetes, with markers of islet autoimmunity, compared with type 1B diabetes where markers are absent (see below).

Operational definition
- Acute symptomatic onset (usually with osmotic symptoms) under the age of 30 in a non-obese, usually white, person.
- Ketonuria and/or metabolic acidosis at presentation.
- Immediate and permanent requirement for insulin (though insulin requirements may be minimal during the 'honeymoon' period, i.e. 6–18 months after diagnosis).
- No evidence of vascular complications at presentation.

Epidemiology
The epidemiology is fascinating, if largely unexplained.
- Type 1 diabetes can occur at any age after about 18 months, but classical type 1 diabetes has a peak incidence in children between 10 and 15 years old, somewhat earlier in girls.
- It has a pronounced seasonal variation, most cases occurring between autumn and spring in the northern hemisphere.
- From puberty onwards there is a consistent excess of cases in males, especially in the age group 25–29 years, where there is a 50% excess, unique for an autoimmune condition.
- Its incidence is rapidly increasing, especially in those under 5 years old. In Finland, which has the highest incidence in the world, cases have doubled in the 15 years between 1980 and 2005, and are projected to double again up to 2020.
- The 'accelerator hypothesis' has been confirmed in most studies: this assumes that β-cell loss is accelerated through insulin resistance, fuelled by increased obesity in youth, and predicts that the age of diagnosis is inversely related to body mass index (BMI).
- Cumulative risk of type 1 diabetes in offspring of type 1 diabetic parents is greater in fathers (up to 14%) than in mothers (up to 6%). The rate of transmission is three times higher (14% vs. 5%) in fathers who developed their diabetes aged under 5 compared with those aged 15–17 years.

Serological markers of islet-cell autoimmunity
These include insulin antibodies (rarely measured), islet-cell antibodies, antibodies to glutamic acid decarboxylase (GADA, specifically GAD_{65}) and antibodies to tyrosine phosphatases IA-2 and IA-2β. Testing for combinations of these markers increases predictive power. Strictly speaking, they predict progression to insulin requirement (rather than being diagnostic tests for type 1 diabetes). This is a similar situation to the

presence of anti-thyroid antibodies, which are not diagnostic of abnormal thyroid function but should increase vigilance for it. Detection of diabetes-associated antibodies should likewise increase vigilance for insulin deficiency, especially ketosis, but not precipitate immediate insulin treatment, though where markers are available, insulin treatment tends to be started sooner in antibody-positive subjects. Outside the research area, they should be requested only if there is a clinical dilemma, in an atypical clinical situation such as older symptomatic patients (e.g. over the age of 30), or in adolescents (remembering that 4% of the background population has positive GADA). The tests are neither completely reliable nor standardized, and must be regarded as an adjunct to careful clinical evaluation. Even those with major expertise in the area caution that the clinical benefit of individual testing has not been established [4]. HLA serotyping cannot be used in this situation; although characteristic alleles occur with high reliability in type 1 diabetes, they are also common in the background population. These include both predisposing (e.g. HLA-DR3 and -DR4) and protective (e.g. HLA-DR2) alleles.

Endocrine associations of type 1 diabetes [5]

Two autoimmune polyglandular syndromes (APS) are associated with type 1 diabetes. The rare autosomal recessive type 1 APS caused by a mutation in the autoimmune regulator gene (*AIRE*) comprises mucocutaneous candidiasis with nail dystrophy, hypoparathyroidism and Addison's disease. Type 1 diabetes occurs in 2–12% of patients. Much more common is type 2 APS, which usually occurs in HLA-DR4-positive females. It comprises, in decreasing order of frequency:

- Addison's disease;
- autoimmune thyroid disease (usually Hashimoto's thyroiditis);
- primary gonadal failure;
- less common associations such as alopecia, vitiligo, pernicious anaemia, hypophysitis, coeliac disease, myasthenia gravis and primary biliary cirrhosis.

However, it is important to recognize that this syndrome does not represent the commonest associations encountered in clinical practice [6]. Hashimoto's thyroiditis occurs in about 25%, of whom at least half are hypothyroid. Patients should therefore be screened regularly, initially at presentation for thyroid function and anti-thyroid peroxidase antibodies. Antibody-positive patients should be screened every 6–12 months, while antibody-negative patients can have tests every 1–2 years. On the other hand, hyperthyroidism, usually Graves' disease, seems to be no more common in type 1 patients than in the general population (prevalence $\sim 1\%$). Coeliac disease is much more common than previously thought; 5–10% of type 1 patients have serological markers, and many units screen newly diagnosed type 1 patients for antibodies to tissue transglutaminase, currently the most reliable marker. Definitive diagnosis with a jejunal biopsy is probably justified in asymptomatic antibody-positive patients; in symptomatic adults, close observation after starting a gluten-free diet is suggested.

Addison's disease and autoimmune hepatitis

Addison's disease is very uncommon in the general population (1 in 10000). Its serological marker, antibodies to 21-hydroxylase, occur in only 1–2% of type 1 patients, and routine screening cannot be justified. However, great clinical vigilance is needed, and the simple short Synacthen test should be requested freely in patients with increased unexplained hypoglycaemia, suggestive biochemistry (hyperkalaemia, mild hyponatraemia) or vague abdominal pain and nausea. (Schmidt's syndrome is autoimmune Addison's disease plus autoimmune hypothyroidism, with or without type 1 diabetes, and like many eponyms is unnecessarily confusing in an already complicated area.) Autoimmune hepatitis occurs infrequently, but is an important association: do not automatically attribute mildly abnormal liver functions to non-alcoholic fatty liver disease, especially in type 1 diabetic patients [7].

Type 2 diabetes (hyperinsulinaemia, insulin resistance, and variable insulin deficiency or secretory defects)

This is not usually difficult to diagnose where the following features are present:

- Onset of osmotic symptoms over a variable period – weeks to years, sometimes, in retrospect, intermittent – in an overweight middle-aged person (mean BMI 28–29 in UK at onset).
- Variable weight loss.
- Ketonuria: trace or absent.
- Positive family history in first-degree relatives.
- Presentation with established complications: the pre-diagnosis duration of hyperglycaemia is 7–10 years, with perhaps a further 10 years of preceding metabolic syndrome, while about 20% have detectable microvascular or macrovascular complications at presentation. Presentation with established myocardial infarction or stroke is more common than moderate or advanced microvascular complications, i.e. visual impairment from advanced retinopathy, neuropathic foot ulceration, stick-positive proteinuria or frank nephropathy.

In practice, there is now considerable difficulty in classifying some patients, particularly at onset. Important clinical types include:
- Latent autoimmune diabetes of adults (LADA).
- Type 2 diabetes presenting with diabetic ketoacidosis (DKA).
- Type 2 diabetes in children and adolescents.

Latent autoimmune diabetes of adults

Also called slowly progressing type 1 diabetes, or type 1.5 diabetes, although there is a great deal of argument about the nomenclature. Clinically it is important, and seems to be increasing. Prevalence is about 5–10% of people diagnosed clinically with type 2 diabetes in northern populations.

An arbitrary definition would include the following:

- diagnosis of non-insulin-requiring diabetes at age 30 or older;
- autoantibody positivity, especially GADA;
- 6 months without insulin treatment after diagnosis (this does not help in making the diagnosis at presentation).

A better clinical definition includes two or more of the following:

- Age at onset < 50 years.
- Acute symptoms (< 6 months): osmotic, unintentional weight loss, but not infections or blurred vision.
- Personal history of autoimmune conditions (thyroid, rheumatoid).
- Family history of autoimmune conditions (thyroid, type 1 diabetes, rheumatoid, coeliac) [8].

LADA appears to be at the end of several spectra of diabetes: it is less strongly genetically determined and has a lower number of antibodies associated with it than type 1 diabetes in childhood; metabolically it shares some features of type 2 diabetes, for example there is a similar high prevalence of the metabolic syndrome (75–85%, compared with about 20% in the background population) [9].

The dominant defect is insulin secretion, but clinically is not so severe that ketonuria is common (nevertheless, test for it at each visit). A sulphonylurea, or possibly a dipeptidyl peptidase (DPP)-4 inhibitor, might be the best initial treatment option. However, sulphonylureas may increase β-cell apoptosis, and the response to them in LADA is often suboptimal and short-lived, despite the relatively low BMI at presentation (mean ∼ 27). Insulin, when required, can be basal or prandial; the regimen should be based on individual diurnal blood glucose profiles.

Type 2 diabetes presenting with diabetic ketoacidosis

In the Aβ classification, this form is Aβ$^+$, i.e. islet-autoantibody negative with variably preserved β-cell function. A few patients were described in Africa during the 1960s and 1970s, but a slightly different syndrome was characterized in the 1990s in a group of obese African-American men in their thirties living in the Flatbush area of Brooklyn, hence its occasional eponym 'Flatbush diabetes' [10].

It is now common in the UK in African and African-Caribbean people, and in African-American youth in the USA. It presents with DKA, sometimes severe. After discharge on insulin (this is mandatory, regardless of the presumed diagnosis) doses fall rapidly, and insulin independence occurs at a mean of 3.5 months. Complete remission (good control on diet alone) is seen in 30–40%, and may last for more than 3 years, even without major weight loss. Recurrence of DKA is recognized but is clinically rare. Autoimmune markers are negative; the pathogenesis is related to acute partial temporary β-cell failure. The long-term natural history is not known, particularly the rate of progression of β-cell loss.

Type 2 diabetes in obese children and adolescents

This was first recognized in the early 1980s in the USA, but with increasing frequency in the form of diabetes in adolescence. In the USA, most cases are from ethnic minorities (especially African-American, but also Hispanic American and Native American). In the UK, paediatricians first reported small numbers of both white and ethnic minority adolescents with type 2 diabetes in 2002, but even then the true incidence must have been higher, particularly in young adults who would not have been under the care of paediatricians. For example, OGTT-diagnosed diabetes was found in about 1% of obese white young people over 12 years of age in Germany.

Ketosis and ketoacidosis are more common in ethnic minorities than in white patients (up to 25% vs. 4%), as is axillary acanthosis nigricans, the classical cutaneous marker of insulin resistance [11]. Like the adults, they are negative for islet-cell autoimmunity, though about 30% of white patients initially diagnosed with type 2 diabetes, and not requiring insulin at 12 months, had anti-GADA or IA-2 antibodies. Long-term follow-up of small numbers of patients in the USA (especially the high-risk Pima Indian population) confirms a high rate of vascular complications and risk factors.
- Microalbuminuria progresses at the same high rates as in adults; renal failure occurs at about the same rate as in type 1 diabetes.
- Retinopathy seems to be less prevalent than in type 1 patients.
- Pregnancy loss is high (poor glycaemic control, multiple associated vascular risk factors).
- Systolic hypertension occurs in about 50%.
- Dyslipidaemia, associated with the underlying metabolic syndrome, is common [12].

Screening for type 2 diabetes in children
There are no recommendations in the UK, but the ADA recommends that overweight children (> 85th percentile for age and sex, or weight above 120% of ideal for height) aged 10 years or above should have fasting glucose tested every 2 years if there are two or more of the following risk factors present.
- Family history of type 2 diabetes in first- or second-degree relatives.
- Race/ethnicity (in the UK: South Asian, African and African-Caribbean origin).

- Features of insulin resistance: acanthosis nigricans, dyslipidaemia, hypertension, polycystic ovarian syndrome.

Other schemes, even more stringent, are proposed, but they are all counsels of perfection (adherence to the standard guidelines is weak). In primary care practice, opportunistic screening, especially of severely obese children and adolescents with one or both parents with type 2 disease, using fasting glucose levels (probably together with HbA_{1c}) might be a good starting point. However, as in adults, the prevalence of abnormal fasting glucose levels is likely to be much lower than other components of the metabolic syndrome, especially elevated systolic blood pressure. Any young person with abnormal glucose levels requires a formal diagnosis to differentiate between type 2 diabetes, early type 1 diabetes, monogenic diabetes (particularly if there is a strong family history) and syndromic diabetes.

Other specific types of diabetes
Type 1B diabetes
This is clinically identical to type 1A, but without the autoimmune markers. One type, almost unique to Southeast Asia (mostly Japan, but also reported from South Korea and China) is well described as 'fulminant type 1 diabetes'. Symptoms in young people in their twenties and thirties develop over a few days, culminating in DKA; β-cell function is absent and, because of the short duration, HbA_{1c} is normal at presentation. Despite better overall glycaemic control during long-term follow-up compared with type 1A diabetes, microvascular complications seem to develop at approximately the same rate up to 10 years' duration.

Monogenic defects of β-cell function
These comprise only 1–2% of all cases of diabetes, but are important to diagnose as they have specific treatments and require genetic counselling.

1 Mitochondrial DNA-maternally-inherited diabetes and deafness.
2 Glucokinase and HNF mutations, characterized from the early 1990s onwards. Previously known as MODY (maturity-onset diabetes of the young), they are now best described by the specific mutation. There are currently six types, including:
   (a) Glucokinase ('glucose sensor') mutation (previously MODY2) comprises about 20% of cases.
   (b) Transcription factor mutations: the most common, *HNF1A*, comprises about 60% of all cases, and is the most frequent in the UK. Most are dominantly inherited, but they occasionally occur spontaneously. The *HNF1B* mutation has extrapancreatic features, for example renal cysts, gout, genital malformations and abnormal liver functions tests.

When these present in teenagers and young adults, they are often misdiagnosed and treated as type 1 diabetes.

Genetic defects of insulin action
Examples include lipoatrophic diabetes, Rabson–Mendenhall syndrome and leprechaunism.

Diseases of the exocrine pancreas
Examples include pancreatitis, pancreatectomy (especially involving the tail of the pancreas, where islets are concentrated), pancreatic carcinoma[1], cystic fibrosis, haemochromatosis and fibrocalculous pancreatopathy. These conditions cause more destruction of glucagon-producing α cells than is seen in type 1 diabetes. Since glucagon excess is a major feature of DKA, patients with pancreatic diabetes are less prone to DKA (see Chapter 2). Genetic haemochromatosis due to C282Y homozygosity in the *HFE* gene is common in people of Northern European ancestry, and is frequently complicated by diabetes. Markers of iron overload, especially serum ferritin, are elevated in both the metabolic syndrome and alcohol use. There is no role yet for routine measurement of ferritin levels in Type 2 patients, unless there are other clinical or laboratory hints of iron overload. Ferritin levels >1000 ug/L should be further investigated.

Endocrinopathies associated with hormones mediating insulin resistance
Examples include acromegaly (growth hormone), Cushing's disease or syndrome (cortisol), phaeochromocytomas (catecholamines, especially noradrenaline) and glucagonoma. Up to 10% of obese patients with poorly controlled ($HbA_{1c} > 8\%$) type 2 diabetes have evidence of hypercortisolaemia, but this is difficult to translate into clinical practice, other than to urge vigilance, especially in difficult-to-control diabetes [13].

Drug or chemical induced
Examples include glucocorticoids, protease inhibitors and some second-generation antipsychotics (especially olanzapine and clozapine).

New-onset diabetes after transplantation
The causes of this important and common form of diabetes are multiple, but include the calcineurin inhibitors (ciclosporin, tacrolimus). A year after renal transplantation, 10–20% of patients have OGTT-diagnosed diabetes, compared with about 5% of non-transplanted patients. Mediated predominantly by insulin resistance, it carries an unfavourable prognosis

---

[1]Patients over 50 years old with recent-onset type 2 diabetes have an approximately eightfold increased risk of pancreatic cancer, by which time the disease is usually advanced. Interestingly, the diabetes is serologically mediated through insulin resistance and not β-cell destruction.

for both organ and patient survival, but optimum management strategy and the impact of treatment have not been prospectively investigated.

Infections
Examples include rubella, cytomegalovirus and hepatitis C.

Uncommon forms of immune-mediated diabetes
Examples include stiff man/person syndrome (associated with high GAD_{65} antibody levels) and anti-insulin receptor antibodies.

Other genetic syndromes associated with diabetes
Examples include Turner's syndrome (markedly increased risk of both type 1 and 2 diabetes), Klinefelter's syndrome, Friedreich's ataxia, Huntington's chorea and myotonic dystrophy.

Gestational diabetes mellitus
Gestational diabetes mellitus (GDM) is diabetes with onset or first recognition during pregnancy. The diagnosis is independent of treatment modality. It is important to distinguish between GDM and pregnancy in patients with pre-existing type 1 or 2 diabetes: substantial and growing numbers of the latter group are now being seen, especially in the South Asian ethnic groups in the UK, and carry a particularly poor perinatal outcome.

The Australian Carbohydrate Intolerance Study in Pregnant Women (ACHOIS, 2005) confirmed that active treatment of GDM (dietary advice, glucose monitoring, insulin treatment where blood glucose targets were not achieved) moderately reduced the risks of significant perinatal complications (but not rates of Caesarean section) and improved maternal postnatal well-being [14]. The HAPO study (2008) established that a similar spectrum of complications (including birth weight above the 90th percentile for gestational age) occurred at continuously increasing rates up to glucose levels that would not at the time have been actively treated; however, the effect of increasing glucose levels on Caesarean section rates was again only slight [15]. Until recently the field has been plagued by lack of international agreement on the diagnosis of GDM, but thresholds based on the HAPO study have been agreed that would give a 1.75-fold increased risk for major outcome measures (birth weight, cord C-peptide level and body fat) above the 90th percentile. The thresholds likely to be agreed worldwide are shown in Box 1.1 [16].

Diagnosis of diabetes in non-pregnant adults

The biochemical diagnosis of diabetes is currently based on laboratory venous glucose values (ADA 2010); whole blood and capillary blood glucose values are no longer quoted. Laboratory measurements of HbA_{1c} are

---

Box 1.1 Risk factors for GDM: diagnostic guidelines and target glucose levels

Risk factors (NICE 2008)
- BMI > 30 kg/m²
- Previous macrosomic baby ≥ 4.5 kg
- Previous GDM
- Family history: diabetes in first-degree relative
- Family origin with high prevalence of diabetes: South Asian (especially India, Pakistan or Bangladesh), Black Caribbean, Middle East

Diagnostic thresholds (IADPSG) for GDM
One or more of the following values (75-g OGTT in the third trimester of pregnancy):
- FPG: 5.1 mmol/L (92 mg/dL)
- 1-hour plasma glucose: 10.0 mmol/L (180 mg/dL)
- 2-hour plasma glucose: 8.5 mmol/L (153 mg/dL)

Diagnosis of overt diabetes in pregnancy
- FPG: ≥ 7.0 mmol/L (126 mg/dL) *or*
- HbA$_{1c}$: ≥ 6.5% (48 mmol/mol) (DCCT/UKPDS standardized)

Tentative diagnosis:
- Random plasma glucose ≥ 11.1 mmol/L (200 mg/dL). Confirm with FPG or HbA$_{1c}$

Glucose targets (self-monitoring, testing glucose levels 1 hour after meals)
- Fasting and preprandial: 3.3–5.9 mmol/L (60–106 mg/dL)
- 1-hour post prandial: < 7.8 mmol/L (140 mg/dL)

---

now so reliable that a Diabetes Control and Complications Trial (DCCT)-traceable HbA$_{1c}$ of 6.5% (48 mmol/mol) or above can be used to diagnose diabetes. The epidemiological evidence for this cut-off point is similar to that for FPG values: the prevalence of moderate non-proliferative retinopathy is vanishingly small at lower HbA$_{1c}$ levels. It is likely to be taken up rapidly in developed countries as it is a simple non-fasting measurement, but has not yet been adopted by WHO, and cautions have been expressed (Box 1.2).

The following four criteria can now be used; no confirmatory tests are needed if there are clear-cut symptoms and random glucose is 11.1 mmol/L (200 mg/dL) or more. Repeat testing is recommended for the remaining criteria (1–3).

1 HbA$_{1c}$ ≥ 6.5% (48 mmol/mol) (using DCCT-aligned assay) *or*
2 FPG ≥ 7.0 mmol/L (126 mg/dL) *or*
3 75-g OGTT: 2-hour glucose ≥ 11.1 mmol/L (200 mg/dL) *or*

> **Box 1.2 Cautions in the use of HbA$_{1c}$ for diagnosing diabetes**
>
> - Use DCCT-traceable assays.
> - Ensure that common haemoglobinopathies (e.g. sickle trait) do not interfere with the method used.
> - Where there is a shortened red-cell lifespan (e.g. haemolytic anaemias), only blood glucose levels should be used.
> - The diagnostic rate for HbA$_{1c}$ is probably lower than when using fasting glucose; this may be offset by the greater convenience of HbA$_{1c}$ testing.
> - For confirmation, repeat the initial test used (FPG or HbA$_{1c}$): if concordant, diagnosis is confirmed; if discordant, repeat the test whose result is above the diagnostic threshold (FPG ≥ 7.0 mmol/L, HbA$_{1c}$ $\geq 6.5\%$); consistent results are more likely for HbA$_{1c}$.

4 random plasma glucose (hyperglycaemic symptoms or hyperglycaemic emergency) ≥ 11.1 mmol/L (200 mg/dL).

Difficulties arise when two different tests give discordant outcomes. Fortunately, the two tests that are likely to be used in clinical practice (HbA$_{1c}$ and FPG) are more reproducible than the 2-hour OGTT. The advice is that the test whose result is above the cut point should be repeated. There is considerable complexity here, especially when diagnosing prediabetes (see below) and how this system will operate in real life has yet to be tested, but if one test is near criterion level, the others are likely to be also. The simplicity of FPG and HbA$_{1c}$ measurements means that interval testing to confirm or refute the diagnosis after 3–6 months is straightforward. HbA$_{1c}$ for diagnostic purposes has often been valuable in the practical setting, for example:

- in hospitalized patients with elevated glucose levels or those taking steroids, where an OGTT would be impractical or unreliable;
- in patients who have deliberately lost weight when they recognize diabetic symptoms, and who then present with normal fasting glucose levels;
- where patients decline an OGTT.

A further level of complexity is emerging from continuous glucose monitoring (CGM) studies. Although diagnostic criteria are a long way off, the findings are important in clinical practice. For example, nearly all non-diabetic subjects with low fasting glucose and strictly normal HbA$_{1c}$ levels spent about 30 min daily at IGT levels (> 7.8 mmol/L, 140 mg/dL). One-tenth were at this level for more than 2 hours in 24 hours, and a similar proportion reached diabetic levels (i.e. ≥ 11.1 mmol/L, 200 mg/dL). These findings confirm a highly dynamic situation and hint that defining 'normal' glucose tolerance will become increasingly difficult [17].

Table 1.2 Interpretation of fasting plasma glucose (FPG) values in asymptomatic patients

	FPG (mmol/L)	FPG (mg/dL)	Comment
Normal (non-diabetic)	≤5.5	≤99	Mean FPG in a lean population is ~4.0 mmol/L (72 mg/dL)
IFG	(5.6–6.9) 6.1–6.9	(100–125) 110–125	Repeated measurements in these ranges should be followed by confirmatory OGTT (see Table 1.3)
Diabetes	≥7.0	≥126	

Random glucose measurements

In practice most patients present without clear-cut symptoms and a random venous glucose that is not diagnostic (i.e. < 11.1 mmol/L). In various studies, random glucose levels between 6.6 and 8.6 mmol/L (119 and 155 mg/dL) result in a high yield of diabetes on definitive tests. There is no agreement on a threshold that warrants further tests, but random glucose levels above 7.0 mmol/L (126 mg/dL) should not be ignored.

Fasting glucose measurements

Fasting glucose measurements are still the simplest and commonest entry into the diagnostic pathway for diabetes presenting without symptoms. Accurate interpretation of these values is important (Table 1.2) and single measurements will be able to classify many patients as non-diabetic (≤ 5.5 mmol/L, 99 mg/dL) or as diabetic (≥ 7.0 mmol/L, 126 mg/dL). Traditionally, those with persistent intermediate values (IFG) have proceeded to an OGTT (Table 1.3); with the additional 2-hour values, subjects can be divided into those with IFG, those with IGT, and those with both IFG and IGT. This complex classification, which combines IFG and IGT in the category of 'pre-diabetes', is not only difficult to remember but probably does not usefully discriminate different risks. An intermediate category of high-risk HbA_{1c} will probably be widely used although it has not yet been formally agreed (see below).

High-risk HbA_{1c} (5.7–6.4%, 39–46 mmol/mol)

IFG and IGT identify a group at high risk of developing diabetes and cardiovascular disease, and there is plenty of epidemiological and randomized controlled trial (RCT) evidence to define a range of HbA_{1c}

Table 1.3 Interpretation of the diagnostic OGTT

	Fasting glucose level (mmol/L)	2-hour glucose level (mmol/L)	Significance/comments [18]
Normal	<5.6/6.1	<7.8	If there are diabetes-like symptoms, consider other causes
Pre-diabetes			
IFG	5.6/6.1–6.9	<7.8	Not normal. Characterized by reduced decreased peripheral insulin sensitivity, predominant genetic contribution, male gender and smoking. Risk of cardiovascular disease not known
IGT	<5.6/6.1	7.8–11.1	See below. Associated with physical inactivity, poor diet and short stature
IFG + IGT	5.6/6.1–6.9	7.8–11.1	Technically not diabetes, but treat as such; characterized by severe combined insulin resistance and progressive loss of β-cell function
Diabetes	≥7.0	≥11.1	The OGTT diagnosis of diabetes is based on *either* the fasting *or* the 2-hour value, so there may be diabetes with FPG < 7.0 mmol/L, so-called isolated post-challenge hyperglycaemia (2-hour value ≥ 11.1 mmol/L). About 3% of cases are diagnosed in this way, and it is an independent risk factor for cardiovascular disease

measurements that is also associated with progression to diabetes and cardiovascular disease, although the populations so identified are not identical. The ADA has tentatively defined this range as 5.7–6.4% (39–46 mmol/mol), and also considers those in this group as having pre-diabetes. However, the risk, as with glucose measures, is continuous and curvilinear, so that HbA_{1c} in the range 6.0–6.4% (42–46 mmol/mol) carries a particularly high risk (Table 1.4).

Table 1.4 Glucose measures defining high-risk categories for progression to diabetes

Glucose measure	SI	Traditional
FPG (IFG)	5.6–6.9 mmol/L	100–125 mg/dL
2-hour measure in OGTT (IGT)	7.8–11.0 mmol/L	140–199 mg/dL
HbA$_{1c}$	39–46 mmol/mol	5.7–6.4%

IGT and clinical trials to prevent progression of IGT to diabetes

People with IGT usually have normal blood glucose levels on casual testing, and it can be diagnosed only on OGTT, although the corresponding HbA$_{1c}$ range is 5.5–6.0% (37–42 mmol/mol). IGT clusters with other components of the metabolic syndrome, and is a high-risk state for coronary artery disease. Annually, about 6% of IGT subjects progress to diabetes, three to eight times higher than the general (USA) population.

Many trials have now reported interventions to prevent or delay the progression of IGT to diabetes. Three broad strategies have been used:
- intensive lifestyle intervention;
- pharmacological intervention with drugs used in the treatment of type 2 diabetes;
- pharmacological intervention with other drugs, especially angiotensin-blocking agents.

Lifestyle intervention
The two best-known studies using intensive lifestyle interventions to reduce weight and increase exercise are the Da Qing (1997) and the Finnish Diabetes Prevention Study (2001). Intensive lifestyle intervention in the 3-year Diabetes Prevention Program (2002), which is the only study to have used lifestyle and medication (metformin and placebo metformin) in three separate arms, reduced the risk of progression by 60%, compared with only 30% in the metformin (850 mg b.d.) arm. (In relation to the question of high-risk HbA$_{1c}$ measurements, mean HbA$_{1c}$ in the Diabetes Prevention Program was 5.9%, 41 mmol/mol.) Similar reductions were seen in the other lifestyle studies. In a 3-year follow-up of the Finnish study there was a continuing 36% risk reduction even when the active lifestyle intervention had finished, an important demonstration of a non-drug 'legacy'

effect [19]. The longest follow-up to date has been 10 years in the Diabetes Prevention Program. The original metformin group continued with medication, while all participants were offered lifestyle intervention. The original lifestyle and metformin groups maintained weight that was consistently 2 kg less than the previous placebo metformin group. This modest but clinically relevant weight loss with metformin has been found in other studies (see Chapter 6). Cumulative incidence of diabetes remained lowest in the lifestyle group, with diabetes onset being delayed by about 4 years, compared with about 2 years by metformin. Very few diabetes complications were detected in these low-risk subjects, but the study plans to continue until 2014, when data similar to the Look AHEAD (Action for Health in Diabetes) study might be available [20]. In the Finnish study, and the Diabetes Prevention Program and its 10-year follow-up, lifestyle intervention was most effective in older people (>60 years).

Drugs used in the treatment of diabetes

Six studies have trialled pharmacological agents in use for people with established type 2 diabetes:
- STOP-NIDDM (2002, acarbose);
- TRIPOD (2002, troglitazone);
- XENDOS (2004, orlistat);
- DREAM (2006, rosiglitazone);
- Voglibose (Japanese) (2009);
- NAVIGATOR (nateglinide, 2010).

NAVIGATOR apart, all slowed progression of IGT to diabetes to a greater or lesser extent. In the Diabetes Prevention Program, the preventive effects of metformin were best seen in younger, more obese subjects. Acarbose reduced the risk of progression by 25% in the STOP-NIDDM study (and also, controversially, possibly reduced cardiovascular events and new-onset hypertension), and a longer-term study of cardiovascular outcomes is in progress (Acarbose Cardiovascular Evaluation, ACE). The glitazones have all been shown to be highly effective; rosiglitazone (DREAM, 2006) and pioglitazone (ACT-NOW) reduced risk by 60 and 80% respectively, although congestive heart failure increased with rosiglitazone. However, concerns about the long-term effects of the glitazones make them unsuitable for clinical use in this situation. In striking contrast, in the NAVIGATOR study, nateglinide 60 mg t.d.s. neither reduced progression to diabetes over 5 years nor (as a primary aim of the study) had any impact on cardiovascular events [21].

Other drugs

In many studies of angiotensin-converting enzyme (ACE) inhibitors and angiotensin receptor blockers (ARBs), the observed incidence of new-onset diabetes was less frequent than in the placebo group, hinting at a clinical correlate of laboratory evidence for the insulin-sensitizing properties of these drugs. However, in the DREAM study (2006), ramipril 15 mg daily did not reduce the incidence of diabetes, although 2-hour post-load glucose values were numerically lower. In the much larger NAVIGATOR study (2010), valsartan 160 mg daily, though reducing the incidence of diabetes by 14%, importantly, like its co-drug in the same study nateglinide, had no impact on a wide spectrum of cardiovascular outcomes (including hospitalization for heart failure and non-fatal stroke) [22].

Practical implications
- When detected, IGT and the associated features of the metabolic syndrome should be actively managed.
- The aims should be to reduce weight by 4–6 kg and increase moderate exercise to 150 min per week.
- Discuss the evidence for using metformin 850 mg b.d. or acarbose, increasing if tolerated to 100 mg t.d.s.

Screening for diabetes

In the UK, firm recommendations are still awaited. The following scheme is based on the 2010 ADA recommendations, in turn derived from the Diabetes Prevention Program results. Screen, using FPG measurements, adults of any age who are overweight or obese (BMI ≥ 25 or ≥ 23 in South Asians in UK) with any of the following additional risk factors [23].
- First-degree relative with diabetes (parents and sibs).
- Previous GDM (or baby weighing > 4 kg) is a very important group for screening. Around 5% of diet-treated white GDM patients progress each year to type 2 diabetes, about 10 times the background rate. The rate is increasing with increasing population obesity. Obese ethnic-minority patients with postpartum IGT are the very highest risk group, especially for development of premature coronary heart disease, and annual screening would seem prudent, though not yet officially recommended.
- Hypertension (twofold to threefold increased risk) or history of vascular disease.
- Dyslipidaemia, especially with insulin-resistant dyslipidaemia: triglycerides > 2.8 mmol/L (250 mg/dL) and/or high-density lipoprotein (HDL)-cholesterol < 0.9 mmol/L (35 mg/dL).
- Conditions associated with insulin resistance, e.g. polycystic ovarian syndrome, acanthosis nigricans, severe obesity.
- High-risk ethnic groups.

The ADA also includes those who are 'physically inactive' as a risk factor, which indeed it is, but including this criterion poses evident practical difficulties. All normoglycaemic individuals should be rescreened at 3-year or shorter intervals, and in the absence of risk factors the ADA suggests commencing screening at 45 years of age.

Prevention of type 1 diabetes

Over the past 20 years many intervention studies have attempted to prevent complete loss of β-cell function immediately after the clinical diagnosis of type 1 diabetes. Most agents have been ineffective or toxic. Less toxic compounds, for example nicotinamide and BCG, also showed no benefit. While a recent trial of oral or parenteral insulin (Diabetes Prevention Trial – Type 1) also showed no benefit, it did demonstrate the practicality of screening large numbers of high-risk first-degree subjects for inclusion in future studies. (Importantly, knowing the antibody status of their children and participating in a clinical trial does not increase parental stress levels.) Currently, the most promising agent is otelixizumab, a chimeric/humanized CD3 antibody (ChAglyCD3). Given as a 6-day course within 3 months of diagnosis, it preserved β-cell function better than placebo over 3 years and delayed the rise in insulin requirements over 4 years, with lower HbA$_{1c}$ measurements. A confirmatory Phase III clinical trial (DEFEND-2) is in progress. The anti-CD20 monoclonal antibody rituximab (intravenous), the tumour necrosis factor (TNF)-α inhibitor etanercept (subcutaneous) and oral interferon (IFN)-α all also preserve C-peptide levels better than placebo. Results with these varied agents are encouraging, though concerns about possible long-term adverse effects may limit their use, especially in children. Non-pharmacological interventions include a new phase of primary prevention trials manipulating putative environmental triggers, for example different infant feed formulae, or supplementing with vitamin D, deficiency of which seems to be closely associated with increased risk of type 1 diabetes. Early studies of autologous stem-cell transplantation are in progress, and almost daily reported in the popular press.

References

1. Tapp RJ, Zimmet PZ, Harper CA *et al*. Diagnostic thresholds for diabetes: the association of retinopathy and albuminuria with glycaemia. AusDiab Study Group. *Diabetes Res Clin Pract* 2006;73:315–21. PMID: 16644057.
2. Selvin E, Crainiceanu CM, Brancati FL, Coresh J. Short-term variability in measures of glycemia and implications for the classification of diabetes. *Arch Intern Med* 2007;167:1545–51. PMID: 17646610.
3. Balasubramanyam A, Nalini R, Hampe CS, Maldonado M. Syndromes of ketosis-prone diabetes mellitus. *Endocr Rev* 2008;29:292–302. PMID: 18292467.

4. Bingley PJ. Clinical applications of diabetes antibody testing. *J Clin Endocrinol Metab* 2010;95:25–33. PMID: 19875480.
5. Eisenbarth GS, Gottlieb PA. Autoimmune polyendocrine syndromes. *N Engl J Med* 2004;350:2068–79. PMID: 15141045.
6. Barker JM. Clinical Review: Type 1 diabetes-associated autoimmunity: natural history, genetic associations, and screening. *J Clin Endocrinol Metab* 2006;91:1210–17. PMID: 16403820.
7. Bell DS, Allbright E. The multifaceted associations of hepatobiliary disease and diabetes. *Endocr Pract* 2007;13:300–12. PMID: 17599864.
8. Fourlanos S, Perry C, Stein MS, Stankovich J, Harrison LC, Colman PG. A clinical screening tool identifies autoimmune diabetes in adults. *Diabetes Care* 2006;29:970–5. PMID: 16644622.
9. Leslie RDG, Williams R, Pozzilli P. Clinical Review: Type 1 diabetes and latent autoimmune diabetes in adults: one end of the rainbow. *J Clin Endocrinol Metab* 2006;91:1654–9. PMID: 16478821.
10. Banerji MA, Chaiken RL, Huey H et al. GAD antibody negative NIDDM in adult black subjects with diabetic ketoacidosis and increased frequency of human leukocyte antigen DR3 and DR4. Flatbush diabetes. *Diabetes* 1994;43:741–5. PMID: 8194658.
11. Brickman WJ, Huang J, Silverman BL, Metzger BE. Acanthosis nigricans identifies youth at high risk for metabolic abnormalities. *J Pediatr* 2010;156:87–92. PMID: 19796772.
12. Pinhas-Hamiel O, Zeitler P. Acute and chronic complications of type 2 diabetes mellitus in children and adolescents. *Lancet* 2007;369:1823–31. PMID: 17531891.
13. Chiodini I, Torlontano M, Scillitani A et al. Association of subclinical hypercortisolism with type 2 diabetes mellitus: a case-control study in hospitalized patients. *Eur J Endocrinol* 2005;153:837–44. PMID: 16322389.
14. Crowther CA, Hiller JE, Moss JR, McPhee AJ, Jeffries WS, Robinson JD for the Australian Carbohydrate Intolerance Study in Pregnant Women (ACHOIS) Trial Group. Effect of treatment of gestational diabetes mellitus on pregnancy outcomes. *N Engl J Med* 2005;352:2477–86. PMID: 15951574.
15. Metzger BE, Lowe LP, Dyer AR et al. Hyperglycemia and adverse pregnancy outcomes. HAPO Study Cooperative Research Group. *N Engl J Med* 2008;358:1991–2002. PMID: 18463375.
16. International Association of Diabetes and Pregnancy Study Groups Consensus Panel. International Association of Diabetes and Pregnancy Study Groups recommendations on the diagnosis and classification of hyperglycemia in pregnancy. *Diabetes Care* 2010;33:676–82. PMID: 20190296.
17. Borg R, Kuenen JC, Carstensen B et al. Real-life glycaemic profiles in non-diabetic individuals with low fasting glucose and normal HbA$_{1c}$: the A1C-Derived Average Glucose (ADAG) study. *Diabetologia* 2010;53:1608–11. PMID: 20396998. See Preface: this is a good example of laudable attempts at simplification resulting in unintentional complexity, with individual practitioners and their patients being caught in the crossfire.
18. Faerch K, Borch-Johnsen K, Holst JJ, Vaag A. Pathophysiology and aetiology of impaired fasting glycaemia and impaired glucose tolerance: does it matter for prevention and treatment of type 2 diabetes? *Diabetologia* 2009;52:1714–23. PMID: 19590846.
19. Lindström J, Ilanne-Parikka P, Peltonen M et al. Sustained reduction in the incidence of type 2 diabetes by lifestyle intervention: follow-up of the Finnish Diabetes Prevention Study. *Lancet* 2006;368:1673–9. PMID: 17098085.

20. Diabetes Prevention Program Research Group. 10-year follow-up of diabetes incidence and weight loss in the Diabetes Prevention Program Outcomes Study. *Lancet* 2009;374:1677–86. PMID: 19878986.
21. The NAVIGATOR Study Group. Effect of nateglinide on the incidence of diabetes and cardiovascular events. *N Engl J Med* 2010;362:1463–76. PMID: 20228403.
22. The NAVIGATOR Study Group. Effect of valsartan on the incidence of diabetes and cardiovascular events. *N Engl J Med* 2010;362:1477–90. PMID: 20228402.
23. American Diabetes Association. Standards of medical care in diabetes 2010. *Diabetes Care* 2010;33(Suppl 1):S11–S61. PMID: 20042772.

Further reading

Definition, diagnosis and classification

American Diabetes Association. Diagnosis and classification of diabetes mellitus. *Diabetes Care* 2010;33(Suppl 1):S62–S69. PMID: 20042775.

Definition and diagnosis of diabetes mellitus and intermediate hyperglycemia: report of a WHO/IDF consultation. 2006 update and revision of the 1999 document. Available at www.who.int/entity/diabetes/publications

National Institute for Health and Clinical Excellence. Prevention of type 2 diabetes. Publication expected June 2011.

Children and adolescents

American Diabetes Association. Type 2 diabetes in children and adolescents. *Diabetes Care* 2000;23:381–9. PMID: 10868870.

Pregnancy and GDM

International Association of Diabetes and Pregnancy Study Groups Consensus Panel. International Association of Diabetes and Pregnancy Study Groups recommendations on the diagnosis and classification of hyperglycemia in pregnancy. *Diabetes Care* 2010;33:676–82.

National Institute for Health and Clinical Excellence. CG63 Diabetes in pregnancy: full guideline (reissued July 2008). Available from www.nice.org.uk

Books of general interest: medical and cultural history of diabetes

Bliss M. *The Discovery of Insulin*, 25th Anniversary Edition. Chicago: Chicago University Press, 2007.

Feudtner C. *Bittersweet: Diabetes, Insulin, and the Transformation of Illness*. Chapel Hill, NC: University of North Carolina Press, 2003.

Tattersall R. *Diabetes: The Biography*. Oxford: Oxford University Press, 2009.

Websites

Diabetes Prevention Program (NIDDK, NIH), study documents website: www.bsc.gwu.edu/dpp/index/htmlvdoc

National Diabetes Information Clearinghouse: www.diabetes.niddk.nih.gov

National Diabetes Education Program: www.ndep.nih.gov

Diabetes in the emergency department

CHAPTER 2

Key points

- Hyperglycaemic emergencies are costly and still carry a mortality, especially the hyperosmolar hyperglycaemic state in older people.
- The underlying cause of diabetic ketoacidosis is insulin deficiency. Ensuring adequate insulin replacement in the face of falling glucose levels is important in rapid resolution.
- The rate of fluid replacement and reduction in glucose levels must be tailored to the clinical situation, especially in patients with severe hyperglycaemia at presentation.
- Severe hypoglycaemia is very common, and increasingly so in type 2 patients, in whom it is a risk factor for mortality, regardless of the level of overall glycaemia. Treat the hypoglycaemia and, where possible, address the underlying problem(s).
- Patients presenting with acute diabetic foot infections require careful assessment, as the underlying severity may not be reflected in symptoms and signs; admission is usually required.

Introduction

Every day many patients with established or newly diagnosed diabetes pass through emergency departments. Few require admission, but all need careful evaluation and management: emergencies in diabetes can develop rapidly, and they carry a risk of mortality. Deciding who needs admission requires clinical skill and experience. Type 1 patients are often young and may look superficially well even though metabolically decompensated, and type 2 patients with, for example, apparently minor foot infections

Practical Diabetes Care, 3rd edition. © David Levy.
Published 2011 by Blackwell Publishing Ltd.

may be severely septic with relatively few symptoms or signs. Those presenting without a primary diabetes problem may be much sicker as a result of poorly controlled diabetes and underlying long-term complications (especially renal and cardiac) that are not always apparent.

Hyperglycaemic emergencies: diabetic ketoacidosis and hyperglycaemic hyperosmolar state

Differentiating between DKA and hyperglycaemic hyperosmolar state (HHS, previously hyperosmolar non-ketotic state or HONK) is not difficult, but is important (Table 2.1). HHS has a different pathogenesis, occurs in a different group of patients (older, type 2, often with significant comorbidities) and carries a worse prognosis, with quoted mortality rates of about 15%. Fortunately, despite increasing numbers of cases, deaths from DKA are now uncommon and in developed countries mortality is around 2%, lower than the 4–10% quoted in the literature, although mortality increases with age, reaching 15% in those aged over 70. In the USA, mortality due to all hyperglycaemic emergencies fell consistently between 1985 and 2002. Nevertheless, even in a cohort of European youngsters diagnosed since 1989, there is a twofold increased standardized mortality rate, and up to one-third of deaths in this relatively early phase of diabetes, before the onset of late complications, may be related to DKA [1]. In the UK, one-quarter of all DKA cases occurs in those under 18.

All true hyperglycaemic emergencies require clinical and biochemical vigilance. They are not 'set-piece' emergencies, especially HHS. Some studies quote up to 30% of DKA patients having a simultaneous hyperosmolar state, though clinically it seems to be much less frequent. Finally, despite hyperglycaemic emergencies being so common, the evidence base for their management is surprisingly slim.

Diabetic ketoacidosis

It is important to distinguish between DKA and hyperglycaemic states that require different, less urgent and less intensive treatment. Writing 'DKA' is easy, because it is a simple acronym, but all three elements must be present to make the diagnosis.
- Hyperglycaemia, though it is not always very marked.
- Ketosis, signifying insulin deficiency.
- Acidosis: other causes of metabolic acidosis that are clinically rare, for example alcohol intoxication or salicylate overdose, can present as ketoacidosis (alcohol intoxication is a frequent precipitant of DKA, but very rarely through its metabolic consequences).

Table 2.1 Clinical features of diabetic ketoacidosis (DKA) and hyperglycaemic hyperosmolar state (HHS)

	DKA	HHS
Patients	Type 1 diabetes (but see Chapter 1 for important exceptions)	Type 2 diabetes
Duration of symptoms	Short, often <24 hours	Longer, often several days, sometimes insidious over weeks
Pathogenesis	Insulin deficiency Glucagon (and other counter-regulatory hormone) excess Abnormal metabolism of non-esterified fatty acids	Insulin deficiency Renal impairment Reduced thirst
Mortality	<< 4%	~ 15%
Complications	Cerebral oedema, especially in the young Respiratory distress syndrome Thromboembolism Rhabdomyolysis	Thromboembolism Rhabdomyolysis
Working biochemical definition	Blood pH < 7.3 (mild 7.25–7.30; moderate 7.00–7.24; severe < 7.0) Blood bicarbonate ≤ 17 mmol/L (in early compensated phase, bicarbonate buffers ketoacids, so bicarbonate is low but pH normal) Urinary ketones ≥ 2+	Arterial pH > 7.3 Plasma osmolality > 320 mosmol/kg Bicarbonate >18 mmol/L

Therefore it is important to distinguish DKA from severe hyperglycaemia and ketosis.
- *Severe hyperglycaemia*: many type 1 patients have occasional blood glucose levels above 20 mmol/L (360 mg/dL), and those in chronically very poor control, e.g. HbA_{1c} above 10% (86 mmol/mol) may occasionally have values in excess of 30 mmol/L (540 mg/dL) without being unwell or ketotic.
- *Ketosis*: high blood glucose levels with ketonuria (≥1+) but no acidosis in an otherwise well patient. Significant ketonuria is quite

uncommon these days in ambulatory practice; always try to find a reason for it, and ensure the patient has a supply of urine test strips (e.g. Ketostix, Bayer; Ketur Test, Roche Diagnostics) to monitor ketonuria two or three times daily, and report back if there are symptoms, or ketonuria does not remit within 24 hours.

The primary problem in DKA is therefore insulin deficiency, not hyperglycaemia. Appreciating this permits efficient and safe management; however, the insulin deficiency is often ignored in preference to treating blood glucose levels, which do not correlate with clinical severity.

Management of the clinically well, newly presenting type 1 patient

Even when there is significant ketonuria ($\geqslant 2+$) and hyperglycaemia, e.g. up to 20 mmol/L (360 mg/dL), an otherwise well younger patient does not routinely require admission, but they need immediate attention, where available, by the hospital diabetes team and a clear plan for close follow-up. Emergency outpatient insulin is straightforward, especially with modern disposable insulin pens, and many patients can learn to inject insulin very quickly. However, for this to be safe, the following are mandatory:

- telephone access to diabetes specialist nurse;
- good home circumstances and support;
- no physical or other disabilities that could impede insulin administration;
- follow-up within 24 hours of discharge, preferably in person.

In general, patients with known type 1 disease and marked hyperglycaemia and ketonuria without acidosis should be admitted at least briefly as there may be compliance problems that make immediate discharge more hazardous. Intravenous rehydration is not routinely required if patients are drinking; where available, measure capillary ketones (see below), and if elevated a brief admission for intravenous fluids and insulin should rapidly resolve the situation.

Precipitating factors

Diabetic ketoacidosis

Immediate precipitating causes include the following.

1 Newly presenting type 1 or type 2 diabetes (10–20%).
2 Infection, most commonly chest, urinary tract or gastrointestinal (30–40%).
3 Other intercurrent medical illness, e.g. myocardial infarction, stroke, occasionally surgical illness (especially acute pancreatitis).

4 Omission of insulin (15–30%):
   (a) Most commonly through failure to implement the sick-day rule not to stop insulin treatment if not eating ('no food, no insulin').
   (b) Accidental, e.g. failure of insulin pump (very rare) or insulin pen, more commonly simply running out of insulin supplies.
5 There are several reports from the USA of recreational drugs, especially cocaine, being associated with DKA (especially if recurrent). Screening has been suggested but poses ethical problems; nevertheless, remember the association and ask [2].
6 Other causes: 'brittle diabetes'; young women with disordered eating and associated insulin omission (see Chapter 13); patients with advanced neuropathy and gastroparesis, leading to recurrent vomiting; and antipsychotic drugs, especially olanzapine and clozapine, are associated with DKA, probably by directly inhibiting insulin secretion.

A common clinical scenario is the young person who drinks too much alcohol, vomits, and fails to take their bedtime insulin and mealtime insulin the following morning and lunchtime because they do not wake up. In up to 40% of cases there is no identifiable precipitating factor.

Hyperglycaemic hyperosmolar state

HHS is much more commonly a presentation of previously undiagnosed type 2 diabetes than is DKA a presentation of type 1 diabetes, though the quoted figure of 30% is 20 years old and it is probably much lower now. Infection, renal impairment, cardiac events and the slow, relentless and sometimes undetected progression of hyperglycaemia that is the hallmark of type 2 diabetes are probably the most important factors, together with the thirst impairment associated with old age.

Ketones in DKA (Fig. 2.1)

Accelerated lipolysis caused by excess catecholamines and insulin deficiency are the major factors generating elevated ketone levels in DKA. The normal plasma ratio of the major ketone bodies, acetoacetate and β-hydroxybutyrate, is 1 : 1 (total concentration about 0.5–1.0 mmol/L), but in DKA may rise to 6 : 1 or more, with β-hydroxybutyrate concentrations up to 12 mmol/L (1.2 mg/dL). To adequately suppress ketogenesis, the key to managing DKA is intravenous insulin at approximately 0.1 unit/kg per hour (see below). Acetone, the minor ketone body, is not dissociated and does not contribute to acidosis, but together with acetoacetate is detected on routine urinalysis for ketones. Many people cannot smell acetone on the breath of DKA patients; others can detect apparently low concentrations.

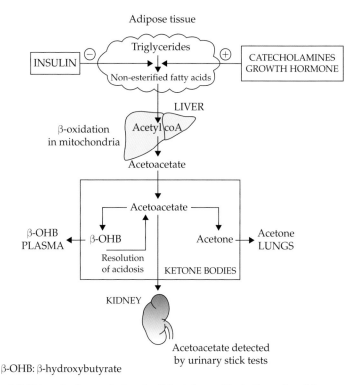

Fig. 2.1 Ketone body metabolism in diabetic ketoacidosis. Reproduced from Levy D (2010) *Type 1 Diabetes*, with permission from OUP

Insulin deficiency in untreated DKA results in excess acetyl-CoA, which condenses to acetoacetate and is reduced to β-hydroxybutyrate; the reverse oxidation occurs once insulin is given, resulting in decreased plasma β-hydroxybutyrate but increased urinary acetoacetate and acetone [3]. Resolution of ketosis is therefore not reliably detected by the use of urinary ketones, which may remain positive long after β-hydroxybutyrate has disappeared from the plasma.

Simple quantitative capillary β-hydroxybutyrate measurements are now available using a standard blood glucose meter with specific strips (Abbott Optium Xceed Meter with Optium β-Ketone Test Strips). The assay range is 0–8 mmol/L; less than 0.6 mmol/L is normal, and significant ketosis is present with values above 1.0–1.5 mmol/L; patients in DKA may have levels in excess of 6 mmol/L. Where meters and strips are available, in DKA blood ketones should be measured frequently, for example every 4 hours, to monitor resolution of ketosis. Because of the delayed resolution of ketonuria compared with blood ketone levels, the measurement is also useful in patients who have positive urinary ketones despite being clinically well. Blood ketones should be normal (<0.6 mmol/L) before discharge. The use of capillary ketone measurements in DKA has been shown to reduce length of hospital stay.

Intensive care unit?

Local policy varies – in some countries all DKA patients are admitted to the intensive care unit (ICU) – but all patients with impaired consciousness should be promptly assessed by the ICU team, as level of consciousness is related to the degree of metabolic derangement. They are at risk of (or may already have) cerebral oedema, particularly common in children and adolescents (up to 5% of cases) and which carries a mortality of up to 25%. The youth and lack of comorbidity of a DKA patient should not influence decision-making: a young person in pre-coma is a high-risk patient. Other groups who should be considered for ICU include those in shock and those with a surgical illness or severe coexisting medical illness, for example sepsis, pneumonia or rhabdomyolysis.

Most patients can be managed well in emergency medical centres/units, where intensified medical, nursing and biochemical supervision can easily be given, especially in the critical first 12–24 hours.

Abdominal pain in hyperglycaemic emergencies

Abdominal pain is common in DKA, its severity related to the degree of acidosis but not to the degree of hyperglycaemia or dehydration; it is particularly likely to be present when serum bicarbonate is less than 5 mmol/L, and with alcohol or cocaine use. Acute pancreatitis secondary to severe hypertriglyceridaemia is more likely to occur in HHS than DKA, but serum amylase measurements correlate also with pH and serum osmolality; even a threefold increase in serum amylase is not a reliable indication of acute pancreatitis, and amlyase cannot be measured in severely lipaemic serum, common in all hyperglycaemic emergencies. Investigate abdominal pain if pH is near-normal or if pain persists after resolution of DKA [4].

Investigations

Do not waste time ordering unnecessary emergency investigations. A biochemical flow chart is invaluable.

Obligatory

- Urinalysis for ketones (and where available capillary β-hydroxybutyrate); write results prominently and clearly in the notes. Urinalysis results should be recorded using the familiar semi-quantitative grades (negative, trace, 1+, 2+, 3+) and not as pseudo-quantitative measurements which may be misinterpreted.

- Plasma glucose, urea, creatinine and electrolytes (blood gas [K^+] measurements can be clinically misleading).
- Blood pH and bicarbonate: in clinically stable patients who are not hypoxic, venous blood is satisfactory and allows frequent sampling.
- Full blood count and C-reactive protein (CRP): ketosis itself causes neutrophilia, but there is no agreement on what constitutes non-specific elevation. Assess for presence of infection clinically and with CRP.
- Place a large intravenous line.

According to circumstances
- ECG in patients over 40 years old (then maintain on cardiac monitor, especially if there is hyperkalaemia or hypokalaemia).
- Chest radiography.
- Cultures: blood, urine, throat, cerebrospinal fluid, septic site (always quickly check the feet for painless infected ulcers). Symptoms of infection can be blunted by acidosis and neuropathy.
- Creatine kinase (CK): rhabdomyolysis can occur in both DKA and HHS. Consider when there is high glucose and osmolality, low phosphate, otherwise unexplained renal impairment (though this is very common in HHS) or clinically dark urine. Measure CK in all patients found collapsed in pre-coma or coma.
- Phosphate and magnesium in severe metabolic disturbance (see below).

Management

The hazards of DKA and HHS include the following.
- Circulatory collapse (hypovolaemia, acidosis, electrolyte disturbance).
- Cerebral oedema, associated with massive fluid over-replacement and rapid changes in osmolality.
- Pulmonary oedema in older people, again associated with fluid over-replacement.
- Hypokalaemia, especially if serum [K^+] is normal or low to begin with.
- Rapid changes in serum [Na^+] (see below): central pontine myelinolysis has been reported in a small number of cases of HHS with very high glucose levels at presentation where treatment caused rapid changes in osmolality.

Fluid replacement
When surveyed, physicians say they aim to replace the fluid deficit of 5–8 L in only 8 hours, although the general view is that this replacement should be over 24 hours, especially in HHS. The traditional approach

of giving one or more 'stat' litres of 0.9% NaCl in the accident and emergency department is potentially hazardous, especially in HHS. Severe prerenal failure is often present in both DKA and HHS, and occult ischaemic heart disease should be assumed in older HHS patients. Hypotension should be treated on its own merits. Insulin is less effective in the hyperosmolar state, so starting fluids before the insulin infusion may have advantages.

Fluid replacement: correcting serum [Na⁺] for prevailing glucose levels

Sodium chloride 0.9% is recommended. However, hypernatraemia (serum $[Na^+] > 150\,mmol/L$) is common in both DKA and HHS. This occurs because severe hyperglycaemia causes initial *hypo*natraemia due to osmotic effects from water moving out of cells: an increase in glucose of $3.4\,mmol/L$ ($60\,mg/dL$) reduces serum $[Na^+]$ by $1\,mmol/L$ (use the approximation of $4\,mmol/L$ for $1\,mmol/L$).

Therefore, a glucose level of about $40\,mmol/L$ ($700\,mg/dL$) depresses $[Na^+]$ by about $12\,mmol/L$, and at presentation HHS glucose values of $80–100\,mmol/L$ ($1440–1800\,mg/dL$) are not uncommon, accounting for serum $[Na^+]$ levels being depressed by $24–30\,mmol/L$. Many patients presenting with severe hyperglycaemia and low or normal serum $[Na^+]$ are therefore at risk of hypernatraemia once the glucose is corrected. Always correct laboratory $[Na^+]$ for prevailing glucose levels. Consider using 0.45% ('half normal') NaCl after the first litre or two of isotonic NaCl in patients with high corrected $[Na^+]$. The clinical impression is that serum $[Na^+]$ continues to climb for several hours after appropriate fluid is given, so anticipate this problem. Triglycerides are not osmotically active, and the often severe hypertriglyceridaemia of uncontrolled diabetes, caused by insulin deficiency (and resulting in 'strawberry yoghurt' venous blood), does not cause hyponatraemia with modern laboratory methods for measuring electrolytes.

In the UK there is a move away from NaCl for routine fluid replacement towards Hartmann's solution (sodium lactate), which has a lower sodium concentration (131 vs. $154\,mmol/L$) and lower chloride concentration ($111\,mmol/L$). However, patients in DKA may already have elevated lactate levels, and the additional lactate in Hartmann's solution could generate higher glucose levels. More practically, Hartmann's solution contains a fixed low potassium concentration ($5\,mmol/L$); restrictions on adding KCl to intravenous infusions could limit flexible and adequate potassium replacement. The advice is that NaCl remains standard intravenous fluid for initial treatment of hyperglycaemic emergencies [5].

Intravenous insulin regimen and blood glucose monitoring
Diabetic ketoacidosis
In severe hyperglycaemia, most glucose disposal is through non-insulin-dependent pathways (e.g. renal). Insulin is used primarily to suppress ketogenesis and glucagon levels, and not to reduce hyperglycaemia (see above). Rehydration and correction of acidosis will cause blood glucose levels to fall independent of the rate of insulin infusion. Current UK guidelines recommend continuing subcutaneous long-acting analogue insulin in the usual dose and at the usual time.

In the UK, insulin is usually given by continuous intravenous infusion through an infusion pump (soluble insulin: 50 units Humulin S or Actrapid in 50 mL 0.9% NaCl), although intermittent intramuscular insulin regimens are effective and still widely used. Ketosis is suppressed with insulin at the usual starting rate of 6 units/hour, but this rate often causes a precipitous fall in blood glucose, especially in HHS. Usual practice is to change from 0.9% NaCl to 5% glucose infusion when capillary blood glucose falls below 14 mmol/L (250 mg/dL), but at this level most so-called 'sliding scale' (variable rate) intravenous insulin infusions specify rates of 1–2 units/hour, too low to suppress ketogenesis but still sufficient to cause hypoglycaemia, especially when given with 5% glucose. Finally, since this point may be reached only a few hours after presentation, substantial rehydration with NaCl is still required. Where possible, therefore, after initial resuscitation and once capillary blood glucose levels are below 14 mmol/L, use a triple infusion regimen (Fig. 2.2):
- 10% glucose at 100 mL/hour (or 500 mL over 4 hours);
- maintain rehydration (and potassium replacement) with 0.9% NaCl (in the UK 10% glucose does not come with pre-added KCl);
- soluble insulin infusion at a constant 6 units/hour with careful capillary blood glucose monitoring.

Perform frequent (4-hourly) capillary ketone measurements (where available) and venous bicarbonate measurements until the acidosis has resolved, in addition to hourly capillary blood glucose measurements. Remember that most near-patient glucose meters read up to a maximum of 33 mmol/L (600 mg/dL), some (those manufactured by Abbott) up to 27.8 mmol/L (500 mg/dL); use laboratory measurements until values are below this level.

Hyperglycaemic hyperosmolar state
HHS patients have residual β-cell function and are not ketotic, so high insulin doses should not be required; clinically, HHS patients are often sensitive to insulin. The risk of rapid osmotic shifts and severe hypernatraemia can be reduced by using low-dose insulin infusions (e.g. 1–2 units/hour), which can be increased if blood glucose levels do not fall,

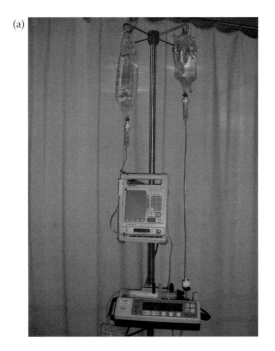

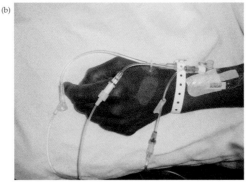

Fig. 2.2 Intravenous infusions in diabetic ketoacidosis. (a) Triple infusion: 0.9% NaCl (left) running at, for example, 1 L 6–8 hourly, together with 10% glucose (right) 500 mL 4-hourly, once blood glucose is < 14 mmol/L (250 mg/dL), and (below) infusion pump delivering soluble insulin at 6 units/hour. (b) Infusion running

together with gentle intravenous 0.9% NaCl (e.g. 1 L every 6–8 hours). Although the metabolic disturbance may not be as evident as in DKA, the high level of comorbidity, especially renal impairment (which may be severe), means that HHS patients, especially the elderly, require careful clinical assessment and management. Very rapid rehydration may be fatal.

Electrolytes

- Measure creatinine and electrolytes at 4 and 8 hours, thereafter according to the clinical and biochemical state.
- Hypokalaemia, rather than hyperkalaemia, is often a problem, because insulin and rising pH both drive extracellular potassium into cells.
- Bicarbonate: do not give unless pH is below 7.0 and patient is gravely ill. There is no indication for bicarbonate in an otherwise well DKA patient even with severe acidosis. Give 700 mL of 1.2% sodium bicarbonate solution over 45 min, together with 20 mmol KCl, and repeat until pH exceeds 7.0. DKA requiring bicarbonate should be managed on the ICU or under intensivist supervision.
- Magnesium and phosphate can both be low in DKA (low phosphate occurs in about 15%), but they are of little clinical importance except in the most severe metabolic disturbances. DKA associated with acute alcoholic intoxication or rhabdomyolysis can cause hypophosphataemia, so measure serum phosphate in these circumstances. Severe hypophosphataemia is associated with respiratory failure, arrhythmias and generalized weakness. Consider intravenous phosphate replacement in critically ill patients in ICU [6].
- Hyperchloraemic acidosis, a transient non-anion gap acidosis, may occur as ketones are replaced by chloride, especially when large quantities of NaCl have been given. This may account for slow resolution of acidosis in some cases of DKA. Move to a high-glucose (10%) and high-insulin infusion regimen with frequent biochemistry and pH monitoring.

Other interventions

- Patients with impaired consciousness should have a urinary catheter and nasogastric tube placed, but these patients should be managed in ICU. There is no need for either in an otherwise clinically well patient; unnecessary use, especially of urinary catheters, may delay discharge and predispose to infection that was not there in the first place.
- Urinary tract and chest infections are frequent precipitants or associations of DKA and HHS. Neutrophilia is a non-specific finding in DKA, neuropathy may blunt pleuritic or ischaemic chest pain and dysuria, and ketosis can suppress fever. After taking appropriate cultures, antibiotics (e.g. co-amoxiclav) should be used freely in these patients.
- Anticoagulation: use prophylactic anticoagulation in HHS patients, and immobile or unconscious DKA patients.
- Keep meticulous fluid balance charts; most hospitals have their own monitoring and prescription charts for hyperglycaemic emergencies.

Follow-up

The first 12–24 hours of a hyperglycaemic emergency are usually managed with few problems, but the transition to discharge can be less smooth. Always involve the inpatient diabetes team as soon as possible after admission: they are likely to know many of the DKA patients.

- *Establish the cause of the emergency.* This can be explored in more detail by the diabetes team. There must be an educational review: DKA should be seen as a failure of integrated diabetes care in the community. Many DKA patients are poor clinic attenders with premature complications, poor long-term glycaemic control and high rates of associated psychiatric problems. A definitive follow-up plan must be formulated and agreed with the patient; organize a further diabetes review (telephone or in-person) within a few days of discharge. Try to remember to request an HbA$_{1c}$ measurement, particularly in poor clinic attenders, as this will help medium-term management planning.
- *Duration of intravenous insulin infusion.* In moderate or severe DKA, most patients will require 24 hours of intravenous insulin, often longer in the sicker HHS patients. As soon as ketosis has resolved, preferably judged by capillary ketone measurement, transfer patients to subcutaneous insulin. If ketonuria persists while the patient is well and eating, confirm the absence of true ketosis by measuring capillary ketones.
- Where possible, discontinue intravenous insulin early in the day. Discontinue intravenous insulin after a subcutaneous dose has been given, just before a meal.

Hyperosmolar patients with persistently negative ketones

Hyperosmolar patients with persistently negative ketonuria can usually be transferred to oral hypoglycaemic agents before discharge.

- Do not use metformin alone: it acts too slowly under these circumstances and impaired renal function may contraindicate its use.
- Start newly diagnosed patients on a low dose of sulphonylurea (e.g. gliclazide 40–80 mg b.d.), together with a low dose of metformin if no contraindications. Unless the patient is thin, regard the sulphonylurea as a temporary glucose-reducing measure that should be discontinued as soon as possible. Ensure the patient has clear straightforward advice on the symptoms of hypoglycaemia, on how to contact the diabetes team if it occurs, and how to reduce or stop the medication.
- Even in ketone-negative patients, err on the side of caution, and discharge patients on insulin if there has been preceding weight loss or if the patient is thin or of normal weight.

- Where possible, observe for 24 hours after starting oral hypoglycaemic agents to ensure reasonable blood glucose levels (e.g. 8–12 mmol/L, 145–220 mg/dL).
- Ask for a dietitian consultation: at this stage of type 2 diabetes, resolve will be at its greatest and a substantial proportion will be well controlled on diet with or without metformin in due course.
- Involve the inpatient diabetes team or diabetes specialist nurses: education is critical, especially about hypoglycaemia, which is perceived by most to be a problem that only occurs in insulin-treated diabetes.
- Ensure that there is good communication with the patient's primary care team, and arrange follow-up within a week with either team.

Known type 1 patients

Re-establish the previous insulin regimen, unless there is good reason to believe that it was itself responsible for the emergency, which would be unusual compared with the much more frequent problem of failing to take the previously agreed insulin dose. Making changes while an inpatient often delays discharge, is often pointless and is potentially hazardous. Changes are much better made in the ambulatory setting shortly after discharge, with inpatient time being used to discuss the reasons for the episode.

Newly diagnosed type 1 patients

Most patients at some stage will be established on a multiple-dose insulin (MDI) regimen. In some countries, newly diagnosed patients remain in hospital for an intensive period of education. In Norway, for example, many start insulin pump treatment immediately after diagnosis. Elsewhere, the major considerations are safety – avoiding hypoglycaemia and suppressing ketogenesis – and this can be achieved with relatively low doses of insulin. There is no agreement about whether patients do better in the early stages with a twice-daily fixed mixture regimen or MDI. Twice-daily biphasic mixtures (e.g. NovoMix 30 or Humalog Mix 25 given with breakfast and the evening meal, or Humulin M3 or Insuman Comb 25 given 30 min before these meals) are easy to teach and use, especially with insulin pens (see Chapter 4). Where there are the educational resources, low-dose MDI is secure and will avoid the need to change insulin preparations.

Newly presenting ketotic patients with initially indeterminate diabetes

The practical rule is simple: newly presenting ketotic patients (i.e. those with initial insulin deficiency), with or without acidosis, should be discharged on insulin treatment. Classical type 1 patients will be clinically apparent, but the heterogeneity of ketosis-prone diabetes (see Chapter 1) means that during an initial hospital admission there can be diagnostic uncertainty, and results of supportive laboratory tests (e.g. GADA) are usually not immediately available. The only safe approach is to discharge on insulin, and review frequently until the clinical course becomes clear.

Initial insulin doses

The widely used rule of adding up the previous 24-hour intravenous insulin requirements and dividing into two or four doses according to the planned number of daily injections may be hazardous: DKA is an insulin-resistant state, and using this rule may result in high insulin doses causing hypoglycaemia. Patients treated with high-dose insulin and 10% glucose will inevitably need large doses. Finally, patients are likely to be moving into 'honeymoon', with partial temporary recovery of β-cell function, and will also be much more active once they return home. Calculate an initial total daily dosage at about 0.5 units/kg body weight, the lower end of the usual range of stable insulin requirements for type 1 patients (i.e. 30–40 units/day).

However, there is no room for complacency over glycaemic control in the period following diagnosis of type 1 diabetes. In the DCCT, about one-third of patients with disease duration of less than 5 years had some residual insulin secretion, and intensive treatment (i.e. $HbA_{1c} < 7.0\%$, 53 mmol/mol) can help sustain endogenous insulin secretion for perhaps another 5 or 6 years, with lower risks of severe hypoglycaemia and of microvascular complications [7]. This is particularly important (and challenging) for adolescents where, because of worse overall glycaemic control than adults, the beneficial long-term 'legacy' effects on retinopathy are much less pronounced (see Chapter 9).

Hypoglycaemia

Every person presenting to an emergency department with impaired consciousness must have a reliable capillary glucose measurement recorded in the notes.

- Hypoglycaemia is the commonest complication of type 1 diabetes.
- Hypoglycaemia is frequent in insulin- and sulphonylurea-treated type 2 patients.
- Hypoglycaemia carries a substantial mortality, either directly through brain damage or indirectly through injuries sustained while hypoglycaemic.
- Hypoglycaemia is frightening and disruptive to family, social and work life, undermines confidence, sometimes in the long term, may have neuropsychiatric consequences (e.g. scholastic achievement), especially in the young, and remains the major barrier to implementing intensive glycaemic control in type 1 patients.

Always try to find a reason for the episode. Where possible, trace a recent HbA$_{1c}$ measurement to assess prior over-tight control (e.g. HbA$_{1c}$ < 6.0%, 42 mmol/mol). Reduce oral hypoglycaemic agents or insulin dosages before discharge (with clear written suggestions, especially for the elderly, the forgetful and those who were admitted with severe hypoglycaemia), emphasize increased frequency of home blood glucose monitoring, and arrange early follow-up with the primary or secondary care diabetes team.

Causes

Singly or in combination, the following factors account for most episodes of hypoglycaemia:

- dietary (missing or delaying a meal);
- too much insulin (inadvertent administration);
- unaccustomed exercise;
- alcohol and other drugs.
  However, consider the more uncommon causes listed below.
- Overdose of insulin or sulphonylurea: factitious sulphonylurea overdosing in patients with documented severe hypoglycaemia is surprisingly common. A wide range of sulphonylureas can be measured in plasma. Factitious insulin overdosing can be diagnosed by detecting high insulin and low C-peptide levels in hypoglycaemic patients. Metformin, glitazones, glucagon-like peptide (GLP)-1 analogues and DPP-4 inhibitors do not cause hypoglycaemia individually or in combination, although mild hypoglycaemia can occur in normoglycaemic people treated with metformin, for example patients with polycystic ovarian syndrome.
- Newly developing endocrine disorders, especially Addison's disease (increased risk in type 1 diabetes) and hypopituitarism. The onset may be insidious: consider Addison's in type 1 patients where insulin dose falls by more than about 20% in response to frequent hypoglycaemia, even if the classical biochemical picture ($\uparrow$ [K$^+$], $\downarrow$ [Na$^+$]) is absent.
- Impaired absorption: gastroenteritis, coeliac disease (check tissue transglutaminase).
- Impaired gastric emptying: gastroparesis.
- Failure to decrease insulin dose postpartum; breast-feeding.
- Early pregnancy: decreased insulin requirements plus nausea/hyperemesis.
  In the appropriate setting, remember the non-diabetic causes of hypoglycaemia: insulinoma (not in type 1 patients), hypothermia, alcohol and drugs.
- Severe hypoglycaemia has been reported in patients taking glibenclamide who are prescribed fluoroquinolone antibiotics (fluoroquinolones inhibit the cytochrome P450 CYP3A4 hepatic system that metabolizes glibenclamide) [8]. There is an isolated case report of severe hypoglycaemia in a type 1 patient taking the anti-smoking drug varenicline.

- Non-steroidal anti-inflammatory drugs (including aspirin) can also potentiate the actions of sulphonylureas.
- Combinations of drugs may contribute to hypoglycaemia in patients already in good control (e.g. beta-blockers, ACE inhibitors), though this is rarely seen in practice.
- Reports surface intermittently of herbal remedies and internet and street drugs being spiked with sulphonylureas. Always take a full drug history.

Operational classification of hypoglycaemia
Biochemical/asymptomatic

Counter-regulation in the non-diabetic person (increased glucagon, reduced endogenous insulin) begins when blood glucose levels fall below 3.8 mmol/L (70 mg/dL) (Fig. 2.3). This value is the basis for the widespread recommendation to avoid blood glucose levels lower than 4 mmol/L (72 mg/dL) – 'four's the floor' is a useful mnemonic, though somewhat less snappy when expressed in traditional units. Educating patients that hypoglycaemia is not necessarily an impairment of consciousness, but is frequently a 'numerical' and almost asymptomatic problem that may nevertheless have serious consequences, is important. Cognitive function becomes impaired at blood glucose levels below 3 mmol/L (54 mg/dL),

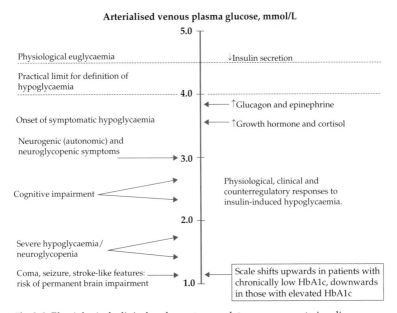

Fig 2.3 Physiological, clinical and counter-regulatory responses to insulin-induced hypoglycaemia

and this level is used by the European drug licensing authority (EMEA) in assessments of adverse effects of diabetes therapies.

Treatment
Patients should take or be offered prophylactic glucose when asymptomatic blood glucose levels below 4.0 mmol/L are detected. It should go without saying that appropriate dose reductions in insulin or oral hypoglycaemic agents should be made if biochemical hypoglycaemia is frequent, with arrangements for monitoring and follow-up, but unfortunately it still needs saying.

Mild (self-treated) symptomatic hypoglycaemia
Most well-controlled type 1 patients have about two mildly symptomatic hypoglycaemic episodes each week [9]. Symptoms are variable, but in individuals they are often stereotyped in nature and sequence.
- Autonomic: sweating, hunger, trembling, anxiety, pounding heart.
- Neuroglycopenic: confusion, odd behaviour, difficulty concentrating. The earliest signs of neuroglycopenia are often very subtle, for example an almost imperceptible slowing or hesitation of speech, and only those who know the patient well (family members, friends, co-workers and sometimes members of the diabetes team) may be able to detect them.
- Motor: incoordination, difficulty walking.
- Sensory: visual disturbance, perioral tingling.
- Others: headache, nausea, difficulty speaking.

Treatment
Take about 20 g carbohydrate, for example:
- two slices of bread;
- two snack-sized chocolate bars;
- 100 mL Lucozade or equivalent glucose sports drink;
- 200 mL non-diet cola drink;
- three cubes of sugar (sucrose);
- in the UK, Glucogel (40% dextrose gel, formerly HypoStop) is available in 25-g tubes (containing 10 g carbohydrate) or 80-g bottles (containing 32 g carbohydrate).

Absorption characteristics for solid and liquid glucose are similar, although liquid is usually recommended. Glycaemic response occurs within 10–15 min, though symptoms improve more rapidly. There is no point in repeating capillary blood glucose measurements after a shorter interval. Do not use nutritional supplements, for example Fortisip (Nutricia), to treat hypoglycaemia in hospitalized patients. These consist mainly of complex carbohydrates (maltodextrins) with only small amounts of free sugars, and are probably not absorbed as quickly as glucose.

Severe hypoglycaemia

An event where blood glucose falls below 2.8 mmol/L (50 mg/dL) and the patient requires the assistance of another person.

- About 10% of type 1 patients have an episode of severe hypoglycaemia every year, rising to about 30% in intensively treated patients. The DARTS/MEMO collaboration in Scotland found that insulin-treated type 2 patients have the same frequency of severe hypoglycaemia as type 1 patients.
- About 3% of type 1 patients have recurrent severe hypoglycaemia but despite concern that this could cause long-term cognitive decline, an 18-year EDIC (Epidemiology of Diabetes Interventions and Complications) follow-up of the DCCT cohort found no evidence for it [10]. The corresponding rate in patients treated with oral hypoglycaemic agents is much lower, about 0.5% per year.
- About 6% of deaths during the DCCT were hypoglycaemia related, similar to the 2–4% rate reported elsewhere. Since DCCT reported in 1993, the rate of severe hypoglycaemia has not decreased, and may have increased; motivation, education and intensive monitoring, as in the DCCT, therefore remain critical in reducing severe hypoglycaemia.
- ACCORD (see Chapter 5) confirmed the link between severe hypoglycaemia and death in type 2 patients, regardless of the intensity of glycaemic treatment (actually the hypoglycaemia rate was higher in the conventional rather than the intensive treatment group) [11].

Most patients are aware of autonomic symptoms at glucose levels of 2–3 mmol/L (36–54 mg/dL) but patients with habitual low blood glucose levels often have a degree of hypoglycaemia unawareness, probably due to a combination of impaired sympathetic autonomic and catecholamine responses, and may apparently be fully alert and responsive at levels of 1–2 mmol/L (18–36 mg/dL). However, demonstrable impairment of cognitive function is invariable at levels below 3 mmol/L. The term 'hypoglycaemia-associated autonomic failure' describes the vicious cycle of hypoglycaemia perpetuating hypoglycaemia by reducing humoral and neurological responses to antecedent hypoglycaemia. Strict avoidance of hypoglycaemia for as little as 2–3 weeks can restore hypoglycaemia awareness. Achieving this is a challenge [12].

Risk factors for severe hypoglycaemia

1 Intensive insulin therapy (multiple dose insulin or insulin pump treatment).
2 Type 1 diabetes: low HbA_{1c}, often in the non-diabetic range (4–6%, 20–42 mmol/mol). Anecdotally, patients tend to be young or middle-aged males without microvascular complications despite long duration of type 1 diabetes. Intensive monitoring of HbA_{1c} levels

with frequent specialist follow-up can be helpful: whether it is beneficial to demonstrate hypoglycaemia objectively with CGM is not yet known.

3 Type 2 diabetes: ACCORD (see Chapter 5) identified the following risk factors:
   (a) female
   (b) African-Americans compared with non-Hispanic whites
   (c) lower levels of education
   (d) the elderly
   (e) insulin-treated patients.

4 In striking contrast with type 1 patients, there was a consistent *decrease* in hypoglycaemia, less marked for intensively treated patients, with lower HbA$_{1c}$ levels. This may account for, though not easily explain, the frequent hypoglycaemia often encountered in insulin-treated type 2 patients with apparently poor HbA$_{1c}$ levels [13].

5 The elderly, often treated with sulphonylureas, and who may not have been sufficiently educated about hypoglycaemia.

6 Alcohol: the conventional view is that moderate alcohol taken alone has little effect acutely on blood glucose but can cause hypoglycaemia the next day. This is not consistent, either clinically or in research studies, but always caution about the possibility of late hypoglycaemia after alcohol, even when taken with food. Moderate hypoglycaemia (e.g. 2.3 mmol/L, 40 mg/dL) combined with low levels of blood alcohol (below the current UK driving limit) severely impair cognitive function; if they are driving, type 1 patients should not drink any alcohol.

7 Exercise: a factor that consistently leads to late hypoglycaemia, characteristically 17–30 hours after moderate exercise. Adolescents have impaired counter-regulation caused by sleep itself, leading to a possible increased risk of hypoglycaemia during the night after exercise [14].

8 Hypoglycaemia unawareness: risk factors include increasing duration of insulin treatment, extremes of age, and previous hypoglycaemia.

9 Established autonomic neuropathy is not consistently a factor, although autonomic neuropathy is associated with long-duration diabetes.

10 Pancreatic diabetes, due to absent glucagon secretion, through destruction of α cells.

11 Social isolation.

Remember the unusual presentations of hypoglycaemia:
- seizure;
- hemiparesis;
- aggressive (possibly criminal) behaviour;

- 'He's been drinking, doctor';
- acute back pain (opisthotonos or rarely crush fracture of thoracic vertebra caused by fits).

Treatment
Intravenous glucose. Give 20–30 mL of 50% glucose (10–15 g) by bolus intravenous injection into a large peripheral vein. Potential problems include the following.
- Viscous solution: may be difficult to inject, especially in a restless patient.
- Phlebitis (with both intravascular and extravascular placement): superficial extravasation, sometimes caused by attempts to give glucose via a small cannula inserted on the dorsum of the hand, can cause severe skin necrosis (Fig. 2.4).
- Gaining venous access in patients who have had repeated previous infusions: avoid using peripheral leg veins, and veins in the antecubital fossa in pre-dialysis patients.
  Where available 20% glucose, 50–75 mL is safer.

Glucagon. A major insulin antagonist hormone, useful in management by paramedics out of hospital, by partners of type 1 patients at risk of hypoglycaemia, especially nocturnal, and as initial treatment in the unconscious or restless patient where there is a delay in gaining venous access. The standard presentation contains 1 mg glucagon in powder form for reconstitution with water for injection in a prefilled syringe (GlucaGen

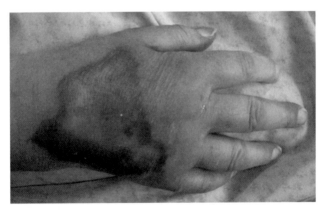

Fig. 2.4 Hazard of hypertonic glucose. Hypoglycaemia during the night in an elderly female inpatient: severe skin necrosis of the back of the hand as a result of extravasated hypertonic glucose through a small intravenous cannula. Where available, use 20% glucose

Hypokit, NovoNordisk). Glucagon acts by directly stimulating hepatic glycogenolysis and is therefore:

- relatively ineffective in the patient with poor hepatic glycogen stores (thin, malnourished, starving, anorectic or alcoholic);
- relatively effective in patients with pancreatic diabetes, who are glucagon deficient;
- usually clinically effective within 20 min;
- usually transiently effective (~90 min) and needs supplementing with oral glucose as soon as the patient is capable of taking it.

Glucagon can be given by intravenous, intramuscular or subcutaneous injection, but intramuscular administration is preferable; subcutaneous administration may be ineffective in vasoconstricted patients and intravenous injection can cause nausea.

Sulphonylurea-induced hypoglycaemia

Admit all patients with sulphonylurea-induced hypoglycaemia because of the risk of late relapse after treatment, especially with long-acting sulphonylureas such as glibenclamide and glimepiride. Both 50% glucose and glucagon stimulate residual insulin secretion and may exacerbate hypoglycaemia. Use continuous intravenous 10% or 20% glucose, with hourly blood glucose monitoring. The somatostatin analogue octreotide inhibits insulin and glucagon secretion (as well as many other hormones) and is of value in severe sulphonylurea-induced hypoglycaemia (50 μg s.c. 12-hourly).

Follow-up of patients with severe hypoglycaemia

- After initial treatment in the emergency department, replenish hepatic glycogen stores with a substantial carbohydrate-containing snack after recovery (three to six biscuits, bread, or sandwiches) to prevent recurrent hypoglycaemia.
- Check blood glucose level after 20 min.
- If the patient has recovered, is fully conscious and has a blood glucose above 7 mmol/L (126 mg/dL) within an hour, admission is not required, but make firm arrangements for prompt follow-up by the diabetes team, especially if there is no obvious reason for the episode. In the meantime suggest at least 10% reduction in relevant insulin dose(s), and stop or halve the dose of sulphonylureas. A few days of moderate hyperglycaemia is much preferable to another possibly even more severe episode of hypoglycaemia.

When to admit

- Patients with residual neurological deficits or prolonged coma after treatment: consider postictal state, cerebral oedema, head injury, intracranial

infection, bleed or infarction, and coexisting poisoning with alcohol or drugs. Obtain an urgent brain CT scan.
- Patients living on their own with no facilities for close supervision over the next 24 hours. In type 1 diabetes, episodes of severe hypoglycaemia seem to cluster, presumably through impairment of hypoglycaemia awareness following the first episode, though other factors are likely to be involved.
- Recurrent hypoglycaemia, despite adequate initial treatment, suggesting liver disease, insulin or sulphonylurea overdose, intentional or otherwise.

The acute diabetic foot

Detailed investigation and management of the patient with diabetic foot ulceration is covered in Chapters 7 and 10. However, lower-limb infections, with or without ulceration, commonly present to emergency departments, and the default should be admission unless:
- the infection is truly minor *and*
- there is a firm immediate management plan in place *and*
- the patient has low-risk, adequate accommodation and social support if sent home.

The reasons for caution include the following.
- Symptoms and signs of infection are likely to be less obvious (impaired inflammatory responses, sensory impairment from neuropathy): patients with known severe neuropathy who describe any symptoms of discomfort in the foot may be harbouring a severe occult infection.
- Seemingly trivial infections can spread very rapidly: diabetes is a risk factor for necrotizing fasciitis.
- Underlying lesions (osteomyelitis, deep abscesses, Charcot neuroarthropathy) may not be clinically or radiologically apparent, and may be difficult to differentiate on plain radiography.
- Antibiotic therapy alone is insufficient; it must be combined with good wound care and bed rest for optimum outcomes.

Many classification systems for diabetic foot ulceration have been devised, but a recent one has been supported by prospective correlation. Admit any patient with a moderate infection associated with ulceration, i.e. more than one of the following:
- >2 cm cellulitis around ulcer;
- lymphangitis;
- spread beneath fascia;
- abscess or gangrene.

Patients with systemic toxicity (fever, hypotension, leucocytosis, impaired renal function) must be admitted [15].

More difficult clinically are patients with cellulitis but without foot ulceration. Again, always err on the side of caution and admit, especially with additional risk factors, for example:

- chronic leg oedema, lymphoedema;
- skin blistering;
- immobility;
- recurrent cellulitis;
- known methicillin-resistant *Staphylococcus aureus* (MRSA) infection;
- presentation on Friday/public holiday.

All that is needed initially is recognition of the need for admission, basic blood tests, a plain foot radiograph and referral to the admitting medical or diabetes team. Many patients will be known to the diabetes and specialist podiatry team.

References

1. Patterson CC, Dahlquist G, Harjutsalo V *et al.* Early mortality in EURODIAB population-based cohorts of type 1 diabetes diagnosed in childhood since 1989. *Diabetologia* 2007;50:2439–42. PMID: 17901942.
2. Nyenwe EA, Loganathan RS, Blum S *et al.* Active use of cocaine: an independent risk factor for recurrent diabetic ketoacidosis in a city hospital. *Endocr Pract* 2007;13:22–9. PMID: 17360297.
3. Wallace TM, Matthews DR. Recent advances in the monitoring and management of diabetic ketoacidosis. *Q J Med* 2004;97:773–80. PMID: 15569808.
4. Umpierrez G, Freire AX. Abdominal pain in patients with hyperglycaemic crises. *J Crit Care* 2002;17:63–7. PMID: 12040551.
5. Dhatariya KK. Diabetic ketoacidosis. *Br Med J* 2007;334:1284–5. PMID: 17585123.
6. Amanzadeh J, Reilly RF Jr. Hypophosphatemia: an evidence-based approach to its clinical consequences and management. *Nat Clin Pract Nephrol* 2006;2: 136–48. PMID: 16932412.
7. The Diabetes Control and Complications Trial Research Group. Effect of intensive therapy on residual beta-cell function in patients with type 1 diabetes in the diabetes control and complications trial. A randomized, controlled trial. *Ann Intern Med* 1998;128:517–23. PMID: 9518395.
8. Mehlhorn AJ, Brown DA. Safety concerns with fluoroquinolones. *Ann Pharmacother* 2007;41:1859–66. PMID: 17911203.
9. Cryer PE, Davis SN, Shamoon H. Hypoglycemia in diabetes. *Diabetes Care* 2003;26:1902–12. PMID: 12766131.
10. Jacobson AM, Musen G, Ryan CM *et al.* Long-term effects of diabetes and its treatment on cognitive function. Diabetes Control and Complications Trial/ Epidemiology of Diabetes Interventions and Complications Study Research Group. *N Engl J Med* 2007;356:1842–52. PMID: 17476010.
11. Bonds DE, Miller ME, Bergenstal RM *et al.* The association between symptomatic, severe hypoglycaemia and mortality in type 2 diabetes: retrospective epidemiological analysis of the ACCORD study. *Br Med J* 2010;340:b4909. PMID: 20061358.
12. Cranston I, Lomas J, Maran A, Macdonald I, Amiel SA. Restoration of hypoglycaemia awareness in patients with long-duration insulin-dependent diabetes. *Lancet* 1994;344:283–7. PMID: 7914259.

13. Miller ME, Bonds DE, Gerstein HC *et al.* The effects of baseline characteristics, glycaemia treatment approach, and glycated haemoglobin concentration on the risk of severe hypoglycaemia: post hoc epidemiological analysis of the ACCORD study. *Br Med J* 2010;340:b5444. PMID: 20061630.
14. Tamborlane WV. Triple jeopardy: nocturnal hypoglycaemia after exercise in the young with diabetes. *J Clin Endocrinol Metab* 2007;92:815–16. PMID: 17341578.
15. Lavery LA, Armstrong DG, Murdoch DP, Peters EJ, Lipsky BA. Validation of the Infectious Diseases Society of America's diabetic foot infection classification system. *Clin Infect Dis* 2007;44:562–6. PMID: 17243061.

Further reading

Hyperglycaemic emergencies
Joint British Diabetes Societies Inpatient Care Group. The management of diabetic ketoacidosis in adults (March 2010). Available at www.diabetes.nhs.uk

Kitabchi AE, Umpierrez GE, Miles JM, Fisher JN. Hyperglycemic crises in adult patients with diabetes. *Diabetes Care* 2009;32:1335–43. PMID: 19564476.

Krentz A. *Emergencies in Diabetes: Diagnosis, Management and Prevention.* Oxford: Wiley-Blackwell, 2004.

Levy D. Presentation and diabetic emergencies. In: *Type 1 Diabetes.* Oxford: Oxford University Press, 2010.

Hypoglycaemia
Frier BM, Fisher M (eds) *Hypoglycaemia in Clinical Diabetes*, 2nd edn. Oxford: Wiley-Blackwell, 2007.

Management of hypoglycaemia in inpatients
Joint British Diabetes Societies Inpatient Care Group. The hospital management of hypoglycaemia in adults with diabetes mellitus (March 2010). Available at www.diabetes.nhs.uk

The acute diabetic foot
Wraight PR, Lawrence SM, Campbell DA, Colman PG. Creation of a multidisciplinary, evidence based, clinical guideline for the assessment, investigation, and management of acute diabetes related foot complications. *Diabetic Med* 2005;22:127–36. PMID: 1566-728.

Management of inpatient diabetes

CHAPTER 3

Key points

- There is no convincing evidence that achieving near-normoglycaemia in hospitalized patients with diabetes improves outcomes.
- Hospital management of people with diabetes is safety-directed, aiming to minimize hypoglycaemia and prevent symptomatic hyperglycaemia.
- Consensus is that glucose levels should be below 10 mmol/L (180 mg/dL) without hypoglycaemia; this includes intensive care and coronary patients.
- In coronary care, glucose/insulin infusions are no better than optimizing existing treatment regimens in terms of important cardiac outcomes, so long as management other than glycaemia is meticulous.
- In patients with symptomatic coronary artery disease, the best initial management strategy is usually maximum medical treatment; insulin treatment confers no benefit over insulin-sensitizing strategies.
- Hypoglycaemia with intensive glucose control in intensive care patients is probably harmful and must be avoided.
- Inpatients should have access to a hospital inpatient diabetes team; at the very least they seem able to reduce length of stay.
- Tailor perioperative management to individual requirements, placing safety above considerations of 'tight' glycaemic control.

Introduction

There has been a recent resurgence of interest in the management of diabetes in hospitalized patients. Guidelines in the USA are well established, and in the UK the 'ThinkGlucose' campaign has highlighted the

Practical Diabetes Care, 3rd edition. © David Levy.
Published 2011 by Blackwell Publishing Ltd.

importance of good diabetes care in hospital. Note that good diabetes care does not simply mean good (i.e. 'tight') glucose control: the criteria for judging this are controversial and there is little RCT evidence, though an abundance of less robust data. Minimizing prescribing errors (especially of insulin), ensuring awareness of diabetes in its entirety for the whole hospital team, aiming where possible for autonomy in self-care and insulin administration, quality improvement and audit are all critical components of good inpatient diabetes care. Equally important is tailoring the level of intensity of glucose management to the patient's clinical need, and this requires clinical acumen and insight.

Many cohort and registry studies have found that new-onset hyperglycaemia in hospitalized patients not known to have diabetes carries a high hospital mortality, higher even than patients with known diabetes, although the findings are not consistent. 'Stress hyperglycaemia' (hospital/acute illness-related hyperglycaemia) – hyperglycaemia in people without known diabetes that settles once the acute admission is over – is a concept with a long history [1] and there are many factors that may contribute to vascular harm and a poor prognosis in this state. Now that tentative agreement has been reached on the HbA_{1c} diagnosis of diabetes (see Chapter 1), both newly diagnosed and stress hyperglycaemia will be easier to diagnose and differentiate, for example using a combination of blood glucose and HbA_{1c} measurements.

- New-onset diabetes: fasting glucose $\geqslant 7.0$ mmol/L (126 mg/dL) *or* random glucose > 11.1 mmol/L (200 mg/dL) *or* $HbA_{1c} \geqslant 6.5\%$ (48 mmol/mol); one measure preferably repeated for confirmation.
- 'Stress hyperglycaemia': blood glucose levels as for new-onset diabetes, *but* $HbA_{1c} < 6.5\%$ (48 mmol/mol).

In specific conditions, for example acute coronary syndromes (ACS) and intensive care, the assumption that 'lower is better' has recently been challenged. However, the basis for good perioperative glycaemic control is reasonably well founded. These are all areas in which best practice is likely to continue to change rapidly.

Acute coronary syndromes (ST-segment elevation acute myocardial infarction, non-ST-segment elevation acute myocardial infarction and unstable angina)

The epidemiology is clear: ACS patients with diabetes have a higher rate of all adverse outcomes (heart failure, renal failure, cardiogenic shock and death). In the USA, mortality rates are higher during admission, at 30 days and at 1 year, although some of these differences may be historical and some related to underuse of proven secondary prevention measures in diabetic patients (e.g. beta-blockers). In the UK between 1995 and 2003, although 30-day mortality improved, and to a similar degree as in non-diabetic patients, the late outcomes (18-month mortality) did not change [2]. Mortality after percutaneous coronary intervention (PCI) undertaken for any reason in diabetic patients is about two-thirds higher than in non-diabetic subjects for at least 4 years after the procedure, highlighting the need for intensive secondary prevention measures (see below) [3].

Several factors are likely to be responsible for the increased risk in diabetes.

- Classical (textbook) ischaemic symptoms are less marked or absent, presumably due to somatic and autonomic neuropathy. Think of cardiac ischaemia in a diabetic patient who describes shortness of breath (diastolic dysfunction), nausea/vomiting, sweating, even non-specific upper body discomfort. Patients are unlikely to use textbook terminology if English is not their first language.
- Hospital presentation is later and coronary interventions delayed.
- The extent of infarction is probably no greater than in non-diabetic patients, but coronary artery disease is more diffuse and more advanced, and associated risk factors more marked.

Prevalence of diabetes in ACS patients and identification of diabetes status

Glucose intolerance is common in patients with myocardial infarction. In a Scandinavian study (2002), prevalence rates immediately after the event and some months later were similar [4]: normal glucose tolerance, 50%; IGT, 30%; diabetes, 20%. Nevertheless, random admission glucose values were unremarkable, typical of pre-diabetes, with a mean blood glucose of only 6.1 mmol/L (110 mg/dL). This increased to 6.9 mmol/L (124 mg/dL) in a mixed-ethnicity group in the UK, comprising 30% South Asians, but with a similar proportion of diabetes and IGT (30% each). Diagnostic HbA_{1c} measurements may help in this situation, but the lability of glucose measurements in stressed medical conditions warns against adoption of simple numerical limits. For example in the Scandinavian study mean admission HbA_{1c} was only 5.0% (31 mmol/mol), yet a level of 5.3% (34 mmol/mol) strongly predicted diabetes on the OGTT – compare the proposed lower limit of 5.7% (39 mmol/mol) for 'pre-diabetes'.

Glycaemic control in ACS – DIGAMI and beyond

Glucose/insulin/potassium (GIK) infusions in the acute phase of myocardial infarction have a long history; the metabolic reasoning includes converting myocardial fatty acid metabolism to more efficient glucose metabolism. Translating the experimental rationale into evidence-based clinical practice has been long and inconclusive. The first DIGAMI study

(1997) [5] showed that 24-hour GIK treatment after admission with transmural myocardial infarction in patients with blood glucose above 11.1 mmol/L (200 mg/dL), followed by 3 months of basal bolus subcutaneous insulin treatment, reduced fatal infarctions by 11%, but there was no effect on total reinfarction rate. Those with newly presenting and known diabetes gained similar benefit, and younger people without heart failure fared particularly well. DIGAMI is still widely cited as justification for this complicated regimen, but it was conducted early in the thrombolysis era; very few had PCI, post-infarction prophylaxis was relatively rudimentary, and BARI 2D (though in patients with stable advanced coronary artery disease) could not find prognostic advantage in the use of insulin. It is difficult to draw conclusions on glycaemic control from the follow-up, DIGAMI 2 (2005) [6], which attempted to separate out the contributions of acute intravenous insulin and longer-term subcutaneous insulin. The study was underpowered and terminated early, and although glycaemic targets were not met, mean admission HbA_{1c} was already low (7.3%, 56 mmol/mol), no significant separation occurred between the three groups, and overall glycaemic control did not change. Perhaps the most important finding was that cardiac outcomes were at least as good as, if not better than, a concurrent non-diabetic registry group, and vigorous management of all factors (of which glycaemic control was one, but only one), including PCI in 40%, is likely to explain the excellent outcome in this otherwise high-risk group.

Further doubt was cast on GIK by the huge CREATE-ECLA study (2007) which recruited about 20 000 patients with ST-segment elevation acute myocardial infarction (STEMI) around the world [7]. Mortality or serious cardiovascular end points were no different in those with and without diabetes, although blood glucose levels were relatively high (8–10 mmol/L, 144–180 mg/dL). An analysis including CREATE-ECLA and another GIK study, OASIS-6 GIK, raised concerns that a higher rate of death or heart failure in the first 2 days after STEMI might be related to hyperglycaemia, hyperkalaemia and fluid overload as a result of the GIK infusion. The usual plea is that maintaining strict normoglycaemia (4–6 mmol/L, 72–108 mg/dL) might reveal cardiac benefits of GIK treatment not apparent in studies using less rigorous glycaemic control, but the practical difficulties and potential risks (particularly hypoglycaemia) of achieving this either in a large RCT or in individual patients using current technology are prohibitive. The practical approach should be to maintain glycaemic control in ACS patients at levels recommended in ambulatory practice (e.g. < 10 mmol/L, 180 mg/dL), which will mean a temporary intravenous insulin infusion for some. Although the level at which it should be initiated is not known, the DIGAMI threshold of 11.1 mmol/L, still widely used, is arbitrary.

Glycaemic control in non-ST-segment elevation acute myocardial infarction and unstable angina

There is no RCT evidence for tight glycaemic control improving outcomes in diabetic patients with non-ST-segment elevation acute myocardial infarction and unstable angina. Conventionally, however, intravenous insulin infusions are used for 24 hours in hyperglycaemic patients, but the warnings of the CREATE/OASIS analysis should be heeded, so minimizing fluid volumes and careful monitoring of serum potassium are important. However, regardless of management during the index event, good glycaemic control (e.g. $HbA_{1c} < 7.0\%$, 53 mmol/mol) in PCI patients is associated with a lower risk of the need for target vessel revascularization at 12 months. The specific regimen used to achieve this level of control is probably not important.

Percutaneous coronary intervention in diabetes and ACS

Primary PCI has replaced thrombolysis in STEMI. It has the same advantages over thrombolysis as for non-diabetic patients and should be undertaken wherever possible, though 30-day mortality is nearly twice as high [8]. Periprocedural glycoprotein (GP)IIa/IIIb inhibitor treatment and 12 months of clopidogrel decrease the risk of longer-term events, but they are still more common in people with diabetes. Although there is controversy over the use of bare-metal versus drug-eluting stents, diabetic patients appear to have a generally better outlook with drug-eluting stents, although secondary prevention medication is more intensive in these patients, and may account for some of the benefit.

Coronary intervention versus optimum medical treatment in stable multivessel disease: BARI and COURAGE

The first BARI study (1996), in the pre-stent era, found that coronary artery bypass graft (CABG) carried a better 5-year survival in diabetic (but not in non-diabetic) patients, and this advantage was maintained up to 10 years. CABG also reduced the risk of fatal reinfarctions. BARI 2D (2009) [9] studied only type 2 patients with stable symptoms and angiographically characterized coronary artery disease. A complex study, it was designed to mimic real-life decision-making and to promote joint clinical decision-making between cardiologists and diabetologists. A decision for either PCI or CABG was made on the angiographic findings, and therefore importantly this was *not* a randomized trial of PCI versus CABG in multivessel disease (the FREEDOM trial is currently addressing this [10]). There were two subsequent randomizations:

- prompt intervention (target within 4 weeks) as decided at angiography (and intensive medical treatment) versus intensive medical treatment alone, reserving the predetermined intervention to a later time if clinically needed;

> **Box 3.1 Findings and conclusions from BARI 2D**
>
> *Findings*
> - 5-year mortality: no difference between revascularization and intensive medical groups; no difference between insulin-sensitizing and insulin-providing groups.
> - Major cardiovascular events: significantly reduced in the early-intervention CABG group compared with the intensive medical group, and by insulin-sensitizing treatment.
> - Quality of life initially improved more in the revascularization group than the medical group, but by 3 years there were no differences.
>
> *Conclusions*
> - Intensive medical treatment alone is the preferred option in type 2 patients with controlled angina and less severe disease on angiography; insulin treatment offers no benefit compared with metformin/rosiglitazone.
> - CABG is preferable in patients with more extensive disease (the first BARI study came to the same conclusion), and the risk of myocardial infarction is reduced with insulin-sensitizing treatment.
> - In this study, insulin-sensitizing treatment had a better overall profile than insulin-providing treatment: lower HbA_{1c} (7.0 vs. 7.5%, 53 vs. 58 mmol/mol), higher HDL-cholesterol, fewer severe hypoglycaemic reactions and less weight gain.
> - The recommendation for maximum medical treatment without the need for additional PCI in stable coronary disease is supported by the COURAGE study (2007) [11], which included about 34% diabetic patients.

- insulin-sensitizing regimen (metformin and rosiglitazone) versus insulin-providing regimen (various insulins, sulphonylureas and meglitinides).

Targets for control of blood pressure and low-density lipoprotein (LDL) were exceeded, though the HbA_{1c} target was not quite reached:

- HbA_{1c} 7.2% (55 mmol/mol), target < 7.0% (53 mmol/mol);
- blood pressure 125/70 mmHg, target < 130/80 mmHg;
- LDL 2.05 mmol/L (80 mg/dL), target < 2.6 mmol/L (100 mg/dL).

The PCI-intended group had, not surprisingly, less advanced coronary artery disease (two versus three significant coronary lesions, 10% vs. 20% proximal left anterior descending artery lesions). The key findings are summarized in Box 3.1.

Post-coronary interventions (adapted from COURAGE, 2007)

These recent studies have reinforced the importance of lifestyle modification and medications after a coronary event.

Lifestyle adjustments

1 *Exercise*: post-myocardial infarction rehabilitation programmes can be effectively and more economically delivered at home than at a formal centre [12]. COURAGE recommended 30–45 min of moderate-intensity exercise five times per week and an increase in daily lifestyle activity.

2 *Smoking cessation*: bizarrely, patients with diabetes appear *less* likely to receive inpatient smoking cessation counselling after myocardial infarction than non-diabetic people. For those who receive counselling, there is a significant mortality benefit [13]. Currently, varenicline is the most effective pharmacological adjunctive treatment, although side-effects, including nausea, headache, sleep disturbance and gastrointestinal symptoms, are common. Because of its pharmacology (partial agonist of the α_4/β_2 nicotinic acetylcholine receptor while competitively inhibiting nicotine binding), there has been concern that it may increase cardiovascular risk factors, but it is probably safe in stable coronary artery disease, though it should not be used in the phase immediately after myocardial infarction. Severe recurrent hypoglycaemia has also been reported in a type 1 patient, so use with caution in this situation.

3 *Diet*: there is limited RCT evidence, but adherence to a portfolio of diet advice and components is likely to be beneficial:
   (a) Weight reduction: target BMI < 25, or 10% weight loss if initial BMI is > 27.5
   (b) 'Mediterranean' diet [14] (see Chapter 5).
   (c) Low total and saturated fat and low dietary cholesterol
   (d) Low salt
   (e) Recommended alcohol intake where appropriate
   (f) Increased soluble/insoluble fibre
   (g) Increased oily fish (two portions per week)
   (h) Avoid 'antioxidant' vitamin supplements
   (i) ?50 g dark ($\geqslant$ 70% cocoa) chocolate/day.

Medication

Glycaemia
- HbA_{1c} ~ 7.0–7.5% (53–58 mmol/mol) without hypoglycaemia; emphasize insulin-sensitizing drugs.
- Avoid glibenclamide.
- Role of GLP-1 analogues in cardioprotection not yet established in RCTs.

Lipids (see Chapter 12)
- LDL target < 1.7–1.8 mmol/L (66–70 mg/dL). Intensive statin therapy started within 14 days of hospitalization for ACS reduces death and

cardiovascular events after 4 months of treatment. Most clinical trials have used high-dose atorvastatin (80 mg daily), which has a good safety record in this situation. Compliance with statin treatment is also higher if it is started in hospital rather than after discharge [15].

- HDL as high as possible; triglycerides < 1.7 mmol/L (150 mg/dL) (consider niacin or pharmacological doses of fish oils).
- Omega (ω)-3 fatty acids: DHA (docosahexaenoic acid) plus EPA (eicosapentaenoic acid) 1 g daily starting within 3 months of event.

Others
- ACE inhibitor (ACE-i) to maximum recommended dose; ARB only if ACE-i side-effects.
- Aspirin with or without clopidogrel.
- Beta-blocker.

Atrial fibrillation

Class 3 obesity (BMI > 40) is associated with an increased risk of sustained atrial fibrillation (AF), and this effect is in part mediated by diabetes. Diabetes is one of the factors in the CHADS risk score (www.mdcalc .com) that identifies aspirin-treated AF patients at increased risk of stroke. Patients with a score of 3 or more have a stroke risk of about 4 per 100 patient-years of aspirin, and long-term warfarin should be considered. In GISSI-AF (2009) the ARB valsartan did not prevent recurrence of AF, but several studies have found that new-onset AF is less frequent in patients treated with ARBs. Although an ARB can be used for other cardiovascular risk factors (albuminuria, hypertension), there is no RCT evidence yet for their routine use in hypertensive patients without ventricular hypertrophy or diastolic dysfunction in the primary prevention of AF [16].

Patients in the intensive care unit

Hyperglycaemia, whether associated with known diabetes or not, carries a poor prognosis in critically ill patients through multiple mechanisms, including vascular disease, polyneuropathy, an increased tendency to infection, dyslipidaemia, and abnormal anti-inflammatory and coagulation responses. Consistent near-normoglycaemia has therefore been a target for surgical patients in the ICU since van den Berghe reported significant reductions in mortality and morbidity by targeting blood glucose levels in the range 4.5–6.0 mmol/L (81–108 mg/dL; achieved mean 6.1 mmol/L, 110 mg/dL) compared with a target of 10–11 mmol/L (180–198 mg/dL) in patients spending more than 5 days in ICU [17]. Similar results were subsequently seen in medical ICU patients, though without the mortality benefits. Two major recent studies replicating van den Berghe's protocol have moderated nearly 10 years of euglycaemic enthusiasm. Both highlighted a significantly increased risk of severe hypoglycaemia, one a possible trend towards longer ICU stays, the other a significantly increased death rate (NICE-SUGAR [18]). The whole field is currently unclear again, but blood glucose levels below 10 mmol/L (180 mg/dL), avoiding hypoglycaemia, are now generally considered reasonable in critically ill patients. Variable-rate insulin infusions are required, especially with enteral or parenteral nutrition.

Non-critically ill patients

There is no RCT evidence in general medical patients for benefits or otherwise of tight glycaemic control, but severe hypoglycaemia must be avoided: inpatient mortality significantly increases with any hypoglycaemic episode with glucose below 1.7 mmol/L (30 mg/dL), and both inpatient length of stay and 1-year mortality increases with increasing numbers of hypoglycaemic episodes where glucose is below 2.8 mmol/L (50 mg/dL) [19]. Although these are not RCT data, the figures are compelling, particularly in the light of other recent RCTs, and certainly more convincing than the evidence for near-normglycaemia in general medical patients. There is no reason for blood glucose targets to be different from those in critically ill patients (i.e. < 10 mmol/L, 180 mg/dL), while rigorously avoiding hypoglycaemia and taking immediate action to prevent further episodes. A blood glucose target below 10 mmol/L is difficult to achieve with non-insulin agents or twice-daily biphasic insulin, but if the patient is eating, a temporary change to a basal-bolus regimen will usually be satisfactory. If not eating, then use a continuous variable intravenous insulin infusion together with 5 or 10% glucose, but this is uncomfortable, labour-intensive and carries risks of hypoglycaemia, hyponatraemia and hypokalaemia. A recent trend in the UK is to alternate glucose or saline infusions depending on an arbitrary blood glucose level, together with a continuous variable intravenous insulin infusion. It has no sound basis, and carries an increased risk of both hypoglycaemia and inadequate volume replacement. Use glucose and insulin for control of blood glucose, and infuse other solutions as necessary for volume replacement, as in hyperglycaemic emergencies (see Chapter 2).

Stroke

The degree of hyperglycaemia at presentation of stroke is related to initial infarct volume, early infarct progression, and poor short- and medium-term clinical outcomes, but as in many aspects of glycaemia and general medicine, these robust observational data are not complemented by RCT evidence. Hyperglycaemia is as common in stroke as in myocardial infarction (40% of survivors have normal glucose tolerance, 40% IGT, 20% diabetes). Studies are in progress to determine the benefits of acute control of hyperglycaemia (target: 4–7 mmol/L, 72–126 mg/dL). Current European guidelines propose glucose levels below 10 mmol/L (180 mg/dL), though caution is required in patients with impaired consciousness. Even without insulin treatment, glucose levels tend to fall in the first 8 hours after admission with stroke, so do not rush to start an intravenous regimen.

Enteral feeding (nasogastric, percutaneous endoscopic gastrostomy)

Malnutrition in hospital is very common, especially in people with diabetes, and renal and neurological impairment, and patients taking less than 60% of their requirements after 7–14 days should be assessed for specialized nutritional support. While the benefits of nutritional support (reduced infection rates and length of stay) are evident, enteral nutrition in people with diabetes may cause marked hyperglycaemia, which may neutralize some of the benefit. Diabetes-specific feed formulations, i.e. low carbohydrate, high monounsaturated fatty acids (up to 30% of total calories) and high fibre, give smaller increases in blood glucose and lower peak values than standard feeds. Overall insulin requirements may be lower, medium-term glycaemia may be better, and where available these formulations should be used [20]. However, the clinical problem remains the rapid rise in blood glucose levels after the start of the feed. Oral agents are usually ineffective, including metformin, the only drug available as a liquid formulation (see Chapter 6). Discuss the feed regimen with the nursing staff, dietitian and the hospital nutrition team, and then devise an appropriate insulin regimen, for example the following two options.

- Isophane insulin (NPH) or the long-acting analogue insulin glargine (Lantus), where the dose of insulin glargine is the same as the total previous insulin dose. This simple regimen is reported to be successful in controlling blood glucose without hypoglycaemia up to 7 days. In patients new to insulin, start at the conservative dose of about 0.5 units/kg body weight per day, but be prepared to increase the dose rapidly.
- A high mixture (e.g. Humalog Mix 50) at the start of the feed, and 8 hourly thereafter.

Many feeding regimens alternate with water for 6–10 hours out of 24; take this into account when planning insulin injection times. High insulin doses are often required, so adjust them every day according to capillary blood glucose (CBG) values. Apart from the few patients requiring parenteral nutrition, avoid intravenous insulin wherever possible.

Glucocorticoid treatment

Acute high-dose glucocorticoid treatment (e.g. prednisolone 20–30 mg daily) or 'neurological' doses of dexamethasone (e.g. 12–16 mg daily) nearly always causes marked and rapid deterioration in glycaemic control in known diabetic patients, especially postprandially. The mechanism is increased peripheral insulin resistance, but this fact is of little practical help, because steroid-induced hyperglycaemia rarely responds to insulin-sensitizing drugs. Sulphonylureas and insulin are the mainstays of treatment, but runaway symptomatic hyperglycaemia is still common, and vigilance is needed. It would be wise to request an HbA$_{1c}$ and perform once- or twice-daily postprandial CBG measurements in people without known diabetes, but at high risk, as soon as the decision is made to start high-dose steroid treatment.

There are no clear guidelines for the management of steroid-induced hyperglycaemia, and it is not known in what proportion of patients it remits once treatment is stopped. The aim in short-term steroid treatment is to avoid severe hyperglycaemia (e.g. blood glucose > 15 mmol/L, 270 mg/dL) and hyperglycaemic symptoms. The usual criteria for good control would apply in long-term treatment.

Patients with known diabetes
Insulin-treated diabetes
Anticipate increased insulin requirements of 25–50% and increase insulin doses immediately steroid treatment starts. Involve the diabetes team as soon as possible.

Diabetes treated with oral hypoglycaemic agents
- Start or increase the dose of sulphonylurea according to CBG measurements. If patients are already taking near-maximum effective doses of sulphonylureas (e.g. glibenclamide 10–15 mg/day, gliclazide 160–240 mg/day, glimepiride 2–3 mg/day), further increases are likely to be ineffective (Chapter 6). Plan for early insulin treatment, and certainly when CBG levels are consistently above 12–15 mmol/L (216–270 mg/dL), at which level symptoms are likely.
- Other glycaemic drugs can be continued, but do not attempt to increase doses: they act too slowly to be effective in this situation.
- Start with twice-daily biphasic insulin (e.g. 12–16 units before breakfast, 8–12 units before evening meal), or Humalog Mix 50 three times daily (e.g. 6 units with breakfast, 8 units with lunch, 8–10 units with the evening meal), and be prepared to increase each dose daily by at least 2 units. Basal bolus regimens may be useful in long-term treatment (add basal bedtime insulin to the 2- or 3-times daily biphasic insulin).

Inpatient screening routine

All people with diabetes should be screened systematically. This is now usually performed at annual review in primary care; where possible, check for recent laboratory tests, and do not repeat them unnecessarily (many laboratories will not permit HbA_{1c} measurements to be repeated within 8 weeks). Be especially vigilant in patients:

- admitted with a hyperglycaemic emergency, particularly type 1 patients with DKA;
- who have limited contact with their primary care team, for whatever reason, including geographical mobility and multiple comorbidities that prevent their attending for primary care reviews.

Clinical examination

1 Weight and BMI.
2 Peripheral pulses.
3 Arterial bruits (femoral, abdominal, carotid).
4 Feet.
5 Urinalysis for ketones and proteinuria.

Laboratory tests

1 HbA_{1c}.
2 Fasting lipids.
3 Thyroid function (if not done within the past year in type 1 patients, within the last 3–5 years in type 2 patients). Remember that sick patients with non-thyroidal illness are likely to have the 'sick euthyroid' picture of low FT_4 and low but not suppressed thyroid-stimulating hormone (TSH), so do not rush into treatment.
4 Early-morning urine for albumin/creatinine ratio (ACR). Although albuminuria increases in infection, fever or severe hyperglycaemia, it will give a broad indication of the likely range of albuminuria out of acute illness.
5 12-lead ECG.
6 Dietetic review, as required.
7 Review insulin-taking patients with diabetes specialist nurse. If possible, identify in advance areas that need addressing, for example:
  (a) The insulin regimen: did it directly or indirectly cause the admission? Can it be rationalized or simplified? Is the patient using up-to-date injection devices?
  (b) Injection technique
  (c) Home blood glucose monitoring: education, technique and equipment
  (d) Employment, school, driving status, family psychodynamics, alcohol, smoking, drugs.

Perioperative management

Metabolic responses to surgery

Surgery induces insulin resistance through several mechanisms including increased secretion of counter-regulatory hormones, especially catecholamines, cortisol and growth hormone. Catecholamines themselves inhibit insulin secretion, and the combination of insulin resistance and reduced insulin secretion, in the presence of perioperative starvation, results in increased lipolysis and ketogenesis, increased protein breakdown, and hyperglycaemia.

Although it is difficult clinically to demonstrate any differences in wound healing in people with diabetes, postoperative infections are more common in poorly controlled diabetes (see Chapter 7), partly as a result of defective neutrophil function.

Aims of diabetes management in surgical patients

Diabetes management in surgical patients aims to avoid:
- excess morbidity and mortality, especially through infection;
- severe hyperglycaemia;
- ketoacidosis in type 1 patients;
- hypoglycaemia during anaesthesia and the postoperative period.

Preoperative diabetic control

Increasing use of minimally invasive and day-case surgery means that patients are less likely, and have less need, to be admitted preoperatively for glycaemic stabilization. Glycaemic control must be optimized before admission, but recognize that mean HbA_{1c} in a hospital diabetes clinic is about 8% (64 mmol/mol), representing an estimated average glucose (eAG) of about 10 mmol/L (183 mg/dL) (95% CI 8–12 mmol/L, 150–220 mg/dL). In many patients, reducing this further is difficult and may not be clinically useful in reducing perioperative complications (while increasing the risk of hypoglycaemia). However, try where possible to improve on HbA_{1c} levels of 9% (75 mmol/mol) or more, representing an eAG of about 12 mmol/L (210 mg/dL) (95% CI 9–14 mmol/L, 170–250 mg/dL). Despite everyone's best efforts some patients remain in very poor glycaemic control ($HbA_{1c} > 10\%$, 86 mmol/mol). Recurrent or prolonged postponement pending improved control is dispiriting for everyone, and this is the group likely to benefit from intensified input from the primary or secondary care diabetes team in the weeks before admission, and from intensive inpatient preoperative management. If admitted preoperatively, start 7-point blood glucose monitoring (before meals, 1.5–2 hours after meals and at bedtime) on the patient's usual insulin regimen. If there is enough time, change temporarily to a basal-bolus regimen if control is very poor, but it may make things worse in the short term. Intravenous insulin infusion from admission may be wise in the chronically poorly controlled. Most hospitals have their own detailed protocols, but bear in mind the following.

General principles of perioperative management

- Wherever possible insulin-treated patients should be first on a morning operating list, a sensible rule that is increasingly not observed. Surgery later in the day puts patients at increased risk because of the need for prolonged preoperative glucose and insulin infusions, and because they may return to the ward late in the day.
- Insulin infusions must always be accompanied by glucose; where necessary for fluid replacement, co-infuse other solutions. Ensure that all infusions keep running during transfer from ward to theatre and back.
- Metformin: omit only on the day of surgery, and restart postoperatively when renal function is confirmed to be normal (or back to preoperative levels). The only caution might be patients taking modified-release preparations with their evening meal; changing to morning dosing for a few days before surgery, especially if there is any renal impairment, would probably be wise.
- Sulphonylureas: omit glibenclamide (glyburide) the evening before surgery because of its long action. The twice-daily injected exenatide is glucose-responsive and does not cause hypoglycaemia, so the evening dose can be taken in the usual way
- Insulin: after the evening meal the day before surgery, do not give further short-acting or biphasic insulin doses. Some recommend continuing long-acting subcutaneous insulin in type 1 patients in order to reduce the risk of DKA if intravenous insulin is interrupted; however, hypoglycaemia while taking long-acting insulin is always a potential problem, and so long as continuity of insulin treatment is assured (which must be an aim of all hospital guidelines), the risks of hypoglycaemia probably outweigh those of DKA. However, maintaining basal insulin treatment during surgery in patients on insulin pumps is strongly recommended where there is sufficient team expertise: basal rates can be rapidly and effectively changed or stopped.
- Minor operations (body surface or endoscopic procedures): wherever possible avoid infusions.
- All other procedures: maintain insulin infusion until normal eating resumes; continue intravenous insulin for 30 min after first subcutaneous injection is given.
- Daily electrolytes: hyponatraemia and hypokalaemia are risks, particularly after orthopaedic and urological procedures.

Colonoscopy is a challenge for people with diabetes, particularly during the 24 hours before the procedure, when only clear fluids are permitted. Frequent blood glucose monitoring, sugary drinks with normal or slightly reduced doses of insulin or oral hypoglycaemic agents, and if necessary emergency contact with the diabetes team are needed; assess carbohydrate content of usual meals and convert to volumes of Lucozade or equivalent sports drink (100 mL contains approximately 20 g carbohydrate, therefore standard 380-mL bottle contains 65 g).

Perioperative intravenous insulin regimens

Single-bag GIK infusions, the simplest and probably the safest for perioperative use, are no longer generally used in the UK because of restrictions relating to additions to infusion fluids (see Chapter 2). Separate 5% glucose infusions and variable-rate intravenous insulin infusions are therefore used; infuse 5% glucose containing 20 mL KCl at 125 mL/hour via an infusion pump, and give soluble insulin via a syringe pump at a variable rate determined by hourly CBG measurements (Table 3.1); 10% glucose is probably better, but in the UK is not available premixed with potassium.

Late diabetic complications in relation to surgery

- Coronary heart disease and congestive heart failure (chest radiography, exercise testing, ECG). Even in type 2 patients without cardiac

Table 3.1 Example of variable insulin infusion for perioperative glucose management

CBG (mmol/L)	CBG (mg/dL)	Insulin infusion rate (units [mL]/hour)
0–4	0–72	0
4.1–7.0	74–126	1
7.1–11.0	128–198	2
11.1–17.0	200–305	4
17.1–22.0	308–396	6 (review regimen)
>22	>396	8 (review regimen)

CBG, capillary blood glucose.

symptoms (Look AHEAD participants), nearly 8% had ST segment depression on routine exercise stress testing, and 1% each angina and arrhythmia; this is a group at high cardiac risk.

- Diabetic nephropathy (anaemia, fluid overload, acute on chronic renal failure).
- Foot ulcers (osteomyelitis, MRSA, systemic sepsis).
- Advanced autonomic neuropathy: increased risk of perioperative cardiovascular events, possibly resulting from arrhythmias or prolonged QTc interval (check postural drop in blood pressure and RR interval variation with deep breathing; see Chapter 10).
- Rare but important: diabetic gastroparesis with delayed gastric emptying (risk of aspiration on intubation).

These patients require very close anaesthetic monitoring.

References

1. Dungan K, Braithwaite SS, Presier JC. Stress hyperglycaemia. *Lancet* 2009;373:1798–807. PMID: 19465235.
2. Cubbon RM, Wheatcroft SB, Grant PJ *et al.* Temporal trends in mortality of patients with diabetes mellitus suffering acute myocardial infarction: comparison of over 3000 patients between 1995 and 2003. *Eur Heart J* 2007;28:540–5. PMID: 17289742.
3. Norhammer A, Lagerqvist B, Saleh N. Long-term mortality after PCI in patients with diabetes mellitus: results from the Swedish Coronary Angiography and Angioplasty Registry. *EuroIntervention* 2010;5:891–7. PMID: 20542773.
4. Norhammer A, Tenerz A, Nilsson G *et al.* Glucose metabolism in patients with acute myocardial infarction and no previous diagnosis of diabetes mellitus: a prospective study. *Lancet* 2002;359:2140–4. PMID: 12090978.
5. Malmberg K. Prospective randomised study of intensive insulin treatment on long term survival after acute myocardial infarction in patients with diabetes mellitus. DIGAMI (Diabetes Mellitus, Insulin Glucose Infusion in Acute Myocardial Infarction) Study Group. *Br Med J* 1997;314:1512–15. PMID: 9169397.
6. Malmberg K, Rydén L, Wedel H *et al.* Intense metabolic control by means of insulin in patients with diabetes mellitus and acute myocardial infarction (DIGAMI 2): effects on mortality and morbidity. *Eur Heart J* 2005;26:650–61. PMID: 15729645.
7. Diaz R, Goyal A, Mehta SR *et al.* Glucose–insulin–potassium therapy in patients with ST-segment elevation myocardial infarction. *JAMA* 2007;298:2399–405. PMID: 18042917.
8. Timmer JR, Ottervanger JP, de Boer MJ *et al.* Primary Coronary Angioplasty vs Thrombolysis-2 Trialists Collaborators Group. *Arch Intern Med* 2007;167:1353–9. PMID: 17620527.
9. Frye RL, August P, Brooks MM *et al.* A randomized trial of therapies for type 2 diabetes and coronary artery disease. BARI 2D Study Group. *N Engl J Med* 2009;360:2503–15. PMID: 19502645.
10. Farkouh ME, Dangas G, Leon MB *et al.* Design of the Future REvascularization Evaluation in patients with Diabetes mellitus: Optimal management of Multivessel disease (FREEDOM) Trial. *Am Heart J* 2008;155:215–23. PMID: 18215589.

11. Boden WE, O'Rourke RA, Teo KK *et al*. Optimal medical therapy with or without PCI for stable coronary disease. COURAGE Trial Research Group. *N Engl J Med* 2007;356:1503–16. PMID: 17387127.
12. Balady GJ, Williams MA, Adex PA *et al*. Core components of cardiac rehabilitation/secondary prevention programs: 2007 update. A scientific statement from the American Heart Association Exercise, Cardiac Rehabilitation, and Prevention Committee, the Council on Clinical Cardiology; the Councils on Cardiovascular Nursing, Epidemiology and Prevention, and Nutrition, Physical Activity, and Metabolism; and the American Association of Cardiovascular and Pulmonary Rehabilitation. *Circulation* 2007;115:2675–82. PMID: 17513578.
13. Van Spall HG, Chong A, Tu JV. Inpatient smoking-cessation counselling and all-cause mortality in patients with acute myocardial infarction. *Am Heart J* 2007;154:213–20. PMID: 17643569.
14. Sofi F, Cesari F, Abbate R, Gensini GF, Casini A. Adherence to Mediterranean diet and health status: meta-analysis. *Br Med J* 2008;337:a1344. PMID: 18786971.
15. Muhlestein JB, Horne BD, Bair TL *et al*. Usefulness of in-hospital prescription of statin agents after angiographic diagnosis of coronary artery disease in improving continued compliance and reduced mortality. *Am J Cardiol* 2001;87:257–61. PMID: 11165956.
16. Disertori M, Latini R, Barlera S *et al*. Valsartan for prevention of recurrent atrial fibrillation. GISSI-AF Investigators. *N Engl J Med* 2009;360:1606–17. PMID: 19369667.
17. Van den Berghe G, Wouters P, Weekeers F *et al*. Intensive insulin therapy in critically ill patients. *N Engl J Med* 2001;345:1359–67. PMID: 11794168.
18. Finfer S, Chittock DR, Su SY *et al*. Intensive versus conventional glucose control in critically ill patients. NICE-SUGAR Study Investigators. *N Engl J Med* 2009;360:1283–97. PMID: 19318384.
19. Turchin A, Matheny ME, Shubina M, Scanlon JV, Greenwood B, Pendergrass ML. Hypoglycemia and clinical outcomes in patients with diabetes hospitalized in the general ward. *Diabetes Care* 2009;32:1153–7. PMID: 19564471.
20. Elia M, Ceriello A, Laube H, Sinclair AJ, Engfer M, Stratton RJ. Enteral nutritional support and use of diabetes-specific formulas for patients with diabetes: a systematic review and meta-analysis. *Diabetes Care* 2005;28:2267–79. PMID: 16123506.

Further reading

Diabetes in hospital

American Diabetes Association. Standards of medical care in diabetes 2010. Section VIII. Diabetes care in the hospital. *Diabetes Care* 2010;33(Suppl 1):S11–S61. PMID: 20042772.
Clement S, Braithwaite SS, Magee MF *et al*. American Diabetes Association Diabetes in Hospitals Writing Committee. Management of diabetes and hyperglycemia in hospitals. *Diabetes Care* 2004;27:553–91. PMID: 14747243.

Website

ThinkGlucose Campaign (NHS Institute for Innovation and Improvement). Available at institute.nhs.uk/quality_and_value/think_glucose/

Type 1 diabetes: insulin treatment

CHAPTER 4

Key points

- However sophisticated MDI treatment becomes, it cannot approach physiological insulin replacement.
- Sensor-augmented insulin pump treatment can approach physiological insulin replacement, as of course can successful pancreas and islet transplantation.
- A realistic target for long-term HbA_{1c} is 7.0–7.5% (53–58 mmol/mol), which in most patients will balance a low risk of vascular complications and an acceptable risk of severe hypoglycaemia.
- Many patients are happy with long-acting insulin analogues; apart from convenience, there is little evidence for the benefit of the short-acting analogues.
- Allow patients to change freely between insulin preparations.
- A trial of insulin pump treatment should be available if MDI is unsuccessful or is causing distress.
- CGM is an important educational and therapeutic innovation.

Introduction

Insulin treatment in type 1 diabetes is substitution/replacement hormone treatment, but replacement is much more variable and difficult to achieve than in other hormone deficiencies (e.g. thyroid, adrenal, gonadal hormones) because of the minute-by-minute variation in insulin secretion by the intact pancreas, which cannot yet be emulated precisely by any subcutaneous insulin regimen. Nevertheless, 24-hour glucose profiles almost

Practical Diabetes Care, 3rd edition. © David Levy.
Published 2011 by Blackwell Publishing Ltd.

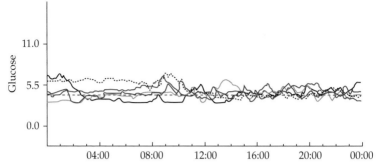

Fig. 4.1 Continuous glucose monitoring study in a non-diabetic person investigated for possible hypoglycaemia. The astonishing consistency and narrowness of the range of normal glucose levels is apparent, with transient slight increases noticeable after breakfast and lunch, but values are never more than about 7 mmol/L (126 mg/dL) and usual values are 3–4 mmol/L (54–72 mg/dL). (In this case, the patient had no significant symptoms, and no glucose levels < 3 mmol/L; continuous glucose monitoring is a valuable technique for the initial investigation of non-diabetic hypoglycaemia.)

indistinguishable from those of non-diabetic people can now be achieved with recent technical innovations in insulin pump therapy; this can only further improve with the long-awaited introduction of closed-loop feedback devices (Fig. 4.1).

Insulin is an anabolic hormone, and results from the DCCT and other studies raise concerns about the following sequence: poor glycaemic control → intensification of insulin treatment (often with increased hypoglycaemia) → increased weight → increased insulin resistance → increased weight and risk factors for macrovascular and microvascular complications, especially nephropathy. For example, intensively treated patients in the DCCT who gained weight had elevated high-sensitivity CRP levels [1].

In clinical practice, therefore, there is a difficult balance to achieve between:
- intensifying insulin treatment in order to reduce HbA_{1c} and thereby vascular complications, but risking increased hypoglycaemia, weight gain and consequent insulin resistance characteristics;
- reducing the risks of recurrent severe hypoglycaemia;
- avoiding persistent hyperglycaemia.

With conventional intermittent subcutaneous insulin treatment compromises are inevitable.

Total daily insulin dose requirements

Total daily insulin production from the pancreas of young insulin-sensitive non-diabetic individuals is about 25–40 units, of which about 50% is basal insulin secretion. Peripheral subcutaneous insulin administration in most type 1 patients requires significantly more, between 0.5 and 1.0 unit/kg body weight daily. Care has to be taken ascribing causality, but long-surviving type 1 patients, for example the 'Golden (50) Years' cohort in the UK, have some characteristics of insulin sensitivity, for example low mean BMI of about 25, elevated HDL-cholesterol (~1.8 mmol/L, 70 mg/dL), and daily insulin doses at the lower end of the usual range (0.52 units/kg) [2]. A similar cohort in the USA with at least 50 years of type 1 diabetes had remarkably similar characteristics.

Patients with long-standing type 1 diabetes therefore often have low total daily insulin requirements similar to those of non-diabetic individuals. Insulin antibodies, which may be produced in response to any insulin preparation (though to a much lesser extent with human and analogue insulins), may act as a 'buffer' to glucose variability. These patients have often used a wide variety of insulin preparations during their diabetic career. It is important to recognize the phenomenon: even if they require only tiny insulin doses, they remain type 1 patients, fully insulin requiring. Do not attempt to withdraw it [3].

Glycaemic targets in type 1 diabetes

Much sought and debated, there is no agreement on a glycaemic 'threshold' for microvascular complications, a sustained level of HbA_{1c} below which microvascular risk is abolished. However, other facts are less in dispute.

- Reduction in HbA_{1c} from any given level will, if maintained for about 6 years (median duration of participation in the DCCT), significantly reduce microvascular risk.
- Glycaemic memory established during this period is maintained for at least a further 10 years, despite slight deterioration in mean HbA_{1c}, and which results in a continued lower risk of developing complications, including macrovascular as well as microvascular events (EDIC).
- HbA_{1c}, and not other glycaemic measures (e.g. glucose variability), overwhelmingly determines microvascular complications.
- Glycaemia alone drives all vascular complications until the emergence of albuminuria, when other factors (blood pressure, lipids, inflammatory factors) become important. The contrast with type 2 diabetes could not be more striking.
- The limits to achieving long-term normoglycaemia are imposed by hypoglycaemia.

HbA$_{1c}$ 7.5% (58 mmol/mol; estimated average glucose 9.3 mmol/L, 169 mg/dL) is a widely accepted and realistic target (the ADA proposes < 7.0% for all adults with diabetes). Pump treatment (and also islet and whole pancreas transplants) offers the possibility of HbA$_{1c}$ levels consistently below 6.0–6.5% (42–48 mmol/mol), at which level the development of microvascular complications is unlikely, and regression of some established complications, especially retinopathy, is possible (see below).

Insulin products

Many insulin products are available, but relatively few are now in common use. The trend has been for manufacturers to progressively slim down their insulin ranges over the past decade, and in the UK only about a dozen preparations are now widely used. There is increasing emphasis on the insulin analogues in preference to the established human insulin preparations, a matter of concern to some practitioners and patients [4], though very recently some manufacturers have started reinforcing their human insulin ranges. It should be remembered that recombinant human insulin preparations began to replace monocomponent (highly purified) pork preparations as recently as the early 1980s, and that the first human analogue insulin (lispro) was introduced only in 1997. Since the mid-1980s insulin for human use has been standardized at 100 units/mL (U100). Insulin vials contains 10 mL (1000 units), cartridges 3 mL (300 units).

Insulin delivery devices (British National Formulary, section 6.1.1.3)

Most UK patients use insulin pens and insulin cartridges, rather than syringes and 10-mL vials, which are still used by the majority of patients in the USA. Many devices are available, and new ones are frequently introduced. While the concept is the same, the details differ, and some are important when discussing the choice of pen device with patients, for example whether they deliver insulin in 0.5, 1- or 2-unit increments, the maximum number of units they deliver (which varies between 40 and 78) and the pressure required to inject the insulin. Specialist teams are usually up to date with delivery devices: ask their advice if you or the patient is uncertain about the precise name. Refillable pens are designed to have a long life, and patients who have not had their injection devices reviewed may be using fully reliable but less convenient devices. There are two basic types: refillable and prefilled disposable pens. (The Monthly Index of Medical Specialities, or MIMS, issued monthly to all GPs in the UK, contains a useful visual guide to all current diabetes devices, including lancets and blood glucose meters.)

Refillable
- NovoNordisk: NovoPen 4, NovoPen Demi (delivers in 0.5-unit increments, useful for children, and adults with low insulin requirements).
- Lilly: HumaPen Luxura, HumaPen Memoir (digital display of the details of the last 16 doses dispensed: date, time and units), Luxura HD (0.5-unit pen).
- Sanofi-Aventis: ClikSTAR.
- Owen Mumford: Autopen 24 (Sanofi-Aventis cartridges), available in 2-unit increment (2–42) and 1-unit increment (1–21) versions. Autopen Classic for Lilly and Wockhardt (animal insulin) cartridges.

Prefilled disposable pens
Increasingly used, these are convenient, and highly suitable for older people and those with dexterity problems.
- NovoNordisk: FlexPen.
- Lilly: KwikPen.
- Sanofi-Aventis: SoloStar.

Insulin prescribing

Errors in prescribing insulin are very common, are frequently more than trivial and are potentially lethal. If there is any doubt, try to corroborate with others, especially GPs and community nurses, and use the expertise of pharmacists before prescribing.
- Generic insulin is not available in most countries; insulin preparations must be prescribed by brand name. Older insulin preparations often had similar-sounding names, but newer insulins are now required to have unique names that are unlikely to be confused. Half-remembered names are dangerous; older patients are apt to recall correctly the names of insulins they used for many years, but which they may not be currently using.
- Analogue (modified human) insulins, on the other hand, also have approved names (see below) based on the amino-acid changes in the molecule, for example insulin glargine is Lantus, insulin aspart is NovoRapid. They are still best prescribed by brand name.
- Write 'units' in full. Do not abbreviate to 'U', which can be misread as '0', or 'IU' (international units), which can be misread as '10'.
- Inpatients: the priority is to prescribe the insulin preparation correctly. If you know the precise name of the device, then it can be added, but it is not critical (compare inhalers). Where protocols are in place, patients should administer their own insulin using their own device.

- Inpatients: indicate the time of administration in relation to meals, as well as by clock time, where necessary. Twice-daily biphasic insulin should not be prescribed in the middle of the day or at bedtime, an alarmingly common practice.

Insulin preparations (Table 4.1)

Basal insulin

Since the first clinical use of insulin in 1922, prolonging the short-lived effect of native hexameric insulin to provide consistent basal insulin levels, especially overnight, has been a pharmaceutical challenge. The first preparation, still widely used, was NPH (Neutral Protamine Hagedorn, 1946). Longer-acting forms with zinc (e.g. lente and PZI) are still manufactured but very little used. Two long-acting human analogue insulins have been introduced over the past decade: glargine (Lantus, Sanofi-Aventis) forms crystals at neutral tissue pH that are slowly absorbed, while detemir (Levemir, NovoNordisk) has a long-chain myristic fatty acid attached to the modified insulin molecule which delays transfer from the subcutaneous tissue and from the circulation by attaching to plasma albumin. It should probably not be used in patients with profound hypoalbuminaemia. Both long-acting analogues are often described as 'peakless', but they are better thought of as having a gentle onset and offset of action that lasts 22–24 hours. This contrasts with the definite peak action of NPH which occurs at about 4–6 hours and which is responsible for its increased risk of nocturnal hypoglycaemia. All are often better given twice daily. Reduction in (but not abolition of) nocturnal hypoglycaemia is the most important effect of the long-acting analogues; any reductions in HbA_{1c} are usually clinically not important. The relative hepatoselectivity of detemir, resulting in less peripheral lipogenesis, may be responsible for the smaller weight gain seen with this insulin compared with NPH and glargine, although the difference is relatively small (e.g. up to 1.5 kg). Very long-acting analogues are in development (see below).

Mealtime insulin

Progressive shortening of the time of onset and offset of short-acting mealtime insulins was achieved initially by changing from beef to highly purified monocomponent pork (1970s), then to biosynthetic human insulin (1980s), and most recently to the rapid-acting human analogue preparations, of which there are currently three. The first, insulin lispro, was introduced in 1997. Various changes to pairs of amino acids in the insulin molecule decrease the tendency to hexamer formation, thereby increasing the speed of absorption from subcutaneous

Table 4.1 Human and analogue insulin preparations in use in the UK (*British National Formulary*, section 6.1.1)

Preparation	Manufacturer	Formulations	Approximate time course of action			Comments
			Onset	Peak	Duration	
Rapid-acting analogues (BNF section 6.1.1.1)						
Insulin lispro (Humalog)	Lilly	Cartridge, pen, vial	30 min	1h	3–4h	Best injected immediately before meals, especially with high glycaemic index carbohydrate meals, but control otherwise not significantly compromised if injected immediately after meals. Glulisine has a more rapid onset of action than aspart; potential (unproven) value in CSII
Insulin aspart (NovoRapid)	NovoNordisk	Cartridge, pen, vial				
Insulin glulisine (Apidra)	Sanofi-Aventis	Cartridge, pen, vial				
Short-acting human (regular/soluble)						
Humulin S	Lilly	Cartridge, pen, vial	30 min	2–3h	6–8h	Slower onset with lower peak serum insulin levels than rapid-acting analogues; similar time course of action after about 3h. Detectable up to about 10h after injection – compare 7–8h for rapid-acting analogues
Actrapid	NovoNordisk	Vial				
Insuman Rapid	Sanofi-Aventis	Cartridge, pen				
Intermediate-acting (NPH/isophane) (BNF section 6.1.1.2)						
Humulin I	Lilly	Cartridge, pen, vial	2–4h	6–7h	12–14h	Marked clinical peak effect at 6–7h, with tendency to hypoglycaemia. Most effectively used twice-daily
Insulatard	NovoNordisk	Cartridge, vial				

Drug	Manufacturer	Form	Onset	Peak	Duration	Comments
Insuman Basal	Sanofi-Aventis	Cartridge, pen, vial (5 mL)				
Biphasic mixtures (human): soluble/NPH						
Humulin M3 (30/70)	Lilly	Cartridge, pen, vial	30min–2h	3–6h	Up to 20–24h	
Insuman Comb 15, 25 & 50 (15/85, 25/75, 50/50)	Sanofi-Aventis	Cartridge (25, 50), pen (15, 25, 50), vial (25–5 mL)				
Biphasic mixtures (analogue)						
Humalog Mix 25 & Mix 50	Lilly	Cartridge, pen, vial (25)	30 min	1–4h	12–16h	Achieved glycaemic control similar to that with human biphasic insulin in type 1 diabetes when used twice daily. Can be used three times daily (with or without bedtime long-acting insulin)
NovoMix 30	NovoNordisk	Cartridge, pen				
Long-acting analogues (BNF section 6.1.1.2)						
Levemir (detemir)	NovoNordisk	Cartridge, pen, vial	1–3h		22–24h	
Lantus (glargine)	Sanofi-Aventis	Cartridge, pen, vial	2h	4–6h (plateau)	22–24h	Once or twice daily administration (see text)

tissue. When given 15 minutes before (though not when given after) meals, they reduce postprandial hyperglycaemia more than soluble/ regular insulin or rapid-acting analogue given at the start of a meal, but comparative trials have not shown consistent improvements in HbA_{1c}. Their benefits vary in different patients: the lower rate of late-morning hypoglycaemia is important to some patients, as is their value in patients who take supplementary doses with snacks between main meals, but their relatively rapid offset of action can lead to pre-meal hyperglycaemia if the interval between meals is more than 4–5 hours, and some patients prefer the longer action of soluble insulin for breakfast and lunch, while using a rapid-acting analogue with a very late evening meal, where a longer-acting soluble insulin might overlap with a long-acting bedtime insulin.

The overall advantages or otherwise of both long- and rapid-acting analogues over their human equivalents continue to be debated; analogue regimens have higher ratings for treatment satisfaction and quality of life measures, but it would be unwise to abandon wholesale a group of insulin preparations that served several generations, including the DCCT cohort, perfectly well.

Basal-bolus/multiple-dose insulin

This is the standard intensive-insulin regimen by which all others in type 1 diabetes are judged. The principle is simple: to provide basal (background) insulin, especially during the night, using a long-acting insulin, and bolus doses of short-acting insulin with meals (Fig. 4.2). Its utility was confirmed in the DCCT (reported 1993) where mean HbA_{1c} values differed very little from those using insulin pumps (7.0% vs. 6.8%, 53 vs. 51 mmol/mol). Interestingly, children and adolescents have lower rates of severe hypoglycaemia with MDI than do adults, though this problem increases again in older adults with very long duration type 1 diabetes (> 30 years).

MDI is physiologically sound, but practical implementation can be complex and requires the following.
• Frequent home blood glucose monitoring.
• An ability to adjust prandial doses in relation to carbohydrate intake, blood glucose levels, prior and anticipated physical activity, previous experience of hypoglycaemia, mental stress and menstruation. This requires detailed continuing education, preferably with specific programmes, for example DAFNE (Dose Adjustment for Normal Eating, UK and Australia).
• Frequent contact with a team experienced in intensive insulin treatment.

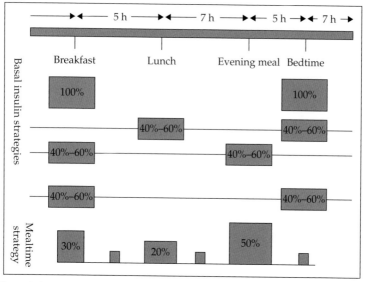

Fig. 4.2 Suggested initial strategies for distribution of basal and mealtime insulin in MDI. Reproduced from Levy D (2010) *Type 1 Diabetes*, with permission from OUP

- Using the simplest, most portable, and robust physical devices for self-testing and injection.
- Recognizing the marked day-to-day and interindividual variation of insulin action, and that the use of MDI *per se* does not confer automatic glycaemic advantage. For example, in 2005 an international survey of young people comparing insulin regimens found that patients using twice-daily free-mixed soluble and isophane insulin, a regimen relatively little used these days, had a significantly lower mean HbA_{1c} (7.9%, 63 mmol/mol) than those using MDI or continuous subcutaneous insulin infusion (CSII) (8.2% and 8.1%, 66 and 65 mmol/mol, respectively) – a good demonstration that the insulin regimen used is less important than the expertise and interest of the diabetes team.

Biphasic (fixed-ratio) mixtures

Usually regarded as inadequate treatment in type 1 diabetes, these are used in about 7% of young people across Europe. Glycaemic control is worse compared with MDI treatment (mean HbA_{1c} 8.6% vs. 8.2%, 70 vs. 66 mmol/mol), but there is no difference in hypoglycaemia rates between human and analogue biphasic preparations. However, analogue mixtures given with meals, as opposed to before meals, are more convenient. Control to target levels is sometimes but not commonly seen, but the regimen may be preferable to MDI where the lunchtime dose (and possibly others) is missed. The 50/50 high-mix preparations are no better than the standard 30/70 mixtures, at least in type 1 diabetes. A variant used in young people, avoiding the often ignored lunchtime injection, is a biphasic mixture with breakfast, soluble or rapid-acting analogue with the evening meal, and a standard long-acting insulin at bedtime, but control is no better than with twice-daily biphasic mixtures, and three different insulins are needed, which probably impedes adherence.

Insulin pump treatment (CSII)

First used at the end of the 1970s, insulin pump therapy is standard treatment for type 1 diabetes, although use varies between countries (e.g. about 1–2% in the UK, probably more now; about 25% in USA, up to 40% in Norway). Only rapid-acting analogue insulin is used, given at a variable low background basal rate, supplemented with mealtime boluses. The technique is used in specialist centres with great success in children and adolescents, and some centres routinely start CSII immediately after diagnosis. In meta-analysis, HbA_{1c} is consistently about 0.3–0.6% lower with CSII than MDI [5].

Indications for CSII (NICE 2008)

The National Institute for Health and Clinical Excellence (NICE) has issued broad guidelines for insulin pump treatment, e.g. disabling hypoglycaemia despite optimized MDI treatment, HbA_{1c} 8.5% (69 mmol/mol) or more despite high level of care in type 1 patients over 12 years old. Other clinical indications might include:

- hypoglycaemia unawareness;
- wide glycaemic fluctuations regardless of HbA_{1c};
- ketosis-prone individuals;
- improvements in HbA_{1c} pre-conception, during pregnancy and where there are potentially reversible microvascular complication (e.g. background retinopathy, microalbuminuria);
- difficulty in managing nocturnal glycaemia (hypoglycaemia, hyperglycaemia, dawn phenomenon);
- irregular shift-work patterns, frequent long-haul travelling;
- intensive exercise (e.g. competitive athletes);
- people requiring either very large or very small doses of insulin.

High levels of motivation and compliance are usually considered necessary, but motivation may improve with treatment, and CSII should be available for a trial period for any patient who is interested and appreciates that the technique, though sophisticated, is not yet a fully automated insulin delivery system.

Pump technology

Advances in pump technology have accelerated recently. They are now very subtly programmable to deliver multiple basal rates at different times of the day and especially night, for example to counteract the dawn phenomenon. Basal rates can be changed temporarily, during periods of inactivity, sports and exercise, menstrual cycles and acute intercurrent illness. Different configurations of boluses can be given, for example spike boluses to correct a high glucose level, extended (square wave) boluses for high fat or high protein meals, combination boluses (immediately followed by an extended bolus), or superboluses (some or all of the basal rate for the next 2–3 hours is borrowed in advance and added to the meal plus correction bolus, to reduce hyperglycaemia before a high glycaemic index meal).

Further refinements are continually being introduced. Software integrated with the pump can calculate and suggest bolus doses, based on estimated carbohydrate intake and prevailing glucose levels (bolus 'wizard'). Sensor-augmented pumps, using a continuous glucose monitor fitted at a different site to the pump, can relay glucose data to the pump display. In one of the largest pump studies to date (STAR 3), nearly 500 children 7 years or older and adults were randomized to remain on MDI or changed to sensor-augmented pump treatment (MiniMed Paradigm REAL-Time System; Fig. 4.3). In pump-treated patients, HbA_{1c} fell by a mean of 0.5–0.6% from a baseline of 8.3% (67 mmol/mol), maintained over a year, with a similar result seen in children and adults. There was a clear relationship between the frequency of sensor use and fall in HbA_{1c}, with the greatest fall (about –1.2%) seen in those using sensors between 81 and 100% of the time [6]. There was no significant weight gain, and hypoglycaemia was no more frequent than in the MDI group. Recently, semi-automated pumps have been introduced that temporarily interrupt basal insulin delivery when glucose levels fall to predetermined levels (e.g. < 4 mmol/L, 72 mg/dL), and the race is on to develop the software to guide the first fully automated closed-loop feedback pump. So far it has been used to safely control glucose levels overnight in children and adults, but the technological hurdle to extend this successfully to daytime use is formidable.

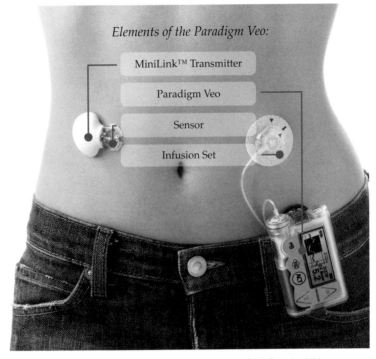

Elements of the Paradigm Veo:

MiniLink™ Transmitter

Paradigm Veo

Sensor

Infusion Set

Fig. 4.3 Sensor-augmented insulin pump. Courtesy of Medtronic, UK

Checklist of practical points whenever there is a problem with blood glucose control

Before discussing radical changes to insulin regimens, always check the following, especially when there has been recent deterioration in control.

- *Adherence.* Ensure that all insulin injections are being given, especially in younger people. Lunchtime, and other, doses of an MDI regimen are often omitted; eliciting this information requires sensitive questioning.
- *Check insulin.* Confirm type and doses of insulin, compatibility of pens and injection needles.
- *Mixing technique.* In the few patients who self-mix insulin, check technique; confirm uniform mixing of any cloudy insulins.
- *Storage.* Modern insulin has an effective shelf-life of about 2 years if refrigerated at 2–8°C, but storage in extreme tropical conditions, hot car interiors, freezer compartments, and airplane holds may cause denaturation. Individual manufacturers' recommendations vary, but

insulin can be kept safely at temperatures below 30°C for about 4 weeks.

- *Check injection sites.* Lipoatrophy, probably an immune complex-mediated inflammatory lesion, is very rare with human and analogue insulins, though a few cases have been described, even with CSII, where a local reaction to the delivery catheters may be responsible. Lipohypertrophy is still common with human insulin, though it may not occur with analogues. Injection into these sites is often less painful, but absorption may be erratic and delayed. Even where there is no lipohypertrophy, absorption from frequently injected sites can be erratic, leading to glycaemic instability.
- *Ensure rotation of injection sites* between thigh, buttock and abdomen (avoiding the immediate periumbilical area). Avoid injecting the upper arm, which may result in intramuscular injection. Absorption is fastest and most consistent from the abdomen, which is the preferred site for injection of mealtime insulin.
- *Injection technique.* Pinch skin and give the injection approximately perpendicular to the skin surface; 6-mm pen needles are satisfactory for most people, and reduce the risk of non-subcutaneous injections. Leave the needle in the skin for up to 10 seconds after the injection, pull it straight out, and gently press on the injection spot, but do not rub it.
- *Home blood glucose monitoring.* Intensify temporarily, concentrating on times of day where blood glucose levels are most erratic. A CGM study is likely to be valuable.
- *Consider new-onset endocrine disorders,* especially Addison's disease, autoimmune thyroid disease and coeliac disease. A short Synacthen test is simple and can be performed non-fasting at any time of day. Take blood for baseline cortisol, inject Synacthen (tetracosactide) 250 μg i.m., repeat cortisol measurement at 30 min and 1 hour; a peak cortisol level above 550 nmol/L is an adequate adrenal response.

Continuous glucose monitoring

This is an invaluable technique that is becoming more widely available as technology improves (wireless, and sensors that can reliably measure glucose levels for 4–5 days, in some cases longer) and costs fall. The subcutaneous sensor measures interstitial, rather than blood, glucose, and there is delay of about 15 minutes, of which half is physiological and half due to instrumental processing delays. This is not critical when CGM is used for diagnostic purposes, but is very important when used in real-time monitoring (Fig. 4.4) or when CGM data are transmitted to insulin pumps (sensor-augmented pumps; see Fig. 4.3). Nevertheless, *patterns* of glycaemia are easier to detect than with even frequent home blood

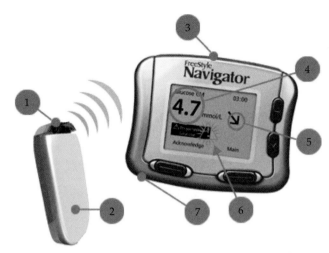

Fig. 4.4 A modern continuous glucose monitoring system (FreeStyle Navigator). 1, Subcutaneous sensor: worn for up to 5 days (arm or abdomen); 2, wireless transmitter (3-m range); 3, receiver; 4, display of glucose value (updated every minute); 5, direction of change of glucose; 6, early glucose alarm (10–30 min in advance of projected highs and lows); 7, built-in glucose meter for calibration and routine measurements. Courtesy of Abbott, UK

glucose monitoring; where there are rapid changes in glucose levels, small differences in timing of insulin injections and fingerprick testing can give an impression of greater variability than there actually is. Long-term use of CGM can lower HbA_{1c} by about 0.5% in adults 25 years or older (though not in children and adolescents), with a simultaneous decrease in severe hypoglycaemia [7].

Associations between CGM and other measures of glycaemia are emerging, and if CGM is now considered the gold-standard test, the reverse correlations with self-monitoring of blood glucose (SMBG) are important for everyday clinical practice.

- CGM and SMBG results are strongly correlated – SMBG is still valuable.
- SMBG 90 min after a meal correlates well with postprandial glycaemic exposure on CGM; we should probably recommend 90-min rather than 2-hour postprandial monitoring.
- Fasting glucose levels are only weakly associated with other glycaemic measures.
- Preprandial glucose measurements impact more than postprandial measurements on HbA_{1c}, especially in type 2 diabetes [8].

A combination of home blood glucose monitoring and CGM frequently identifies characteristic patterns (Fig. 4.5).

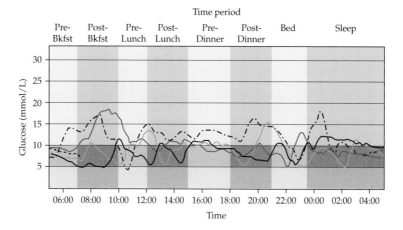

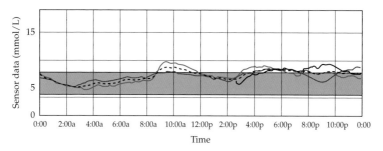

Fig. 4.5 Continuous glucose monitoring (CGM). (a) CGM study over 4 days in a 19-year-old male with diabetes for 4 years. Basal bolus: NovoRapid 8–10 units with breakfast, 10–13 units with lunch and evening meal, Lantus 42 units bedtime. HbA_{1c} 9.1% (76 mmol/mol). Three meals plus bedtime snack. No hypoglycaemic episodes (but unblinded glucose read-out and hypoglycaemia alerts probably account for this). Typical extended postprandial surges; more prandial insulin probably required but risk of inter-meal hypoglycaemia. Stable mild hyperglycaemia overnight with long-acting analogue insulin. Insulin pump treatment or extended trial of CGM? The patient preferred the latter. (b) Three-day CGM study (Medtronic Guardian Real-Time): 26-year-old male, 3 weeks after starting CSII; 30% daily insulin dose reduction compared with previous basal-bolus regimen. No hypoglycaemia, significant weight loss. Courtesy of Laila King and London Medical

Nocturnal hypoglycaemia

This is very common. In a large-scale study of CGM, nocturnal hypogly-caemia (glucose < 3.3 mmol/L, 60 mg/dL) was equally frequent with CSII and MDI, and increased with decreasing HbA_{1c}. Episodes lasting 20 min

or more occur about every 14 days, and nearly one-quarter of all episodes last 2 hours or more. This is another caution against the automatic
assumption that 'modern' insulin technology automatically reduces the
most serious complication of type 1 diabetes [9]. Encourage patients to
reduce their bedtime long-acting insulin, especially where there has been
previous physical activity or alcohol intake. Small changes can have dramatic effects.

Fasting hyperglycaemia

Abolishing nocturnal hypoglycaemia may still not help fasting hyperglycaemia, or high variability of fasting glucose levels. Poorly controlled
type 1 diabetes (and puberty) is associated with the dawn phenomenon,
exaggerated surges of growth hormone in the early hours of the morning,
leading to delayed insulin resistance and fasting hyperglycaemia. This is
easily corrected in pump-treated patients. Declining insulin levels from
an inadequate dose of long-acting bedtime insulin, which will give a similar glucose pattern, is uncommon but easily correctable.

Where there is no evidence for nocturnal hypoglycaemia and the dawn
phenomenon, encourage slow up-titration of bedtime long-acting insulin. Modest dose increases (about 10–15%) often significantly improve
control.

Postprandial hyperglycaemia

This is difficult to manage with MDI. The action of even rapid-acting analogues is too slow to counteract peak postprandial glucose levels, and
increasing the dose may simply increase the tendency to early postprandial hypoglycaemia. The slower onset but longer action of soluble/reg-
ular insulin may help some people at particular times of day, and taking
prandial insulin 15–30 mins before a high-carbohydrate meal may help,
even though this may be considered old-fashioned practice. A more rigorous approach to carbohydrate counting and flexible insulin dosing
can be of real value, and modern insulin pumps have several ingenious
strategies to help manage postprandial peaks, for example dual-wave
boluses. For really motivated patients taking high glycaemic index carbohydrate meals, about one-third of the mealtime bolus can be taken before
the meal, the remainder after.

New developments

New-generation long-acting insulin analogues are in clinical trials.
Insulin degludec (NN1250, NovoNordisk) is a soluble insulin basal analogue suitable for three-times weekly dosing, and gives glycaemic control

and hypoglycaemia rates similar to once-daily glargine. A combination of degludec with aspart (NN5401, a soluble insulin analogue combination, SIAC) may have a basal-bolus profile. SAR161271 (Sanofi-Aventis) will be given daily.

References

1. Schaumberg DA, Glynn RJ, Jenkins AJ *et al.* Effect of intensive glycaemic control on levels of markers of inflammation in type 1 diabetes mellitus in the Diabetes Control and Complications Trial. *Circulation* 2005;111:2446–53. PMID: 15867184.
2. Bain SC, Gill GV, Dyer PH *et al.* Characteristics of type 1 diabetes of over 50 years duration (the Golden Years Cohort). *Diabetic Med* 2003;20:808–11. PMID: 14510860.
3. Fineberg SE, Kawabata TT, Finco-Dent D, Fountaine RJ, Finch GL, Krasner AS. Immunological responses to exogenous insulin. *Endocr Rev* 2007;28: 625–52. PMID: 17785428.
4. Holleman F, Gale EA. Nice insulins, pity about the evidence. *Diabetologia* 2007;50:1783–90. PMID: 17634918.
5. Pickup JC, Sutton AJ. Severe hypoglycaemia and glycaemic control in Type 1 diabetes: meta-analysis of multiple daily injections compared with continuous subcutaneous insulin infusion. *Diabetic Med* 2008;25:765–74. PMID: 18644063.
6. Bergenstal RM, Tamborlane WV, Ahmann A *et al.* Effectiveness of sensor-augmented insulin-pump therapy in type 1 diabetes. STAR 3 Study Group. *N Engl J Med* 2010;363:311–20. PMID: 20587585.
7. The Juvenile Diabetes Research Foundation Continuous Glucose Monitoring Study Group. Effectiveness of continuous glucose monitoring in a clinical care environment: evidence from the Juvenile Diabetes Research Foundation Continuous Glucose Monitoring (JDRF-CGM) Trial. *Diabetes Care* 2010;33: 17–22. PMID: 19837791.
8. Borg R, Kuenen JC, Carstensen B *et al.* Associations between features of glucose exposure and A1c: the A1c-Derived Average Glucose (ADAG) Study. *Diabetes* 2010;59:1585–90. PMID: 20424232.
9. Juvenile Diabetes Research Foundation Continuous Glucose Monitoring Study Group. Prolonged nocturnal hypoglycemia is common during 12 months of continuous glucose monitoring in children and adults with type 1 diabetes. *Diabetes Care* 2010;33:1004–8. PMID: 20200306.
10. Luijf YM, van Bon AC, Hoekstra JB, DeVries J. Premeal injection of rapid-acting insulin reduces postprandial glycemic excursions in type 1 diabetes. Diabetes Care 2010;33:2152-5. PMID: 20693354.

Further reading

Insulin pumps

National Institute for Health and Clinical Excellence. NICE Technology Appraisal Guidance 151: insulin pump therapy, July 2008, review 2011. Available at www. nice.org.uk/TA151

Pickup J (ed.) *Insulin Pump Therapy and Continuous Glucose Monitoring.* Oxford: Oxford University Press, 2009.

Rodgers J. *Using Insulin Pumps in Diabetes: A Guide for Nurses and Other Health Professionals.* Oxford: Wiley-Blackwell, 2008.

Websites

Insulin preparations available in the UK (updated): www.mims.co.uk/Tables/882439/Insulin-Preparations/

Insulin preparations available in the USA: www.diabetes.niddk.nih.gov/dm/pubs/medicines_ez/insert_C.htm

Artificial Pancreas Project (Juvenile Diabetes Research Foundation): www.artificialpancreasproject.com. The target date for completion of this project, in association with the FDA, is 2014.

Type 2 diabetes: general introduction

CHAPTER 5

Key points

- β-cell failure and progressing hyperglycaemia are characteristic of type 2 diabetes, but the natural history differs widely between individuals.
- Lifestyle intervention (weight loss and increased activity) is the key to management, but qualitative changes to diet (e.g. higher protein) may help sustain weight loss; pharmacology to help weight loss has been almost uniformly unsuccessful.
- Vitamin and mineral supplements have shown no benefit in randomized controlled trials and their use should not be encouraged; however, vitamin D is widely deficient in many people with diabetes and should be supplemented for their bone health.
- In clinical trials glycaemic responses to medication are strongly related to baseline glycaemia, but most drugs have weak dose–response effects on HbA_{1c}, and the sustainability of drug effects is variable and sometimes weak.
- Intensive intervention in glycaemia after about 10 years of diagnosed diabetes has limited benefits on outcomes that are important to patients; earlier intervention sustained over many years carries microvascular and macrovascular advantages.
- Intensive intervention with multiple medications in patients with poor glycaemic control ($HbA_{1c} \geqslant 8.5\%$, 69 mmol/mol) may be hazardous (ACCORD).
- Severe hypoglycaemia is strongly associated with adverse vascular outcomes, but may be a marker of susceptibility rather than directly causally related (ADVANCE).

Practical Diabetes Care, 3rd edition. © David Levy.
Published 2011 by Blackwell Publishing Ltd.

Introduction: type 2 diabetes as a progressive condition

Glycaemia in type 2 diabetes progressively deteriorates with time, usually thought to be related to progressive β-cell failure. This was demonstrated dramatically in the United Kingdom Prospective Diabetes Study (UKPDS 1998), but the glycaemic trends have been less marked in more recent studies and even in non-treat-to-target studies (e.g. PROactive, 2005) deterioration in control was barely discernible. Some agents, for example the sulphonylureas, give less sustainable control than others, for example metformin and the glitazones, due to more rapid depletion of progressively β-cell function.

The mean preclinical duration of significant hyperglycaemia is between 7 and 10 years, and 20% of type 2 patients have microvascular complications at diagnosis, most commonly retinopathy and microalbuminuria. A similar proportion has subclinical or clinical macrovascular disease as a result of the even longer duration, perhaps 20 years or more, of insulin resistance/metabolic syndrome, hence the high proportion of newly diagnosed type 2 patients presenting with ACS (see Chapter 3). The concepts of 'early' and 'late' type 2 diabetes, increasingly emphasized in discussing the results of the surge of clinical trials reported in 2008 and 2009, becomes even more important yet increasingly elusive to define. Further complexity was added by the widely quoted studies that used increasing HbA_{1c} levels as a surrogate for progression from 'early' to 'late' diabetes: an orderly progression of hyperglycaemia, initially postprandial, followed by deterioration in control in the first part of the day and finally persistent overnight hyperglycaemia [1]. However, behind this scheme lie both enormous individual variation and the continuously changing phenotypic spectrum of type 2 diabetes. Guidelines emphasizing the homogeneity of type 2 diabetes will therefore progressively fail to reflect the type 2 diabetic population presenting to the clinician. In our present state of knowledge, polypharmacy with continued emphasis on sustainable lifestyle changes, as we are accustomed to practising in hypertension, is the best way to manage the hyperglycaemia of type 2 diabetes (Fig. 5.1).

The general approach to the newly diagnosed type 2 patient

Most patients are overweight or obese at diagnosis, for example BMI 31–33 (women higher BMI than men), but perhaps 20% will be normal weight or overweight. These patients may have late-onset type 1 diabetes (see Chapter 1) and a reasonable initial response to oral hypoglycaemic agents, but control may subsequently deteriorate rapidly. Patients with persistent 1+ or more ketonuria, especially in the presence of continuing weight loss or failure to regain lost weight with medication, should be considered to have type 1 diabetes (or LADA) and insulin treatment considered. GADA may be helpful in confirming immune-mediated diabetes and the likelihood of more rapid progression to insulin requirement (see Chapter 1).

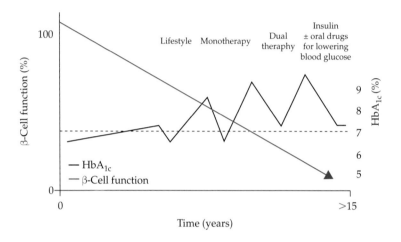

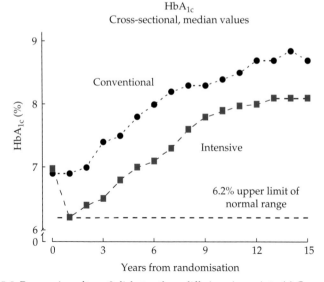

Fig. 5.1 Progression of type 2 diabetes: three differing viewpoints. (a) General schema (Reproduced from Heine RJ *et al*. *Br Med J* 2006;333:1200–4 with permission from British Medical Association). (b) The famous glycaemic 'tick' in UKPDS (1998). (c) Flat-lining in the non-treat-to-target PROactive study (2005)

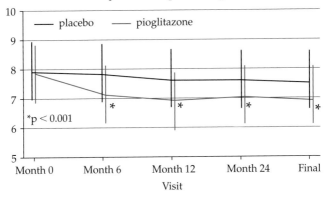

Fig. 5.1 (Continued)

Initial evaluation

Initial examination should include:
- height, weight and BMI;
- blood pressure;
- urinalysis for protein and ketones;
- examination of peripheral pulses (listen for carotid, femoral and renal bruits) and for peripheral neuropathy (see Chapter 10).
  Laboratory tests should include the following.
- Creatinine and electrolytes, HbA_{1c}.
- Liver functions, including gamma-glutamyltransferase.
- Fasting lipids (though mixed hyperlipidaemia, sometimes severe, at presentation of type 2 diabetes is common; see Chapter 12).
- Thyroid function: note the high prevalence of subclinical hypothyroidism (up to 1 in 12) in white female type 2 diabetic patients.
- Resting 12-lead ECG.
  Defer investigation of abnormal liver functions and lipids until glycaemic control has stabilized. Although most patients will have 'usual' type 2 diabetes in association with obesity, always bear in mind other underlying diagnoses, especially in non-overweight patients:
- pancreatic causes, especially alcohol, and underlying pancreatic carcinoma in the over fifties;
- genetic haemochromatosis;
- late-onset type 1 diabetes;
- syndromic type 2 diabetes, suggested by multisystem involvement, family history of diabetes/deafness, consanguineous parents, and insulin resistance in the absence of obesity.

At diagnosis, all patients should see a dietitian, a nurse practitioner/practice nurse/community diabetes specialist nurse, and a podiatrist. They should be offered a structured educational programme and entered into the local retinopathy screening service and, where appropriate, smoking cessation programme. The DESMOND group education and self-management programme, now widely available in the UK, has been formally evaluated; at 12 months, compared with usual care, weight loss and smoking cessation were greater, as were understanding of diabetes and positive beliefs about illness. Depression scores were lower, though there was no difference in HbA$_{1c}$ [2].

Lifestyle intervention: diet and exercise

Retarding the progression of IGT to type 2 diabetes through intensive lifestyle intervention, with some evidence for a long-term legacy effect, is now established through many formal clinical trials (see Chapter 1). With perhaps the exception of the glitazones, which are not used in this situation, lifestyle interventions are more effective than drug treatment, though in practice both approaches are likely to be used. Whether these interventions translate into reduced cardiovascular events will not be known for several years.

Similarly, there is no evidence at present that intensive lifestyle intervention in people with established type 2 diabetes reduces cardiovascular outcomes but the Look AHEAD trial is a huge prospective 12-year study powered to demonstrate any such benefits [3]. Although not completed, it has already yielded much valuable information on intermediate outcome measures (Table 5.1). The interventions and methods are similar to those of the Diabetes Prevention Program, but even more ambitious:

- individual weight loss target, 10% (mean 7% for the intensive intervention group), with mean weight loss 8.6 kg after 1 year;
- activity goal, 175 min/week.

Aims of dietary therapy in type 2 diabetes
- Weight loss that is usually described as modest (5–10%, i.e. about 4–8 kg). However, weight regain usually starts from a nadir at 3–6 months, although sustaining this degree of weight loss over a long period is possible in a clinical trial with intensive input (see below).
- Limit postprandial glucose excursions.
- Achieve a healthy evidence-based balance of macronutrient and micronutrient intake, avoiding those that might do harm.
- Combine judiciously with exercise therapy, rational pharmacotherapy and, in some cases, bariatric surgery.

Table 5.1 One-year results of Look AHEAD: effects of about 8 kg weight loss and intensified activity

Glycaemic control	FPG ↓1.2 mmol/L (22 mg/dL) HbA$_{1c}$ ↓0.6% Diabetes medication use ↓10%
Blood pressure	↓7/3 mmHg (systolic/diastolic)
Lipids	HDL ↑0.09 mmol/L (3.4 mg/dL) LDL ↓0.1 mmol/L (5.2 mg/dL) Triglycerides ↓0.3 mmol/L (30 mg/dL) Lipid-lowering drug use ↓12%
Albumin/creatinine ratio	Rate of normalization ↑15%
Others	Improved objective measures of quality of life Slight improvement in erectile dysfunction Improvement in measures of obstructive sleep apnoea, especially with weight loss > 10 kg Overall reduction in medication use (estimated monthly cost saving $30–50)

Role of anti-obesity agents

A worthy goal, to safely reduce weight significantly using pharmacological agents in patients with type 2 diabetes, has remained largely elusive. Rimonabant, a cannabinoid receptor antagonist, was withdrawn in 2008, and sibutramine in 2010, leaving only orlistat, a lipase inhibitor. In RCTs orlistat 120 mg t.d.s. results in modest weight loss (about 3–5 kg), and in clinical practice it is most effective when used as part of a comprehensive weight-management programme. Where this is not available, success is more limited; the fat malabsorption induced by orlistat hinders compliance in the early stages of treatment. Orlistat may have a limited role in delaying progression of IGT to diabetes (see Chapter 1).

In future, the GLP-1 analogues may have a role in managing obesity, whatever the degree of glucose tolerance (see Chapter 6). Liraglutide, given at 1.2–3.0 mg/day with a 500 kcal/day energy-deficit diet, causes moderate weight loss (2.0–4.4 kg, placebo-corrected) over a short period in people with normal glucose tolerance or pre-diabetes. Even at the lowest dose, 1.2 mg daily, weight loss was significantly greater than with orlistat. Much longer studies (e.g. similar to Look AHEAD) will be required to demonstrate any useful effect on cardiovascular end points and progression to diabetes [4].

In recent years the concept of the obese individual who is nevertheless metabolically 'healthy' (the 'fit fat') has, not surprisingly, gained popularity. At any given BMI, low or high, individuals may be very insulin resistant or sensitive, or any point in between; of those with high insulin sensitivity, many do not, at least in cross-sectional studies, have associated hypertension, hyperglycaemia or high visceral fat mass, a key component of unhealthy obesity. Perhaps 10–25% of obese people fall into this category [5]. However, over a 30-year follow-up, overweight and obese Swedish men without the metabolic syndrome had a similar cardiovascular event rate and total mortality to those with the metabolic syndrome. 'Fit fat' may be a product of collective wishful thinking; certainly all obese people require follow-up for the development of the characteristics of the metabolic syndrome and associated cardiovascular risks.

Qualitative aspects of diet

While consistent reductions in calorie intake are inevitably required for sustained weight loss, there has been a great deal of interest over the past decade in whether diets of specific composition can more successfully maintain weight loss. Long-term adherence to the traditional Mediterranean diet has been shown to reduce risks of cardiovascular disease and of cancer by up to 50%, with presumably similar or greater benefits in people with diabetes compared with the general population (Fig. 5.2) [6]. Both Mediterranean and low-carbohydrate diets are more effective than the traditional high-carbohydrate low-fat diet (better glycaemic control with the Mediterranean diet, more favourable lipid profile with the low-carbohydrate diet, better sustained weight loss with both), and were safe and effective in a 2-year clinical trial [7]. These options should be offered to type 2 patients at diagnosis, where determination and adherence are at their greatest.

General recommendations on macronutrients
Carbohydrate
- Recommended daily allowance is about 130 g.
- Low glycaemic index foods (e.g. barley, oats, beans, lentils, rye bread) can reduce HbA$_{1c}$ by about 0.4% (4 mmol/mol) compared with high glycaemic index foods. More importantly, high whole-grain, cereal fibre, bran and germ intake was associated with lower cardiovascular and all-cause mortality in women with diabetes in the Nurses Health Study.
- Fibre intake: similar to that in non-diabetic people, i.e. 14 g per 1000 kcal as high-fibre foods ($\geqslant$ 5 g fibre/serving). A daily fibre intake of about 50 g (difficult to maintain) improves glycaemia in both type 1 and 2 diabetes and bran intake was independently associated with lower mortality in the Nurses Health Study. However, the soluble fibre guar gum supplements

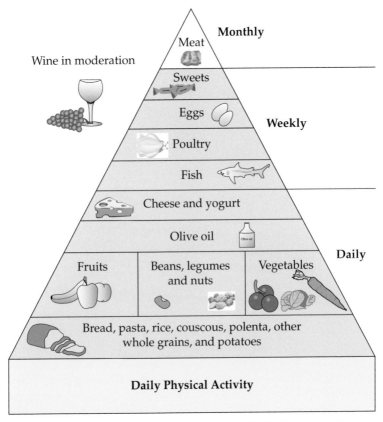

Fig. 5.2 Food pyramid reflecting the traditional healthy Mediterranean diet (Source: Hu FB. *N Engl J Med* 2003;348:2595–6)

in vogue in the mid-1990s have fallen out of use because of their weak and inconsistent glycaemic effects, though they more consistently improve lipids and seem to improve hepatic extraction of insulin.

Sweeteners
- Sucrose need not be excluded from the diet of diabetic patients: it yields similar blood glucose levels as starch.
- Fructose is increasing rapidly in the diet, mostly as the ubiquitous high-fructose corn syrup used in soft drinks and many prepared foods, rather than in fruit, which contains relatively small amounts. Fructose does not stimulate insulin secretion, and raises very low-density lipoprotein (VLDL) and urate levels, both components of the metabolic syndrome; there is concern that it is a significant promoter of population obesity [8].

Protein

The usual recommendation is 15–20% of total energy intake. High protein diets (~30%) seem to be safe and more effective in achieving sustained weight loss than low-fat, high-carbohydrate diets, though the inevitable increase in fat should be as monounsaturated fatty acids rather than saturates.

Fats and fatty acids

- The ADA and the American Heart Association recommend less than 7% of total calorie intake as saturated fat, and limiting cholesterol intake to less than 200 mg/day. However, moderate intake of prawns and eggs, widely believed to be high in cholesterol, does not affect lipid profiles in non-diabetic subjects [9].
- Minimize *trans* fatty acid intake; their use is banned in some countries.
- Take two or more portions per week of oily fish (ω-3 fatty acids, DHA and EPA).
- Increase *cis*-monounsaturated fatty acid intake as, for example, olive and rapeseed (canola) oils.

Micronutrients

Many people with diabetes take vitamin and mineral supplements, but there is almost no evidence for their benefit. Several RCTs have included additional arms of micronutrient supplementation, but neither HOPE (vitamin E 400 IU/day) nor HOPE2 (folic acid, vitamins B_6 and B_{12}) found any benefit on cardiovascular or renal outcomes, and folic acid 1 mg plus vitamin B_{12} 1 mg daily for 7 years did not reduce vascular outcomes in patients recovering after myocardial infarction in the SEARCH study, despite substantial reductions in homocysteine levels, a putative cardiovascular risk factor much in vogue a few years ago [10]. Folic acid and vitamin B_6 and B_{12} supplements are harmful in diabetic nephropathy (see Chapter 8). Vitamin D deficiency has often been linked epidemiologically with insulin resistance, and vitamin D insufficiency and deficiency is common, especially in obesity and in dark-skinned people. However, there is no conclusive evidence that it clinically improves insulin resistance or glycaemic control. Nevertheless, because of its critical role in the skeleton (both type 1 and type 2 patients are at increased fracture risk), where detected or clinically likely, active vitamin D supplementation is important. The current recommendation is a daily intake of 800–1000 IU (20–25 μg). There is no consensus on optimum blood 25-hydroxy-vitamin D levels or the daily intake of vitamin D_3 needed to achieve them. However, levels of 37.5 nmol/L (15 ng/mL) or more are widely recommended, and some suggest levels in excess of 75 nmol/L (30 ng/mL) or even 90–100 nmol/L (35–40 ng/mL). Supplementation with 1000 IU (25 μg) daily will raise serum vitamin D levels by about 25 nmol/L (10 mg/mL), and will be required in the high proportion of UK patients with inadequate sun exposure (see extensive review by the Office of Dietary Supplements, National Institutes of Health, http://ods.od.nih.gov/factsheets/vitamind.asp#en12).

Chromium, especially as chromium picolinate, has long been regarded as an insulin-sensitizing factor. Clinical studies have shown inconsistent glycaemic benefits, but there may be minor improvements in dyslipidaemia. High-cocoa content chocolate ($>70\%$, e.g. 50 g/day) has been shown to have short-term vasodilator and hypotensive effects; definitive trial results are very eagerly awaited, though British milk chocolate (cocoa content $\sim20\%$, sugar $\sim55\%$) is unlikely to figure prominently in current or future dietary recommendations.

Exercise

The Diabetes Prevention Program, studying people with IGT, set an activity goal of 150 min/week, now a widely adopted target. These values lie within the evidence-based range of 150–250 min/week (energy expenditure of 1200–2000 kcal/week) to *prevent* weight gain in most non-diabetic adults. For weight loss, current recommendations are as follows:

- <150 min/week leads to minimal weight loss;
- >150 min/week leads to modest weight loss (about 2–3 kg);
- >225 to 420 min/week leads to 5–7 kg weight loss.

'Lifestyle' physical activity (e.g. walking during commuting), often promoted as beneficial, but difficult to define or quantify, may contribute to prevention of weight gain, but even when done for long periods is unlikely to result in significant wight loss. However, exercise and calorie restriction are invariably linked in 'lifestyle' approaches to weight reduction. Combining moderate calorie restriction (500–700 kcal/day) with physical activity results in greater weight loss than diet alone; interestingly, this does not seem to be the case with more restricted calorie intakes. Even with calorie restriction, resistance training does not promote weight loss, though it may increase lean mass and loss of body fat and improve blood pressure and lipid profiles [11].

Drug treatment of type 2 diabetes

The many classes of drugs now available for the treatment of type 2 diabetes operate through largely independent mechanisms. Most have been introduced in the past decade (Fig. 5.3). There are several hundred theoretical combinations of these classes, but even allowing for functional duplication and evident incompatibilities, only a handful have been subjected to RCTs, and no studies so far have systematically studied combinations beyond triple therapy. There is a strong analogy with antihypertensive agents, three or more of which are needed for control of blood pressure in many patients, most combinations unlicensed because

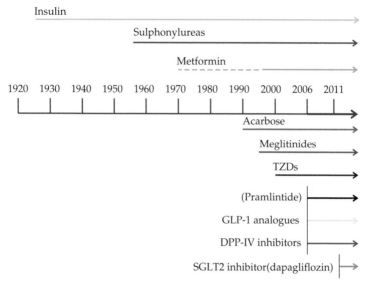

Fig. 5.3 The increasing pace of introduction of drugs for type 2 diabetes over a 90-year period

untrialled in formal RCTs. This difficulty is reflected in current guidelines (e.g. NICE 2009), which includes about 11 licensed combinations, quite sufficient options for establishing glycaemic control in the majority of patients but probably inadequate for the 10–20% of patients in persistently poor control, many of whom will have, or be at risk of developing, vascular complications.

Glycaemic responses

1 Strongly related to baseline glycaemia: the higher the initial fasting glucose/HbA_{1c}, the larger the initial fall. With a maximum dose of an additional agent (including insulin) expect:
   (a) A fall in HbA_{1c} of about 1.5% (17 mmol/mol) from a starting value of about 8.5% (69 mmol/mol); the corresponding fall in FPG is about 3 mmol/L (54 mg/dL).
   (b) A fall in HbA_{1c} of about 2% (21 mmol/mol) from an initial value of about 10%.
   (c) *Exception* is acarbose, where maximum doses result in lower falls in HbA_{1c} (e.g. up to 0.5%, 5 mmol/mol).
2 Nadir glucose levels are usually reached at 16–24 weeks with active dose titration.
3 Dose–response relationships: moderately strong for metformin, relatively weak for other agents, especially sulphonylureas.

4 Sulphonylureas give a larger initial fall in glucose levels compared with metformin or the glitazones, but thereafter the long-term rise in glucose is faster than with metformin or the glitazones.

5 Individual responses to the GLP-1 analogues, DPP-4 inhibitors and the glitazones are highly variable, and there is a null-response rate that is evident in clinical practice.

6 For all agents except metformin, invest in slow and careful dose titration with 2 to 3-monthly HbA_{1c} monitoring

7 Above all, explain the variability of response in advance with patients; assuming good adherence, a weak response or non-response is likely to be related to the agent and not the patient.

Implications for glycaemic management of type 2 diabetes in studies reporting in 2008 and 2009

Summary of UKPDS glycaemic study

The glycaemic arm of UKPDS (1998) concluded that intensive glycaemic control from diagnosis with insulin or sulphonylureas (mean HbA_{1c} 7.0% vs. 7.9%, 53 *vs.* 63 mmol/mol, over 10 years):

• significantly reduced the risk of serious microvascular end points (e.g. renal failure, vitreous haemorrhage, laser treatment);

• had a borderline significant effect on incidence of acute myocardial infarction;

• had no effect on diabetes-related deaths.

Outcomes were similar with sulphonylureas (chlorpropamide or glibenclamide) and insulin, which had to be maintained for 6 years for improvements in retinal complications and 9 years for improvements in microalbuminuria. Intensive treatment with metformin in a small group of obese subjects:

• had no beneficial effects on microvascular end points;

• reduced myocardial infarction (this finding, one of the major headlines from UKPDS, may not be as clear-cut as widely believed) [12];

• reduced diabetes-related deaths.

Metformin thereby became first-line management, along with lifestyle intervention; intensive glycaemic control established at diagnosis improved microvascular and macrovascular outcomes and glycaemic targets were set at 7.0% (53 mmol/mol) or less by most international bodies. Epidemiological evidence consistently linking increasing HbA_{1c} levels, even within the non-diabetic HbA_{1c} reference range, with macrovascular events supported the progressive lowering of HbA_{1c} targets to 6.5% (48 mmol/mol) or less despite a signal of increased cardiovascular event rates in intensively controlled long-standing diabetes (HbA_{1c} 7.2% vs. 9.2%, 55 vs. 77 mmol/mol) in the Veterans Administration feasibility study (1995). The full Veterans Affairs Diabetes Trial (VADT) study [13], and two others, ACCORD [14] and ADVANCE [15], were performed specifically in the light of the equivocal UKPDS outcomes to address the question of whether intensive glycaemic control improved cardiovascular outcomes. They were all treat-to-target studies in patients at high cardiovascular risk (either with a previous macrovascular event or several risk factors for it) designed to maintain stable glycaemic differences between intensive and conventional control arms over several years. ACCORD patients were widely treated with rosiglitazone, ADVANCE with modified-release gliclazide. In VADT, patients with BMI above 27 were started with rosiglitazone and metformin, those with BMI below 27 with rosiglitazone and glimepiride, though additional agents were permitted in order to achieve target HbA$_{1c}$ levels. The final study in this group was the natural history follow-up of the UKPDS cohort, 10 years after randomization had ceased.

Late intensive glycaemic control: conclusions from ACCORD, ADVANCE and VADT

Broad characteristics of the study populations (see Table 5.2 for more details)
- Mean age: 60–66 years.
- Mean known diabetes duration at study entry: 8–11.5 years.
- Mean HbA$_{1c}$ at baseline: 7.2–9.4% (55–79 mmol/mol).
- Difference in mean HbA$_{1c}$ at end of trial: 0.7–1.5% (8–17 mmol/mol)
- Mean duration of follow-up: 3.5–5.6 years.

Cardiovascular outcomes
From year 1 onwards in ACCORD, all-cause mortality was significantly increased in the intensive treatment group (mean achieved HbA$_{1c}$ 6.4%, 46 mmol/mol); the glycaemic arm of the trial was terminated prematurely, while the lipid and blood pressure randomizations in the same study continued (see Chapters 11 and 12). There has been much post-hoc analysis in an attempt to discover the reasons for, or characteristics of those with, the increased mortality in the intensively treated group. Severe symptomatic hypoglycaemia (blood glucose < 2.8 mmol/L, 50 mg/dL) was an early suspect, as was the rate of glucose lowering, weight gain, and the treatments themselves. Later analyses exonerated these factors; severe hypoglycaemia was associated with increased mortality in both treatment groups. To a certain extent counter-intuitively, those intensively treated patients with high baseline HbA$_{1c}$ ($\geq$ 8.5%, 69 mmol/mol) had increased mortality. It is not yet clear whether the patients in this group actually achieved target HbA$_{1c}$ on inevitably multiple medications, or whether they remained poorly controlled despite intensive treatment. Regardless, it is difficult to translate into a practical approach, other than to urge caution when embarking on intensive treatment in poorly controlled patients. There is a hint, so far unexplained, that aspirin use and

Table 5.2 Summary of recent major studies

Trial	No. in study	Follow-up (median) (years)	Mean age at trial entry (years)	Duration diabetes (years)	Mean baseline HbA$_{1c}$ (mmol/mol)	HbA$_{1c}$ during trial	Prior CV event (%)	Micro benefit?	Macro benefit?	Comments
UKPDS Follow-up	3277	17	53	0	7.1% (54)	8.5% (69) post trial to 7.7% (61) 5 years post trial (2002)	6	Yes (composite: vitreous haemorrhage, laser treatment, renal failure)	Yes	
ACCORD	10 251	3.5	62	10	8.1% (65) (median)	6.4% (46) (int) 7.5% (58) (conv)	35	Yes (some secondary outcome measures, but not advanced outcomes)	No	Glycaemic randomization stopped early due to increased CV deaths; 10% treated with four or five classes of agents including insulin

ADVANCE	11 140	5	66	8	7.2% (55) 6.3% (45) (int) 7.0% (53) (conv)	32	Decreased progression of albuminuria. No effect on retinopathy	No	Low overall macrovascular event rate (2.2% vs. anticipated 3.0%)
VADT	1791	5.6	60	11.5	9.4% (79) 6.9% (52) (int) 8.4% (68) (conv)	40	Decreased progression of albuminuria. No effect on retinopathy	No	Borderline benefit for autonomic neuropathy ($P = 0.07$); no benefit peripheral neuropathy

CV, cardiovascular.

self-reported history of neuropathy may contribute weakly to mortality, but they may just be indicators of patients already at high cardiovascular risk [16].

There was no excess of cardiovascular deaths in the intensive arms of ADVANCE and VADT, though cardiovascular events were significantly lower in the ACCORD intensive group without previous cardiovascular disease and HbA$_{1c}$ below 8% (64 mmol/mol) at baseline, i.e. 'earlier' diabetes. Intensive glycaemic control in VADT reduced events in those patients with less coronary calcification (Agatston scores ≤ 100) compared with those who had heavier calcification, again suggesting that patients with less advanced diabetes might benefit from intensive glycaemic control, but this is not a practical method to stratify risk and allocate treatment intensity. The situation is further complicated by the continuous gradation of risk across the whole range of coronary calcification scores [17].

Severe hypoglycaemia as a risk factor of death continues to be a concern. In ADVANCE, such episodes were associated with a nearly three-fold increased risk of cardiovascular events and deaths, and with almost a doubling of the risk of microvascular events. However, serious non-vascular outcomes were also increased, suggesting that hypoglycaemia may be marker of severe comorbidity, rather than a direct causal factor. Nonetheless, the message is clear [20].

Microvascular outcomes
While the focus of these trials has been on the primary outcome of cardiovascular events, they also investigated microvascular outcomes. Broadly, advanced microvascular end points were not reduced with intensive glycaemic intervention, including the following.
- *Retinopathy*: clinically significant macular oedema, progression to proliferative retinopathy and ophthalmological procedures, e.g. vitrectomy.
- *Renal*: dialysis, transplantation and advanced renal impairment.

However, progression of albuminuria was slowed by intensive treatment in ADVANCE, and ACCORD Eye (see Chapter 9) found some slowing of progression of retinopathy; however, the retinopathy findings are inconsistent between these trials, and may relate to differential effects of intensive glycaemic control on proliferative retinopathy versus maculopathy. There was a non-significant benefit of intensive treatment on autonomic neuropathy in VADT, and some measures of peripheral nerve function were improved in ACCORD. These mixed results are fascinating, but they do not help therapeutic decisions in the individual case, where the balance will have to be taken on possible benefits on microvascular complications, likely beneficial in younger patients, contrasting with the essentially negative findings on macrovascular outcomes, important in older people without microvascular complications [18].

Box 5.1 Practical implications of recent glycaemia studies

- HbA$_{1c}$ sustained at about 7% for 6–9 years from diagnosis will have microvascular and macrovascular benefits (UKPDS). No trials have been conducted to show the benefit of sustained levels lower than this from diagnosis; beyond 10 years after diagnosis, apart from variable benefits on progression of microvascular complications and neuropathy, no macrovascular or microvascular benefits can be seen from sustained values as low as 6.3% (45 mmol/mol; ADVANCE).
- Once macrovascular disease is apparent or cardiovascular risk factors are established, HbA$_{1c}$ up to 8.5% (69 mmol/mol) does not carry macrovascular disadvantage, providing lipids, blood pressure and smoking are rigorously controlled.

Conclusions about specific agents
- Metformin may reduce risk of myocardial infarction.
- Other agents, including insulin and rosiglitazone, do not positively or negatively impact on microvascular or macrovascular outcomes.

UKPDS: long-term follow-up

The 10-year UKPDS [19] provided more optimistic data. Despite convergence of mean HbA$_{1c}$ levels at 8.5% (69 mmol/mol) immediately after the trial, falling in both groups to 7.7% (61 mmol/mol) 5 years later, there was a 'legacy' effect of good glycaemic control, with continuing benefits for the previous intensive control groups, the effects on myocardial infarction and all-cause death being more marked in the intensively treated metformin group compared with the insulin/sulphonylurea group. However, in this long-term follow-up, microvascular complications were not reduced with metformin treatment. Squaring the results of the UKPDS and the three more recent studies has been the subject of extensive discussion, broadly summarized in Box 5.1.

References

1. Monnier L, Colette C, Dunseath GJ, Owens DR. The loss of postprandial glycaemic control precedes stepwise deterioration of fasting with worsening diabetes. *Diabetes Care* 2007;30:263–9. PMID: 17259492.
2. Davies MJ, Heller S, Skinner TC *et al*. Effectivenes of the diabetes education and self management for ongoing and newly diagnosed (DESMOND) programme for people with newly diagnosed type 2 diabetes: cluster randomised controlled trial. *Br Med J*. 2008;336:491–5. PMID: 18276664.
3. Pi-Sunyer X, Blackburn G, Brancati FL *et al*. Reduction in weight and cardiovascular disease risk factors in individuals with type 2 diabetes: one-year results of the Look AHEAD trial. *Diabetes Care* 2007;30:1374–83. PMID: 17363746.

4. Astrup A, Rössner S, Van Gaal L *et al.* Effects of liraglutide in the treatment of obesity: a randomised, double-blind, placebo-controlled study. *Lancet* 2009; 374:1606–16. PMID: 19853906.
5. Blüher M. The distinction of metabolically 'healthy' from 'unhealthy' obese individuals. *Curr Opin Lipidol* 2010;21:38–43.
6. Trichopoulou A, Costacou T, Bamia C, Trichopoulos D. Adherence to a Mediterranean diet and survival in a Greek population. *N Engl J Med* 2003;348:2599–608. PMID: 12826634.
7. Shai I, Schwarzfuchs D, Henkin Y *et al.* Weight loss with a low-carbohydrate, Mediterranean, or low-fat diet. Dietary Intervention Randomized Controlled Trial (DIRECT) Group. *N Engl J Med* 2008;359:229–41. PMID 18635428.
8. Hu FB, Malik VS. Sugar-sweetened beverages and risk of obesity and type 2 diabetes: epidemiologic evidence. *Physiol Behav* 2010;100:47–54. PMID: 20138901.
9. Isherwood C, Wong M, Jones WS, Davies IG, Griffin BA. Lack of effect of cold water prawns on plasma cholesterol and lipoproteins in normo-lipidaemic men. *Cell Mol Biol (Noisy-le-grand)* 2010;56:52–8. PMID: 20196970. This intriguing trial involved eating 225 g cold-water prawns daily for 12 weeks, with a crossover arm of fish ('crab') sticks. Griffin (*Nutr Bull* 2006;31:21–7) is the author of a memorable quote: 'The idea that dietary cholesterol increases risk of coronary heart disease by turning into blood cholesterol is compelling in the same way that fish oil improves arthritis by lubricating our joints'.
10. Study of the Effectiveness of Additional Reductions in Cholesterol and Homocysteine (SEARCH) Collaborative Group. Effects of homocysteine-lowering with folic acid plus vitamin B12 vs placebo on mortality and major morbidity in myocardial infarction survivors: a randomized trial. *JAMA* 2010;303:2486–94. PMID: 20571015.
11. Donnelly JE, Blair SN, Jakicic JM, Manore MM, Rankin JW, Smith BK. American College of Sports Medicine Position Stand. Appropriate physical activity intervention strategies for weight loss and prevention of weight regain for adults. *Med Sci Sports Exerc* 2009;41:459–71. PMID: 19127177.
12. Home P. Impact of the UKPDS: an overview. In: Holman RR, Watkins PJ (eds) *UKPDS: the first 30 years*, chapter 15. Oxford: Wiley-Blackwell, 2008.
13. Duckworth W, Abnraira C, Moritz T *et al.* Glucose control and vascular complications in veterans with type 2 diabetes. *N Engl J Med* 2009;360:129–39. PMID: 19092145.
14. Gerstein HC, Miller ME, Byington RP *et al.* Effects of intensive glucose lowering in type 2 diabetes. Action to Control Cardiovascular Risk in Diabetes Study Group. *N Engl J Med* 2008;358:2545–59. PMID: 18539917.
15. Patel A, MacMahon S, Chalmers J *et al.* Intensive blood glucose control and vascular outcomes in patients with type 2 diabetes. ADVANCE Collaborative Group. *N Engl J Med* 2008;358:2560–72. PMID: 18539916.
16. Calles-Escandón J, Lovato LC, Simons-Morton DG *et al.* Effect of intensive compared with standard glycemia treatment strategies on mortality by baseline subgroup characteristics: the Action to Control Cardiovascular Risk in Diabetes (ACCORD) trial. *Diabetes Care* 2010;33:721–7. PMID: 20103550.
17. Reaven PD, Moritz TE, Schwenke DC *et al.* Intensive glucose-lowering therapy reduces cardiovascular disease events in Veterans Affairs Diabetes Trial participants with lower calcified coronary atherosclerosis. *Diabetes* 2009;58:2642–8. PMID: 19651816.
18. Ismail-Beigi F, Craven T, Banerji MA *et al.* Effect of intensive treatment of hyperglycaemia on microvascular outcomes in type 2 diabetes: an analysis of the ACCORD randomised trial. *Lancet* 2010;376(9739):419–30. PMID: 20594588.

19. Holman RR, Paul SK, Bethel MA, Matthews DR, Neil HA. 10-year follow-up of intensive glucose control in type 2 diabetes. *N Engl J Med* 2008;359:1577–89. PMID: 18784090.
20. Zoungas S, Patel A, Chalmers J et al. ADVANCE Collaborative group. Severe hypoglycemia and risks of vascular events and death. *N Engl J Med* 2010; 363:1410–8.

Further reading

ADA position statement
Skyler JS, Bergenstal R, Bonow RO *et al.* Intensive glycaemic control and the prevention of cardiovascular events: implications of the ACCORD, ADVANCE, and VA diabetes trials: a position statement of the American Diabetes Association and a scientific statement of the American College of Cardiology Foundation and the American Heart Association. *Diabetes Care* 2009;32:187–92. PMID: 19092168.

NICE Guideline/National Collaborating Centre for Chronic Conditions
Type 2 diabetes (update): National Clinical Guideline for Management in Primary and Secondary Care (2008). Available at www.rcplondon.ac.uk/pubs/brochure.aspx?e-247 and www.nice.org.uk/CG66fullguideline

UKPDS 30 years on
Holman RR, Watkins PJ (eds) *UKPDS: the first 30 years*. Oxford, Wiley-Blackwell, 2008. A brilliant confection of scientific summary, the tribulations and limitations of clinical trials, and personal reminiscences and viewpoints, sometimes trenchant, about this remarkable British clinical study, initiated, almost on the back of an envelope, by Robert Turner in 1976, who died at the age of 61, the year after the publication of the main study findings in 1998.
Krentz AJ, Bailey CJ. *Type 2 Diabetes in Practice*, 2nd edn. London, Royal Society of Medicine Press, 2005.

Dietary management
Cheyette C, Balolia Y. Carbs & Cals. A visual guide to carbohydrate counting & calorie counting for people with diabetes. Chello Publishing, 2010.
Frost G, Dornhorst A, Moses R (eds) *Nutritional Management of Diabetes Mellitus*. Oxford, Wiley-Blackwell, 2003.
Collins Gem Carb Counter: a Clear Guide to Carbohydrates in Everyday Foods. London, Collins, 2004.

Exercise
Nagi DK. *Exercise and Sport in Diabetes*. Oxford, Wiley-Blackwell, 2005.

Websites
UKPDS: www.dtu.ox.ac.uk/ukpds (valuable slide sets not only of UKPDS, 1998 and 2008, but also 4-T, ADOPT, DREAM and NAVIGATOR studies).
ADVANCE trial: www.advance-trial.com (includes slide sets).
Slide presentations of all four major studies (VADT, ACCORD, ADVANCE, UKPDS) available at www.diabetesbestpractices.com/slides.aspx

Type 2 diabetes: pharmacological treatment of hyperglycaemia

CHAPTER 6

Key points

- Metformin is universally agreed as foundation treatment for type 2 diabetes.
- All currently used agents have approximately the same glucose-lowering effects for a given baseline glycaemic level.
- Beyond metformin there is now little agreement on next steps; basal insulin, progressing to MDI, is still considered by some the best option, but patients are not enthusiastic for early insulin treatment.
- Sulphonylureas are safe, apart from the risk of hypoglycaemia, but failure can be relatively rapid; the short-acting meglitinides are useful alternatives.
- The injectable GLP-1 analogues are increasingly used in triple therapy with metformin and sulphonylurea in obese patients because they can cause variable weight loss. Glycaemic durability and long-term side-effects are not known, and vomiting and poor glycaemic and weight responses can limit treatment. Several compounds are in the developmental pipeline, some designed for weekly administration.
- A DPP-4 inhibitor (gliptin) can be given a trial at any stage where hypoglycaemia and/or weight gain could be troublesome; long-term efficacy and safety need to be determined.
- The cumulative side-effect profile of the glitazones, especially rosiglitazone, no longer available in Europe, has demoted them from their place in routine triple oral therapy, though paradoxically they both seem to be safe and beneficial in patients with advanced vascular

Practical Diabetes Care, 3rd edition. © David Levy.
Published 2011 by Blackwell Publishing Ltd.

disease. They are also durable treatments, and pioglitazone is of value in patients failing on high-dose insulin.
- Insulin improves glycaemia rapidly, and stable control can often be achieved, but at the cost of increasing injection frequency, hypoglycaemia and weight. Even MDI rarely reduces HbA_{1c} to below 7.0% (53 mmol/mol), and some patients again end up in poor control.

Introduction

The pharmacological management of blood glucose in type 2 diabetes remains the most contentious area of diabetes management, and although until relatively recently in the USA the only agents to treat blood glucose were insulin and sulphonylureas, this limited repertoire in no way inhibited the controversy, which started with the University Group Diabetes Project (UGDP) conclusions about the possible hazards of sulphonylureas in the late 1960s [1]. Perhaps scarred by the UGDP experience, and certainly by the disastrous introduction elsewhere of phenformin, metformin was available in many countries for a long time before it was licensed in the USA as recently as 1995. UKPDS, reporting in 1998, used only metformin, sulphonylureas and insulin (with a small acarbose substudy). Multiple classes of agents are now available, and these are likely to increase further, though certainly at a much slower pace than over the past decade.

The furious rate of pharmacological innovation has not been matched by RCTs powered to study significant diabetes outcomes that are important to patients. Until recently regulatory requirements were limited to acute safety and demonstration of glycaemic non-inferiority, and very few studies lasted over 6 months, always contentious in a condition that spanned decades, not months. In 2007 the controversy over the cardiovascular safety of rosiglitazone stimulated the Food and Drug Administration in the USA to require demonstration of cardiovascular safety before drug approval, but this is quite different from the widespread practice of claiming potential non-glucose benefits on the basis of small, often mechanistic studies. Other than the tentative UKPDS data relating to the cardiovascular advantage of metformin (and recent epidemiological evidence of its possible cancer-reducing properties), there is even now little evidence for the benefit of specific medication in relation to significant diabetes outcomes. The recent glycaemic/ macrovascular studies reviewed in Chapter 5 have reinforced this view, and moreover have relegated glycaemic control in established type 2 diabetes from the position of primacy it enjoyed for decades to be replaced by a more comprehensive view of the metabolic disorder. Unfortunately, however, because we do not have agents that impact on multiple metabolic problems we necessarily end up considering glycaemia in isolation.

Nevertheless, the drugs available to treat blood glucose levels in type 2 diabetes work through independent mechanisms. In a heterogeneous condition such as type 2 diabetes, which can be intercepted along a time continuum of more than 50 years, from pre-diabetes to advanced tissue complications, with different contributions of insulin deficiency and insulin resistance, the availability of these different agents should be regarded as a positive challenge to match where possible patients to medication and not vice versa. The discussion below attempts to discuss pharmacological treatments in this way, rather than using a guidelines-based approach; the controversies here too frequently revolve around the guidelines themselves, rather than the risks and benefits of specific agents.

Metformin (*BNF*, section 6.1.2.2)

A development of the plant-derived guanidine (occuring in goat's rue/ French lilac, *Galega officinalis*), metformin was first used clinically in the late 1950s. Established as a first-line treatment for overweight type 2 diabetes patients in the UKPDS, it has been formally trialled and is licensed for use in dual therapy with all other agents, including insulin; with the sulphonylureas, it has become the standard against which all new agents are initially subjected to RCTs.

Mechanism of action and non-glycaemic effects

Metformin has peripheral effects only, and does not stimulate insulin secretion, though it requires some insulin for its peripheral actions. It suppresses hepatic glycogenolysis and gluconeogenesis, and stimulates insulin-mediated muscle and adipose tissue glucose disposal. There has been much interest recently in its cellular actions, in particular its effect on AMP-activated protein kinase (AMPK), an important component of an intracellular energy-sensing cascade. The intriguing and consistent epidemiological link between metformin use and decreased risk of developing some cancers, for example breast cancer, may be AMPK-mediated (against a background of generally increased cancer risk in type 2 diabetes patients). Metformin also has minor but beneficial effects on the following.

- Lipids, especially lowering triglycerides, VLDL, and fatty acids (a significant effect only in people with poor glycaemic control).
- Blood pressure (not consistent).
- Coagulation factors (e.g. decreased plasminogen activator inhibitor 1).
- Weight: metformin use in UKPDS was associated with weight gain of about 2 kg, compared with about 5 kg in insulin- or sulphonylurea-treated patients. ADOPT (2006) found modest weight loss, about 3 kg

over 5 years, most occurring in the first year. Metformin attenuates the weight-increasing effects of sulphonylureas.

It is safe in adult doses in children with type 2 diabetes, and at a dose of 750 mg daily, with or without intensive lifestyle intervention, reduces weight without hypoglycaemia in non-diabetic patients with schizophrenia starting on antipsychotic medication [2]. It does not cause hypoglycaemia in monotherapy and perhaps this, together with its relatively slow onset of action, certainly in comparison with sulphonylureas, has led to the view that it is a 'weak' antihyperglycaemic agent; there is, however, no evidence that it is any less potent than other drugs used in type 2 diabetes. Metformin treatment should always be maintained or added to existing insulin therapy: a recent trial over 4 years showed that it:

- prevented weight gain (3.1 kg loss);
- reduced mean HbA_{1c} by 0.4% (4 mmol/mol);
- reduced insulin requirements by 20 units/day;
- reduced macrovascular events by 40%, partly accounted for by the weight loss (though there was no effect on microvascular events, outcomes echoing those of UKPDS) [3].

Dose

Metformin is effective in the dose range 500–2000 mg daily. There is little evidence for increased efficacy at doses over 2 g/day, and although it is frequently prescribed at 3 g/day, side-effects are more likely. This practice also illustrates the general point that once maximum doses of a drug are being approached, serious consideration must be given to choosing the next. Even the immediate-release forms require only twice-daily dosing. Unlike several other agents, metformin has a good dose–response relationship, and even if taken at only 500 mg/day, for example in people who suffer gastrointestinal side-effects at higher doses, it can be expected to reduce HbA_{1c} by about 0.5% (5 mmol/mol). Modified-release preparations (e.g. Glucophage SR in the UK) are designed for once-daily dosing, and clinically markedly reduce gastrointestinal side-effects in patients intolerant of immediate-release metformin. In the UK there are fixed-dose combinations of (immediate-release) metformin with pioglitazone and the DPP-4 inhibitors vildagliptin and sitagliptin. The fixed-dose sulphonylurea/metformin combinations available in the USA are not generally used in the UK.

Metformin should be taken with or immediately before meals, starting at 500 mg once or twice daily, and titrated to maximum effect, using once or twice-weekly fasting home blood glucose monitoring. Gastrointestinal side-effects (dyspepsia, nausea, diarrhoea and flatulence) are common in the first 1–2 weeks of treatment, but fewer than 5% of patients cannot tolerate metformin at any dose, and this proportion may be even lower with the use of modified-released preparations. Delayed side-effects are occasionally seen with immediate-release metformin, even after a period during which it has apparently been well tolerated. Stop treatment for a short time, or replace with modified-release metformin before embarking on gastrointestinal investigations. It has a slow onset of action, with a maximum effect around 4 months, and a sulphonylurea should be used initially with metformin in a newly diagnosed patient with symptomatic hyperglycaemia.

Contraindications

Drug accumulation occurs in renal impairment, but there is currently a widespread erroneous view that metformin itself causes renal impairment (Box 6.1). Not many years ago, metformin would have been withdrawn when serum creatinine exceeded about 120 μmol/L (1.4 mg/dL), but this criterion had no evidence base, and it has become clear with wider use that adverse effects due to moderate renal impairment itself are extremely uncommon. The current consensus is that it should be withdrawn if estimated glomerular filtration rate (eGFR) is below 30 mL/min (e.g. serum creatinine ~ 200 μmol/L in a white male aged 60), but can be used safely, though with caution and at minimum effective dosage, if eGFR is 30–60 mL/min (60 mL/min is equivalent to serum creatinine of about 115 μmol/L (1.3 mg/dL) in the same patient).

The potency of metformin as an antihyperglycaemic drug, especially in patients with renal impairment, should not be underestimated. The clinical impression is that HbA$_{1c}$ can increase by up to 3% (33 mmol/mol) if a substantial dose of metformin is abruptly withdrawn. It is the responsibility of the practitioner who withdraws metformin to ensure a plan is in place to manage the resulting, possibly severe, hyperglycaemia. Transient deterioration in renal function in acutely ill hospitalized patients is very common, often precipitating abrupt withdrawal of

---

Box 6.1 Unfounded beliefs about metformin

- It causes renal impairment.
- It is contraindicated in any degree of renal impairment.
- It frequently precipitates lactic acidosis.
- It is contraindicated in people with ischaemic heart disease.
- It should not be used in people who have had an uncomplicated myocardial infarction.
- It should be stopped 48 hours before investigations using intravenous contrast.

metformin, but there is no reason for it not being restarted when renal function improves, though it often is not.

Severe hepatic impairment, and poorly controlled heart failure, are both considered contraindications (though many heart failure patients are treated with metformin, and 45% of them were taking metformin alone), but mildly abnormal liver function tests, very common in people with diabetes as a result of non-alcoholic fatty liver disease, are not a contraindication, and metformin (like the glitazones) may well cause a drop in transaminase levels. It is not contraindicated in patients who have had an uncomplicated myocardial infarction.

Lactic acidosis and vitamin B$_{12}$ levels

Lactic acidosis usually occurs in the context of multiorgan failure, and it is often difficult to ascribe it to metformin use alone. Its incidence relative to metformin use overall is vanishingly small, and a systematic review concluded that there was no true increase in incidence in metformin-treated compared with non-metformin-treated diabetic patients [4]. Vitamin B$_{12}$ metabolism is subtly disturbed with long-term metformin treatment, but simple serum vitamin B$_{12}$ levels have usually been normal. However, a large RCT over 4 years found that vitamin B$_{12}$ deficiency (<150 pmol/L, 203 pg/mL) was 10% more common than in placebo-treated patients, with an associated increase in homocysteine levels. There was no increase in folate deficiency. Since B$_{12}$ deficiency is simple to treat, there is now a strong case for measuring vitamin B$_{12}$ levels every few years in patients taking long-term metformin treatment [5].

Radiological contrast medium-induced lactic acidosis

The conventional, but non-evidence-based, view is that metformin should be withheld 48 hours before and after a procedure involving an intravenous contrast agent, because of the increased risk of lactic acidosis (both agents are renally excreted unchanged). Cases nearly always occur in those with impaired renal function. Where possible, review previous laboratory results to establish trends in renal function, rather than using individual measurements.

- In patients with normal renal function (eGFR > 90 mL/min), continue metformin but ensure adequate hydration.
- Where there is renal impairment, withhold metformin for 48 hours after the procedure. Some patients will require alternative diabetes treatment over this period. Ensure adequate intravenous periprocedural hydration, and check renal function before restarting metformin.

Treatment failure with metformin: early use, or lifestyle first?

Measuring treatment failure with any agent is difficult, as the criteria for failure (often called 'secondary failure') have not been established. In

ADOPT (2006) the failure rate for metformin treatment (defined as FPG > 10 mmol/L, 180 mg/dL) was only about 4% per year, similar to that with rosiglitazone, but lower than glibenclamide. However, in clinical practice the failure rate is much higher –17% per year judged by HbA_{1c} exceeding 7.5% (59 mmol/mol) after treatment with metformin that reduced HbA_{1c} to less than 7.0% (53 mmol/mol). Although many guidelines continue to propose diet and lifestyle first, progressing to metformin treatment only if the non-drug strategy fails (e.g. NICE 2009), where acceptable to patients metformin should be offered at diagnosis, together with intensive lifestyle intervention on the basis that lifestyle effects are likely to wane after 3–6 months in the real-life setting [6].

Sulphonylureas and meglitinides (prandial insulin regulators) (*BNF*, section 6.1.2.1)

Sulphonylureas have been workhorses of diabetes therapy for over 40 years. The short-acting meglitinides, operating through similar mechanisms, are much more recent. Neither should be used as first-line treatment in normal weight, overweight or obese patients, or in those with multiple insulin resistance characteristics, where first-line metformin is preferable (Table 6.1).

Action

Sulphonylureas stimulate pancreatic insulin secretion by binding to the sulphonylurea receptor (SUR1) on the β cell. This closes Kir 6.2 (K-ATP) channels, resulting in calcium influx, stimulating release initially of pre-formed insulin granules (first-phase insulin secretion), and thereafter increasing release and formation of insulin-containing granules (second-phase insulin secretion). It is the prolonged stimulation of insulin release, independent of ambient glucose levels, that increases the risk of profound and long-lasting hypoglycaemia with these drugs. The only truly short-acting agent, tolbutamide, is no longer widely used (though apart from the necessary multiple daily dosing, its demise has been largely dictated by general usage and fashion) and the distinction between the remaining members of the class as either intermediate or long-acting is pharmacokinetic and does not reliably characterize their clinical duration of action, nor the likelihood of their causing severe hypoglycaemia. They are highly protein-bound and can interact with warfarin and salicylates, increasing the risk of hypoglycaemia.

Potential adverse cardiovascular effects

Some sulphonylureas, especially glibenclamide, cross-react with and close cardiac potassium channels and experimentally reduce protective

Table 6.1 Sulphonylureas and meglitinides

Drug	Effect duration (hours)	Daily dose range (mg)	Maximum effective dose (mg)	Doses/day	Comments
Sulphonylureas					
Glibenclamide (USA: glyburide)	20–24	2.5–20	10–15	1–2	No longer a first-line choice (hypoglycaemia), but safe in pregnancy
Gliclazide	10–15	40–320	160–240	Divide doses above 160 mg/day	Modified release (once-daily) available, e.g. Diamicron MR, dose range 30–90 mg (~80–240 mg non-modified release)
Glimepiride	24	1–6	4	1 at all doses	Possible lower risk of hypoglycaemia than with other long-acting sulphonylureas
Glipizide	12–14	2.5–20	20	Divide doses above 15 mg/day	Little used in UK; m/r available in USA
Meglitinides (prandial glucose regulators)					
Repaglinide (introduced 1998)	Few	1.5–16	12–16	0.5–4 mg at each main meal	Take 15–30 min before meals
Nateglinide (introduced 2001)	Few	540	540	60–180 mg at each meal	Take 15–30 min before meals; licensed with metformin, not as monotherapy. Relatively little used

cardiac ischaemic preconditioning. Whether this effect is clinically relevant is not clear, but it is not likely to be a major consideration. Gliclazide, the sulphonylurea most used in the UK, does not have this potential cardiac effect; neither does glimepiride, nor the meglitinides. Though there are few long-term studies, RCT evidence is reassuring: in ADOPT (2006), newly diagnosed patients treated with glibenclamide up to 15 mg daily had a lower cardiac event rate than those treated with metformin or rosiglitazone monotherapy, and there was no excess of cardiovascular events in UKPDS with either glibenclamide or the very long-acting chlorpropamide, no longer used.

Dosing

Initial doses should be low (e.g. gliclazide 40 mg b.d.), with slow and gradual titration while monitoring glucose, HbA_{1c} and, most importantly, hypoglycaemia (see below). Dose–response relationships are weak and maximum glycaemic effect is often seen at doses lower than the recommended maximum; conversely, increasing doses in the face of limited further improvement is not worthwhile. While the maximum effect of sulphonylureas is thought to be in the early stages of type 2 diabetes, when β-cell reserve is at its maximum, it can sometimes be worthwhile reintroducing them later, for example when trying to discontinue insulin treatment using the newer agents; responses can sometimes be surprising. There is consistent evidence from UKPDS, ADOPT and RECORD studies that although the initial glycaemic response to sulphonylureas is more dramatic than with either metformin or glitazones, with lower nadir HbA_{1c} levels, the subsequent failure rate (secondary or sulphonylurea failure) is higher. In ADOPT (Fig. 6.1), using an arbitrary monotherapy failure threshold of 10 mmol/L (180 mg/dL), the approximate annual failure rates were 3% for rosiglitazone, 4% for metformin, and 7% for glibenclamide.

Weight gain is common, UKPDS and ADOPT (the latter using glibenclamide 15 mg daily) reporting about a 2-kg gain, mostly in the first year of treatment.

Meglitinide analogues

The meglitinide analogues (repaglinide and nateglinide) bind to a different site of the sulphonylurea receptor, and have a much more rapid onset and offset of action. They are therefore suitable for taking immediately before a meal and for controlling predominant postprandial hyperglycaemia (possibly beneficial – one study showed that for similar HbA_{1c} reductions, increase in carotid intima–media thickness (CIMT) was less pronounced after repaglinide compared with glibenclamide [7]). Note, however, that in the NAVIGATOR study (2010) nateglinide if anything increased postload glucose levels (in subjects with IGT, where the biochemical problem is

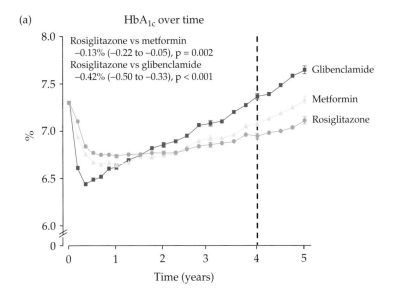

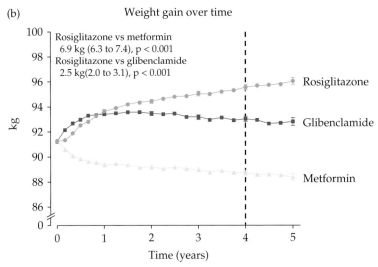

Fig. 6.1 (a) Fasting plasma glucose (FPG) in newly diagnosed patients treated with metformin, glibenclamide (glyburide) or rosiglitazone monotherapy in the ADOPT study showing the lower nadir reached with sulphonylurea treatment but subsequent more rapid rise in FPG. (b) Early weight gain is substantial but stabilizes after about a year. (Adapted from Kahn *et al*. New Eng J Med 2006; 355: 2427–43)

predominantly post load), though it reduced fasting glucose levels. Mild hypoglycaemia can occur with both agents but severe events are uncommon, and importantly they are unlikely to be prolonged, the major hazard with sulphonylureas. Weight gain is about the same as with sulphonylureas. They are suitable for patients with renal impairment, and the flexible dosing may be helpful during Ramadan fasting. The disadvantage is the need for multiple daily doses, which is likely to be less appropriate for the elderly who might particularly benefit from their short action. Repaglinide has similar glucose-lowering effects as sulphonylureas, though nateglinide is less potent (up to about 0.6% HbA$_{1c}$ lowering, 7 mmol/mol). Nonetheless, they are valuable agents that are probably underused in clinical practice.

Sulphonylurea-induced hypoglycaemia

Hypoglycaemia occurs with any sulphonylurea (0.4–0.6% per year in UKPDS; 0.6% of patients in ADOPT had a serious hypoglycaemic event, and nearly 40% reported hypoglycaemia). Clinically it occurs about 4 hours after a morning dose, often in late morning after mild exertion and omitting any mid-morning snack (e.g. on shopping or golfing days). There is an impression that as glycaemic targets continue to be driven down, significant sulphonylurea-related hypoglycaemia is becoming more common. Discuss in detail the possibility of hypoglycaemia when starting sulphonylurea therapy, outline the likely symptoms, and indicate clearly what procedure the patient must follow if hypoglycaemia does occur (dose reduction, stopping treatment).

Profound and prolonged hypoglycaemia, sometimes resulting in death or brain damage, can occur in the elderly, in those with intercurrent illness, malnutrition or alcoholism, and in those with impaired renal function. Admit, especially the elderly, and treat with a prolonged infusion of 10–20% glucose. Bolus injections of glucose and glucagon can stimulate residual insulin secretion in type 2 patients, hence the need for continuing glucose infusion with careful blood glucose monitoring. Monitor serum potassium frequently; it may fall with the high circulating insulin levels. Octreotide may be of value in very severe and prolonged hypoglycaemia, and a bolus subcutaneous injection of 75 μg on admission, in addition to standard treatment, reduces the risk of relapsing hypoglycaemia [8].

Thiazolidinediones (glitazones) (*BNF*, section 6.1.2.3)

No drugs in diabetes have caused more controversy or been more scrutinized than the glitazones. Starting in 2007, the glitazone controversy, especially concerning rosiglitazone, caused a major rethink not only of the fundamental reasons for treating hyperglycaemia in type 2 diabetes, culminating in the trials reporting in 2008 and 2009, but at least in the USA major changes in approval of antihyperglycaemic agents, which are now required to demonstrate cardiovascular safety before licensing. This is not the place to recount the details of the controversy, but a meta-analysis of studies with rosiglitazone published in 2007 had suggested that both myocardial infarction and cardiovascular deaths were increased with this agent. Further studies and analyses confirmed that cardiovascular deaths were not increased, and the recent major glycaemia trials confirmed overall the cardiovascular safety of rosiglitazone though other studies, for example the aborted RECORD study, are less persuasive. The PROactive study using pioglitazone (2005) had shown that major cardiovascular events were significantly reduced with this agent, but the primary outcome, a composite of cardiovascular events and arterial interventions, was unchanged. Perhaps underlying all this was the reversal of the widespread expectation that because of the mode of action of the glitazones, cardiovascular events would be consistently reduced by these agents. More generally, short-term studies in humans or experimental animals that demonstrate improvements in markers of cardiovascular risk cannot be translated into clinical benefit until definitively proven in large-scale RCTs. Redefining the position of the glitazones in the management of type 2 diabetes has been difficult because of the long-term resonances of these studies and expectations, and also history.

The prototype glitazone, troglitazone, was introduced very briefly in the UK during 1997, but withdrawn because of rare but serious hepatic side-effects. It was withdrawn in the USA in 2000. Both the successor compounds, rosiglitazone and pioglitazone, have no adverse hepatic effects. On the contrary, glitazones consistently improve mildly abnormal liver function test results (see below). Although the non-response rate is significant overall they are no less potent antihyperglycaemic agents than any other agents. Nevertheless, after detailed re-evaluation, rosiglitazone was withdrawn in Europe in late 2010 because of continued anxiety over increased myocardial infarction rates, and although it remains marketed in the USA, new use is restricted to those where all other medication options, including pioglitazone, have been exhausted. Pioglitazone is therefore the sole agent available in this group.

Action

Glitazones are agonists of the peroxisome proliferator-activated receptor (PPAR)-γ, acting at nuclear receptors to stimulate various insulin-sensitive genes. They have multiple actions in insulin-sensitive tissues (muscle, liver and adipose tissue), for example increasing glucose uptake, decreasing gluconeogenesis and glycogenolysis, and increasing fatty acid uptake, lipogenesis and differentiation of adipocytes. Like metformin, they require insulin for their glucose-lowering effects, and are antihyperglycaemic rather than hypoglycaemic, so used in monotherapy carry a low risk of hypoglycaemia. Direct and indirect markers of insulin sensitivity are consistently improved, but despite good experimental evidence for improved β-cell function, in the ADOPT study after 5 years there was no significant difference in β-cell function compared with glibenclamide or metformin. Although those with phenotypic features of insulin resistance might be thought to benefit from a glitazones, clinical response cannot be predicted clinically or on the basis of any simple laboratory tests. A carefully observed therapeutic trials in individual patients is therefore important, as with any agent. Onset of glucose lowering is slow and does not maximize until 4–5 months, so pioglitazone should not be used in symptomatically hyperglycaemic patients.

Additional effects

A large portfolio of consistently demonstrated biochemical benefits (including significant reductions in high-sensitivity CRP, white count, various other inflammatory markers, including the plaque-disrupting matrix metalloproteinases, and microalbuminuria) has not translated in large-scale RCTs to a reduction in cardiovascular events. However, smaller studies in well-defined groups with advanced vascular disease are more encouraging.

- A post-hoc analysis of PROactive found that the risk of recurrent stroke was reduced by about 50%, although there was no benefit in primary prevention of stroke.
- Coronary stent restenosis in both diabetic and non-diabetic subjects is reduced with both agents over the medium term in small studies (a bigger study is in progress). However, a large-scale intravascular ultrasound study (APPROACH) found that rosiglitazone had no clear advantage over glipizide in reducing the volume of coronary atheroma over 18 months.
- CIMT is rapidly reduced, independent of glycaemic benefits, again with both agents, though the CHICAGO study with pioglitazone hinted that this effect attenuated with time.
- BARI 2D (2009): cardiovascular outcomes improved in coronary bypass patients treated with metformin/rosiglitazone compared with insulin.

Currently, however, these potentially intriguing uses are largely contraindicated.

Pioglitazone and insulin

A licensed combination of clinical importance. In PROactive, addition of pioglitazone reduced the likelihood of requiring permanent insulin treatment by 50% over 3 years. There was also a consistent 0.5% (5 mmol/mol) HbA_{1c} benefit in the pioglitazone-treated group, including the 30% who were already using insulin; 9% of patients were able to discontinue insulin. The need for multiple insulin injections was reduced as was the number of coadministered oral agents. Not unexpectedly, those in poor glycaemic control and needing higher doses of insulin benefited most from the addition of pioglitazone [9]. While reducing insulin doses or even discontinuing insulin are not considered by academics to be important outcomes, patients are likely to hold a different view.

Glycaemic durability

This is an important consideration. The glitazones consistently show more stable glycaemic control than sulphonylureas and, to a lesser degree, metformin, up to 5 years. In the PROactive study, triple therapy (sulphonylurea, metformin and pioglitazone) was well tolerated and delivered stable glycaemic control over 3 years.

Non-alcoholic steatohepatitis

Many small studies have hinted at improvement in liver histology with glitazone treatment, but in a large 2-year study, while the antioxidant vitamin E (800 IU daily) improved overall histology, pioglitazone 30 mg daily did not. Importantly, neither agent seemed to improve fibrosis scores, though transaminases, as frequently seen in clinical practice, fell with both. Pioglitazone does not seem to consistently improve all histological outcomes in this important condition, and it is unlikely to be licensed for it [10].

Adverse effects

- *Weight gain*: as with other agents, weight gain, largely adipose, can be rapid in the first year but may continue up to 5 years. In ADOPT, the mean weight difference between the rosiglitazone and metformin groups at the end of the study was nearly 7 kg. Although weight gain may be peripheral rather than abdominal, waist and hip circumferences both increase. The weight gain is broadly related to the glycaemic benefit. Ankle oedema is common and occasionally troublesome.
- *Exacerbation of heart failure*: glitazones are contraindicated in any degree of heart failure, and adjudicated cases of heart failure and hospitalization for heart failure, though not mortality, are increased
- *Normochromic anaemia* with a decrease in haemoglobin (Hb) of about 1 g/dL, sometimes greater, may be seen. It may be due to a mild bone marrow effect. Since anaemia occurs early in diabetic nephropathy, and significant renal impairment (eGFR > 30 mL/min) is not a

contraindication to glitazone treatment, the degree of anaemia may be significant in some patients.
- *Fractures*: PPAR-γ inhibits bone formation by diverting mesenchymal stem cells to the adipocyte lineage, and may also stimulate osteoclasts. Distal limb fractures are increased in premenopausal and post-menopausal women taking glitazones compared with those taking sulphonylureas or metformin, and men may also be at increased risk. Typical osteoporotic spine and femoral neck fractures are not increased.
- *Macular oedema*: there have been some case reports associating thiazoli-dinediones with macular oedema. Cohort studies have found a slightly increased risk with both drugs, but there was no association in a cross-sectional analysis of the ACCORD study [11]. Nevertheless, be alert to the possibility, especially in patients with known retinopathy.

Preparations
- Pioglitazone: 15 mg, 30 mg, 45 mg.
- Fixed-dose combinations: 15 mg pioglitazone/850 mg metformin twice daily.

Dose–response relationship is weak; this, together with the variable and gradual glycaemic response, reinforces the importance of the start-low, go-slow approach.

Use
Pioglitazone is no longer licensed as monotherapy. The 2009 NICE guidelines propose the following possible combinations:
- as second-line treatment added to metformin rather than a sulphonyl-urea, when there is a risk of hypoglycaemia or in the rare case of sulphonylurea intolerance (a minor indication with the introduction of DPP-4 inhibitors);
- as third-line treatment added to metformin and sulphonylurea when insulin is not desirable or desired;
- pioglitazone with insulin if glycaemic control is poor on high-dose insulin or if there previously has been a good glycaemic response to a glitazone (see below).

The logical combination of exenatide and a glitazone (with or without metformin) improves glycaemic control and causes significant weight loss, at least in a short study [12]. Another similar potential, but unlicensed, scenario for glitazones would be addition to GLP-1-containing regimens, where weight loss has been substantial but glycaemic improvement limited.

Glitazone use has fallen markedly since 2007. However, in patients who respond without significant adverse effects, durability of glycaemic control can be clinically striking. The trial results in secondary prevention patients – the likely benefit of pioglitazone in PROactive and that of metformin plus rosiglitazine in BARI 2D – contrasts with the limitations of their use in real life in these patient groups.

α-Glucosidase inhibitors (*BNF*, section 6.1.2.3)

Action

These drugs, in vogue in the early 1990s but much less used now (they do not figure in the current NICE guidelines), inhibit enzymes that break down polysaccharides and sucrose in the small intestine, resulting in delayed absorption of glucose and lower postprandial peaks, though the total amount of glucose absorbed is unchanged. In addition, postprandial lipaemia is improved. Although early studies suggested they stimulate incretins, this is probably not a significant clinical effect.

Acarbose was used in a UKPDS substudy, where it reduced HbA_{1c} levels by about 0.5% (5 mmol/mol). This value is consistent across several studies, though in a head-to-head monotherapy comparison with the DPP-4 inhibitor vildagliptin both achieved reductions of about 1.3% (15 mmol/mol) from a mean baseline of 8.6% (70 mmol/mol), but acarbose caused greater weight loss (1.3 kg) [13]. However, its perceived low glycaemic impact, together with significant gastrointestinal side-effects, especially flatulence, has limited its use. The STOP-NIDDM trial (2002) demonstrated a powerful effect of acarbose in reducing progression of IGT to type 2 diabetes, though only while the drug was taken, a consistent finding in pharmacological compared with lifestyle interventions. Voglibose also reduces the risk of progression from IGT to diabetes. STOP-NIDDM controversially also found a reduction in cardiovascular events and new-onset hypertension. Acarbose is the only agent in use in the UK; elsewhere, voglibose and miglitol are available. Dose escalation should be slow, for example acarbose 25–50 mg with the main meal of the day, increasing to 50 mg t.d.s. (100 mg t.d.s. is the maximum recommended dose and has been associated with abnormal liver function tests). Gastrointestinal side-effects decrease over the first 4–6 weeks of treatment, and do not appear to be greater even when acarbose is combined with metformin. Complete neglect of these agents is probably not justified, especially acarbose and voglibose, which are not significantly absorbed systemically; they can be added to combination therapy.

Therapeutic targets in the incretin system (entero-insular axis)

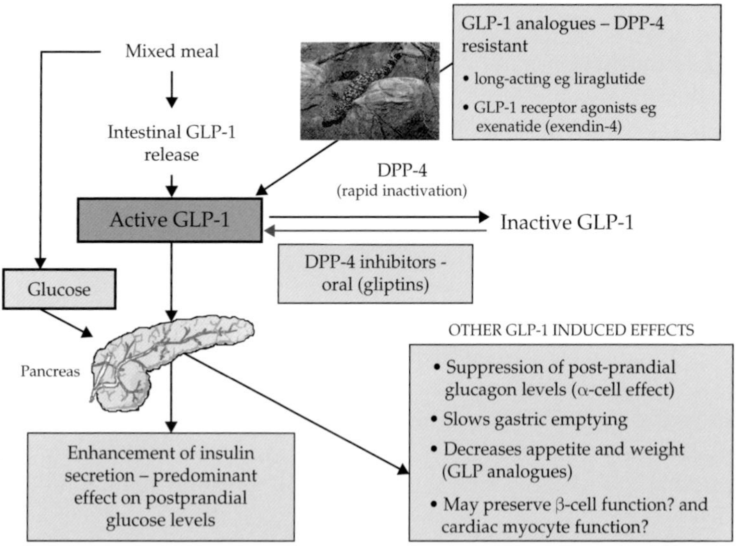

Fig. 6.2 Incretin system (entero-insular axis) and current and future therapeutic targets. The systemic effects are well documented in humans, but the β-cell-preserving effects and actions in other tissues are supported only by animal studies and, in the case of the heart, by limited human clinical studies

Drugs acting on the incretin system (entero-insular axis) (Fig. 6.2)

The incretin effect

Bayliss and Starling inferred the existence of gut-derived substances affecting carbohydrate metabolism more than a century ago, but the incretin effect was not described until 1969: the observation that for a given achieved level of plasma glucose, oral glucose produced a higher insulin concentration than intravenous glucose (Fig. 6.3). In the same year, the term 'entero-insular axis' was coined – the broader concept of all stimuli coming from the small intestine and influencing release of islet hormones. GIP (now named glucose-dependent insulinotropic hormone) was the first incretin to be sequenced in 1970, and the main therapeutic target in diabetes, GLP-1, in 1983.

The incretin system is critical in stimulating postprandial insulin secretion in response to nutrients entering the gut; about 50% of secretion is thought to be mediated by incretins and therefore is at least as important as glucose itself. In type 2 diabetes, the incretin effect is reduced, through a combination of GLP-1 deficiency and defective GLP-1 signalling, and

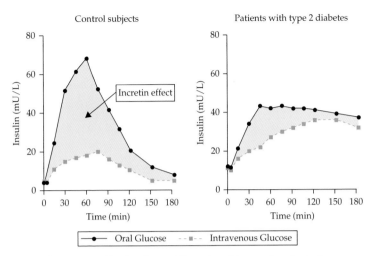

Fig. 6.3 The incretin effect is substantially reduced in type 2 patients. In non-diabetic subjects there is a markedly increased insulin response to oral compared with intravenous glucose (ensuring that the achieved blood glucose levels are the same). This is shown by the shaded area, which is reduced in type 2 subjects. Adapted from Nauck *et al. Diabetologia* 1986;29:46–52

possibly reduced islet responsiveness to GIP (Fig. 6.3). However, there is currently nothing to suggest that abnormalities of incretins themselves contribute to type 2 diabetes [14]. GIP itself does not appear to be deficient, does not lower glucose levels and may even augment postprandial glucose excursions. However, its therapeutic potential continues to be studied, particularly in obesity, for example, using GIP receptor antagonists.

GLP-1 is clearly deficient in type 2 diabetes. It is secreted from L cells situated mostly in the ileum and colon. In non-diabetic individuals, plasma GLP-1 levels increase within 10–15 min of starting to eat, and remain elevated for several hours, due to different populations of L cells being sequentially stimulated [15]. Native GLP-1, which has a circulating half-life of only 1–2 min, cannot be used clinically, though continuous intravenous infusions have been used to beneficial effect in pilot studies in myocardial infarction and heart failure, where GLP-1 may increase myocardial glucose uptake and be anti-apoptotic for cardiomyocytes.

The dominant effect of GLP-1 is therefore on postprandial glucose levels, and two additional mechanisms are important here: (i) decreasing postprandial glucagon secretion (an important factor in type 2 diabetes) and (ii) slowing gastric emptying. In addition, it decreases food intake and weight through a direct hypothalamic effect. Established and more speculative aspects of GLP-1 action are shown in Fig. 6.2.

Two strategies have been used pharmacologically to prolong the therapeutic effects of GLP-1:

- development of GLP-1 analogues/receptor agonists (incretin mimetics) that directly act at the β cell;
- development of drugs (incretin enhancers) that boost endogenous GLP-1 by inhibiting the enzyme DPP-4, which rapidly degrades GLP-1 in plasma.

GLP-1 analogues, like insulin analogues, are GLP-1 molecules modified in various ways, but primarily to resist degradation by DPP-4. Since these are all peptide molecules, they require subcutaneous injection. DPP-4 inhibitors, not themselves peptides, are orally active.

GLP-1 receptor agonists and GLP-1 analogues (*BNF*, section 6.1.2.3)

GLP-1 receptor agonist: exenatide (synthetic exendin-4)

This remarkable substance was discovered in a trawl for bioactive agents in reptiles. Exendin-4 occurs in the saliva and venom of the rare binge-eating gila lizard (*Heloderma suspectum*) and beaded lizard (*H. horridum*) of the southwestern USA, though its unclear role in reptile physiology is not the same as in mammals. In its modified synthetic form, exenatide, it was introduced therapeutically in the USA in 2005. Exenatide is detectable in plasma up to 10 hours after injection, and therefore requires twice-daily administration (Box 6.2). HbA$_{1c}$ reductions of about 1%, sustained up to 3 years, are reported, but in practice individual glycaemic changes are highly variable. Weight loss in trials is progressive and meaningful (about 2 kg at 6 months increasing to about 5 kg at 3 years), but like glycaemic improvement is highly variable in practice, and there is a weak relationship between weight loss and change in HbA$_{1c}$. Cases of good glycaemic results with virtually no weight change, and vice versa, are frequently seen (approximate rates of response: weight loss and glycaemic improvement, 72%; weight loss and glycaemic deterioration, 9%; glycaemic improvement and weight loss, 9%; glycaemic improvement and weight gain, 14%). In RCTs, HbA$_{1c}$ reaches a nadir at about 12 weeks, while weight loss continues for much longer. Consequently, in individual patients tolerating exenatide treatment, a clinical trial of about 4 months should be offered before discontinuation. However, this decision can be difficult; some patients report consistently decreased satiety, while objectively showing minor changes in both weight and glycaemic control. Minor improvements in blood pressure, lipids (especially HDL-cholesterol) and liver function tests have been seen, probably mostly due to weight loss.

Box 6.2 Practical aspects of exenatide treatment

- Licensed indications: with metformin, sulphonylurea or the combination. NICE 2009 limits it to triple therapy with metformin plus sulphonylurea if BMI (European patients) ⩾ 35 or BMI < 35 and insulin treatment is not acceptable because of occupation or if weight loss would be beneficial. In the USA exenatide is licensed as monotherapy with diet and exercise.
- Injections should be taken within 60 min of a meal; in practice, advise subcutaneous injection about 30 min before a meal (injection sites: abdomen, upper arm or thigh).
- Start at 5 μg b.d.; increase to 10 μg b.d. after a month (each 5- or 10-μg pen will last a month). If the twice-daily initial regimen is not tolerated, move to 5 μg with the main meal. Do not compensate for any missed doses.
- Review monthly for weight and adverse effects, and 2-monthly for HbA_{1c} and routine biochemistry.
- Renal impairment: safe where eGFR > 30 mL/min.
- Liver impairment: safe.
- Other medications: gastroresistant formulations (e.g. proton pump inhibitors), oral contraceptive and antibiotics should be taken an hour before or 4 hours after exenatide.
- A long-acting exenatide preparation (exenatide LAR) will soon be available; 2 mg weekly appears to have the same effect on blood glucose as the twice-daily preparation, with more weight loss and less nausea.

Adverse effects
- *Nausea,* usually described as 'mild to moderate' occurs in most patients (~60%) for a short time after each injection, over the first 8 weeks of treatment, declining thereafter. Weight loss with exenatide is independent of gastrointestinal side-effects. Vomiting is described in 17% of patients; rarely it is severe and recurrent, and very rarely it can destabilize diabetes control sufficiently to require admission. Advise patients to stop exenatide immediately if there is any vomiting. In trials, about 5% of patients discontinue treatment because of gastrointestinal side-effects. Avoid in patients with known gastroparesis, and use with great care in patients with advanced peripheral neuropathy (e.g. foot ulceration), where clinically inapparent gastroparesis may be uncovered.
- *Hypoglycaemia.* Increased in patients taking metformin/sulphonylurea or sulphonylurea; reduce sulphonylurea dose.
- *Acute pancreatitis.* About 40–50 cases have been reported so far. Although a rare complication, and a causal link has not been confirmed, patients with a past history of pancreatitis, or risk factors for it (e.g. severe hypertriglyceridaemia), should not have exenatide treatment.

Exenatide vs. insulin in triple therapy with metformin and sulphonylurea
In trials comparing exenatide and insulin (usually basal glargine) added
to metformin plus sulphonylurea, changes in glycaemia are similar,
though some studies have been criticized for not optimizing insulin doses.
Patients in very poor control on metformin plus sulphonylurea (HbA$_{1c}$
about 10%, 86 mmol/mol) have a better glycaemic response to even low-
dose biphasic insulin (12 units twice daily) than to twice-daily exenatide
10 μg over 6 months. A contentious study found that replacing insulin
treatment with exenatide prevented significant deterioration in glycaemic control, but this was also criticized for its 'futile' attempt to replace
an established treatment with a new one [16]. NICE (2009) strongly supports insulin treatment in patients failing on dual therapy, rather than
adding a third drug, 'unless there is strong justification not to'. However,
the benefits of GLP-1 treatment over insulin (weight loss, reduced clinic
time because of less intensive education and simple dosage titration, and
lower risk of hypoglycaemia) mean that outside the RCT setting, in the
overweight or obese patient failing on dual oral therapy, a trial of GLP-1
treatment with careful clinical supervision should often be considered,
with insulin a pre-discussed alternative if unsuccessful. Local practice
is likely to vary on this difficult question; expertise of the team, close
monitoring, and intensive support and education are probably as important as the specific pharmacological approach adopted.

Combined insulin and exenatide treatment
This unlicensed combination is in widespread use where additional oral
agents have failed, and glycaemic control and weight are deteriorating
despite large daily doses of insulin. Prospective studies are needed, but in a
retrospective 2-year study in patients taking a mean total daily insulin dose
of 100 units, adding exenatide reduced HbA$_{1c}$ by 0.5%. Prandial insulin
doses fell by more than 50%, although there was no change in basal insulin
doses. Nadir weight (6-kg loss) occurred at 18 months, climbing again in
the last 6 months [17]. Another option in this situation, addition of pioglitazone to insulin, gives similar glycaemic results but weight increases.

GLP-1 analogue: liraglutide
Liraglutide is a GLP-1 analogue with high homology to human GLP-1.
It gained a European licence in 2009, and was approved in the USA in
2010, but with a caution relating to a possible increased risk of medul-
lary thyroid cancer in non-human studies. The molecule is linked to a
fatty acid–albumin complex, similar to the long-acting insulin analogue
detemir, adding to its DPP-4 resistance and conferring 24-hour duration
of action (Box 6.3).

Box 6.3 Practical aspects of liraglutide treatment

- Current licensed combinations:
  - Dual therapy added to metformin or sulphonylurea.
  - Triple therapy added to metformin plus sulphonylurea or metformin plus pioglitazone.
- Once-daily administration, at approximately the same time each day, not necessarily in relation to meals.
- Injection sites and technique as for exenatide.
- Injection pen: marked for delivery of 0.6 mg (sufficient for 30 days), 1.2 mg (15 days) and 1.8 mg (10 days).
- Start at 0.6 mg daily for 1 week, increasing to 1.2 mg daily. Although the dose can be increased to 1.8 mg after another week, glycaemic and weight benefits of the 1.8-mg dose over the 1.2-mg dose are not clear, and it is not approved by NICE.
- Review: as for exenatide. Because peak levels of nausea are similar for both exenatide and liraglutide, be cautious in recommending a trial of liraglutide where there has been intolerance of exenatide leading to discontinuation. Nausea overall remits more rapidly with liraglutide than with exenatide.
- Renal impairment: use only when eGFR > 60 mL/min; do not use in hepatic impairment.
- There are no known significant drug interactions, and there is no 'no-go' period for drug administration around the time of injection.

There were multiple Phase III trials involving liraglutide (LEAD studies). In summary it is more effective than maximum-dose glimepiride (8 mg daily) in monotherapy, more effective than rosiglitazone 4 mg daily when added to glimepiride 2–4 mg daily, and improved HbA_{1c} by 1% (11 mmol/mol) when added to metformin 2 g daily and rosiglitazone 4 mg daily.

A 6-month head-to-head study comparing exenatide 10 μg twice daily with maximum-dose liraglutide 1.8 mg daily found slightly better glycaemic control with liraglutide (treatment difference 0.3% HbA_{1c}), but similar weight loss (~ 3 kg). Nausea with liraglutide occurred for a shorter time, 2–4% of patients reporting nausea by 16 weeks compared with 14% at onset of treatment. There was no difference in major hypoglycaemic events. The two agents are therefore similar in clinical practice, though the clinical impression is that liraglutide is somewhat better tolerated. Cases of acute pancreatitis have been linked to liraglutide use.

Other GLP-1 receptor agonists and analogues

Several agents are in various stages of development.

- Albiglutide, a GLP-1 dimer fused to human albumin, with a very long half-life suitable for weekly administration
- Lixisenatide, a modified exendin-4 molecule (daily)
- Taspoglutide (weekly; rare hypersensitivity reactions have been reported)
- Semaglutide (weekly)
- Nasally administered form of exenatide.

DPP-4 inhibitors (gliptins) (*BNF*, section 6.1.2.3)

These are once- or twice-daily orally active drugs which are weight neutral, with overall similar or slightly less powerful glycaemic effect compared with other medications for type 2 diabetes. Like the injectable GLP-1 analogues, they are glucose-sensitive and do not cause hypoglycaemia when used as monotherapy or with agents that themselves do not cause hypoglycaemia. Although it is assumed they act by increasing endogenous GLP-1 levels by inhibiting its breakdown, GLP-1 levels rise only modestly with DPP-4 treatment, and other mechanisms may be relevant, for example improved GLP-1 signalling and insulin processing, and effects on other neuropeptides.

RCTs have involved patients in good-to-fair glycaemic control (typically HbA_{1c} 7.5–8.0%, 59–64 mmol/mol) and show a fall in HbA_{1c} of 0.5–1.0% (5–9 mmol/mol). However, like all agents the glycaemic effect is proportional to baseline HbA_{1c} and a mean decrease of 2% has been demonstrated in people with poor initial control ($HbA_{1c} \sim 9\%$, 75 mmol/mol). They are generally well tolerated, with no specific side-effects, other than occasional mild nausea. Pancreatitis has been reported with sitagliptin, but there is no confirmed association.

Three agents, sitagliptin, vildagliptin and saxagliptin, are currently licensed in the UK, with several more in late-stage development. Sitagliptin has the broadest licensed indications.

- Monotherapy in the rare situation where metformin is not tolerated or contraindicated.
- Dual therapy with metformin, or a sulphonylurea, or pioglitazone.
- Triple oral therapy: sulphonylurea plus metformin even in moderate renal impairment (eGFR > 50 mL/min); pioglitazone plus metformin.
- Added to insulin with or without metformin: HbA_{1c} reduction 0.6% from baseline 8.6% (70 mmol/mol), even in long-duration diabetes.

Vildagliptin and saxagliptin are licensed for use only in dual therapy with metformin, a sulphonylurea or a glitazone. Vildagliptin and sitagliptin can be used in moderate renal impairment (eGFR > 50 mL/min). Vildagliptin has been rarely associated with liver dysfunction, and baseline alanine aminotransferase should be less than three times the upper limit of normal; 3-monthly liver function tests are suggested during the first year of treatment, annually thereafter.

The dosages of these agents are as follows.

- Sitagliptin: 100 mg daily as monotherapy; in fixed-dose combination with metformin (1000 mg), 50 mg twice daily.
- Vildagliptin: 50 mg b.d. (fixed-dose combinations with metformin 850 mg and 1 g are available).
- Saxagliptin: 5 mg daily.

The practical use of these agents within license, apart from sitagliptin, is currently limited, but the low risk of hypoglycaemia (except when combined with insulin) makes them attractive alternative second-line agents either when a sulphonylurea has caused hypoglycaemia or in others at high risk of hypoglycaemia, for example the elderly. Although well tolerated, they are expensive and need frequent review for efficacy.

Pramlintide

Pramlintide is synthetic amylin, a β-cell hormone co-secreted with insulin. It is therefore relatively lacking in type 2 diabetes, and absent in type 1. Since it is derived from the pancreas and not the gut, it is not a true incretin, and has no significant direct pancreatic effects. For such an abundant hormone, little is known of amylin's true physiological functions, but pramlintide has been licensed in the USA for use in type 1 and insulin-treated type 2 diabetes. Like the GLP-1 analogues, it slows gastric emptying, suppresses postprandial glucagon and glucose levels and increases satiety, but has no effects on peripheral insulin action. In intensively treated type 1 patients, pramlintide 15–60 μg s.c. with meals reduces weight by about 2 kg and HbA_{1c} by about 0.5%. Hypoglycaemia, sometimes severe, can be avoided by reducing prandial insulin doses by 30–50%. In type 2 diabetes, it is as effective in reducing HbA_{1c} as titrated prandial rapid-acting insulin, and is weight neutral. Nausea is a frequent side-effect. Pramlintide is unlikely to be introduced in Europe.

Combination non-insulin treatment

Many bodies have issued guidelines and consensus documents on combination treatment in type 2 diabetes, but there is surprisingly little common ground among them, other than the initial steps of lifestyle intervention and metformin. The ADA/EASD consensus (2009) makes a valuable distinction between 'well-validated core therapies' and 'less well-validated therapies' (but unlike the NICE guidelines does not include many licensed combinations in this latter group). The number of combinations might therefore be considered conservative, DPP-4 inhibitors are not included, and exenatide appears in only one combination

Well-validated core therapies (all pharmacological treatments are combined with intensive lifestyle intervention)
- Metformin
- Metformin plus basal insulin
- Metformin plus sulphonylurea
- Metformin plus intensive insulin.

Less well-validated therapies
- Metformin plus pioglitazone
- Metformin plus exenatide (insufficient evidence for safety)
- Metformin plus sulphonylurea plus pioglitazone.

Insulin treatment in type 2 diabetes

Insulin has always been a mainstay of treatment for type 2 diabetes. Indeed, until the 1950s, it was the only treatment available and, until the mid-1990s, the only combination treatment available in the USA was insulin with a sulphonylurea. In these simple historical facts lie the problems of objectively assessing insulin treatment in type 2 diabetes, which naturally has not been subjected to the same comparative large-scale RCTs as more recently introduced agents (Box 6.4). The first comparison of insulin treatment against other therapies (other than the fraught University Group Diabetes Program in the early 1960s) was UKPDS, but this aspect of the trial was somewhat overlooked in comparison with the novel intensive versus conventional treatment strategy and its effect on complications. However, UKPDS indicated that insulin treatment:
- was not more effective in glycaemic control than intensive treatment with sulphonylureas or metformin;

Box 6.4 Unresolved questions concerning insulin treatment in type 2 diabetes

- Is it best used early or late in the natural history of the condition?
- Is it more effective than other agents?
- Does it confer vascular or other advantages compared with other agents?
- What is its long-term efficacy?
- How can we predict response and duration of response to insulin treatment?
- If used intensively and in sufficient doses, can good glycaemic control always be established?

- did not confer microvascular or macrovascular advantages over sulphonylureas (there was anxiety at the time that hyperinsulinaemia with insulin treatment might accelerate atheroma);
- carried a consistently higher risk of any and major hypoglycaemia than intensive sulphonylurea treatment (see www.dtu.ox.ac/ukpds for more information).

Since then, countless large-scale RCTs have compared different insulin regimens for short- and medium-term glycaemic control. Many have explored insulin as an early intervention in type 2 diabetes, concluded that it is effective, safe and associated with no detrimental effects on quality-of-life measures, and in many instances seem to have improved it, and have increasingly recommended it in clinical practice. Most RCT protocols require frequent and intensive patient contact and education with algorithmically driven titration regimens and treat-to-target objectives; the result can be long-term glycaemic stability, in contrast with, for example, the near-continual upward glycaemic drift seen in all treatment arms of the UKPDS, which probably more closely resembles what happens in real life.

Mandatory insulin in type 2 diabetes

While much of the discussion and all the trials of insulin treatment in type 2 diabetes relate to overweight or obese subjects failing on routine combined oral hypoglycaemic agents, the relatively small proportion, but large absolute number, of patients with late-onset type 1 diabetes must be recognized (see Chapter 1). While insulin deficiency is rarely complete, and ketonuria therefore uncommon, the persistent presence of urinary ketones should be a warning that insulin treatment may be needed; occasionally patients will be ketonuric during an intercurrent illness that uncovers insulin deficiency. Remember to be alert to the need at some stage, sometimes urgent, for insulin treatment in:

- normal-weight or thin patients, and those with progressive weight loss and persistently poor control on non-insulin agents;
- GAD antibody-positive people;
- those with a personal or first-degree family history of other autoimmune disorders;
- subjects who respond poorly to oral hypoglycaemic agents, especially sulphonylureas;
- the uncommon patient with proximal femoral neuropathy (neuropathic cachexia; see Chapter 10).

Insulin regimens in these patients should be the same as those in type 1 diabetes with the same intensity and targets. Discontinue sulphonylureas; metformin may still be of value in normal-weight patients. The remaining discussion relates to the much more contentious question of insulin treatment in overweight or obese patients.

Glycaemic effects and limitations of insulin treatment

'The potential for glucose lowering with insulin is unlimited' [18]. Statements like this are common, and continue to be made even after the recent trials implicating hypoglycaemia as a serious adverse prognostic factor, and suggesting that HbA_{1c} levels below 7.0% do not meaningfully improve the vascular prognosis in many patients. Nevertheless, it is still widely believed that insulin is a more potent and more effective treatment than other agents.

However, there is little contemporary evidence to support this notion, when insulin (usually with metformin) is compared with combination treatment. In a 6-month trial comparing twice-daily biphasic insulin and metformin with triple oral therapy (glitazone, sulphonylurea and metformin), both reduced HbA_{1c} eventually by 2.1% (9.7% to 7.6%, 83 to 60 mmol/L), though the initial fall was quicker with insulin. This phenomenon is of no long-term importance, but the very rapid fall in glucose levels often seen in the early stages of insulin treatment may be one factor contributing to an impression that insulin treatment is more effective (compare sulphonylurea treatment in newly diagnosed symptomatic patients).

Only in very few studies, whatever the design, are HbA_{1c} levels below 7.0% (53 mmol/mol) consistently achieved, never mind near-normoglycaemia.

- In the ATLANTUS study (2005), HbA_{1c} fell from 8.9 to 7.8% (74 to 62 mmol/mol) over 6 months with basal glargine at a mean dose of 43 units [19].
- More intensive treatment in the 3-year 4-T Study (2009) resulted in a fall in HbA_{1c} of about 1.5%, from a baseline of 8.5% to about 7.0% (69 to 53 mmol/mol), with well-maintained stable control (see below).
- Basal glargine at a lower mean dose (24 units) and liraglutide 1.8 mg daily both reduced HbA_{1c} by about 1.1–1.3% (11–15 mmol/mol) to 7.0–7.2% (53–55 mol/mol; slightly lower with liraglutide); hypoglycaemia rates were similar, but there was a 3.4-kg weight difference between the two groups [20].

Of the recent major outcome studies, only BARI 2D can guide long-term practice, though only in the broadest sense, and patients were in fairly good baseline control (mean HbA_{1c} 7.7%, 61 mmol/mol). After 3 years, the insulin provision group (insulin and sulphonylureas) had significantly higher HbA_{1c} (mean 7.5%, 59 mmol/mol) than those treated with the insulin-sensitizing regimen of metformin and rosiglitazone (7.0%, 53 mmol/mol) and had more severe hypoglycaemia (9% vs. 6%). From this admittedly non-random selection of studies, it is difficult to conclude that insulin treatment, however intensive, gives consistently better glycaemic control than judiciously chosen regimens using other agents (Box 6.5).

Box 6.5 Summary of insulin treatment in overweight/obese type 2 patients failing on dual oral therapy

- In clinical trials, regardless of the initial degree of glycaemic control, insulin used in usual doses and regimens seems to have similar glycaemic benefits as combination treatments with non-insulin agents.
- The unlimited capacity of insulin (with metformin) to improve glycaemic control is not often seen in clinical practice, and even in treat-to-target RCTs final HbA_{1c} values are typically 7.0–7.5% (53–59 mmol/mol).
- Insulin doses genuinely do not seem to be pushed as high as they might, both in trials and in clinical practice, but whatever the reasons (there are likely to be several), it is such a consistent finding even in algorithmically driven RCT protocols that it should be regarded as a true limitation of insulin treatment.
- Increased hypoglycaemia rates and weight gain (e.g. 3–6 kg, see below) are consistent problems.

Early versus late treatment with insulin

Insulin improves glycaemia at any stage of type 2 diabetes. The rationale behind its early use is that it preserves β-cell function better than other agents, but there are no long-term data to support this. It is simpler to achieve good glycaemia in the early stages of diabetes with insulin, but this goes for other treatments; in the LANCET study, insulin and metformin were equally successful in reducing HbA_{1c} from 6.9 to 6.1% (52 to 43 mmol/mol) [21]. The rationale for using it later is that it is the logical agent in patients with depleted β-cell function, though if this were the only mechanism operating it should be simple to achieve the kind of glycaemia we target in type 1 diabetes. Some studies show improved quality of life with insulin therapy (usually together with metformin) compared with multiple non-insulin agents, but outside the clinical trial setting, individualization of treatment, often involving changes of therapy where necessary, is the best option. Insulin does not improve microvascular or macrovascular outcomes compared with other regimens of approximately similar glycaemic effectiveness, whether used early (e.g. UKPDS) or late (e.g. VADT, BARI 2D). Cardiovascular risk factors, including inflammatory markers (e.g. high-sensitivity CRP), do not significantly improve with insulin (LANCET study), in contrast to some studies with metformin treatment (or, as in the Diabetes Prevention Program, intensive lifestyle intervention).

Practical insulin regimens

While there is still controversy surrounding the indications for insulin treatment in patients with type 2 diabetes, earlier studies progressively

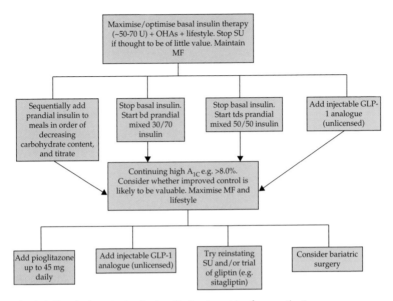

Fig. 6.4 Practical strategies for insulin treatment in obese patients

supported the use of basal insulin with continuing oral hypoglycaemics as the most effective initial insulin regimen. The most recent study is the long-term follow-up of the 4-T, in typical overweight patients (e.g. BMI 30, weight 85 kg) failing on dual sulphonylurea and metformin treatment (mean HbA$_{1c}$ 8.5%, 69 mmol/mol) after 10 years of diagnosed diabetes [22]. The trial randomized patients to twice-daily biphasic insulin, basal bedtime insulin or prandial rapid-acting insulin three times daily with meals, targeting HbA$_{1c}$ 6.5% (48 mmol/mol) or less (unfortunately a full MDI regimen was not included at the start, but many starting with basal insulin progressed to MDI; see below). Metformin was continued, but the sulphonylurea discontinued if HbA$_{1c}$ was consistently 8% or more within the first year, or above 6.5% after the first year, and replaced with:

- lunchtime prandial insulin 4–6 units in patients taking twice-daily biphasic insulin;
- mealtime insulin (×3) 4–6 units in those taking basal insulin;
- basal insulin 10 units was added in those taking prandial insulin.

Basal insulin treatment carried the lowest risk of hypoglycaemia and the least weight gain. This study confirms others (e.g. the APOLLO study [23]) that basal insulin with oral hypoglycaemic agents is an effective and simple starting insulin regimen (Fig. 6.4; Boxes 6.6 and 6.7), though in a shorter 6-month study (INITIATE, 2007) biphasic aspart 30/70 was more effective than basal glargine.

Box 6.6 Starting and managing insulin treatment

- Maintain metformin (maximize to 2 g daily where tolerated) and sulpho-nylurea (reduce to maximum effective dose). Maintain other agents where they have previously shown benefit.
- Start basal (bedtime) insulin at a fixed dose (e.g. 10 units) or at the same dose as a mean fasting glucose level (in mmol/L), usually 10–16 units. Final HbA_{1c} is the same using basal analogue or human isophane insulin, though nocturnal hypoglycaemia is lower with analogue preparations.
- Titrate insulin, either at a fixed rate (e.g. 2 units/week) or a percentage (e.g. 10% of existing dose). Two principles are well established: self-titration is more effective than directed titration, and the number of contacts with the clinical team (this is from RCT data) strongly relates to the improvement in HbA_{1c} [24].
- Target fasting glucose about 5.5–6.0 mmol/L (100–110 mg/dL) but individualize targets according to the clinical situation, especially when there is cardiovascular disease.
- Telephone contact is probably more beneficial than clinical visits, possibly because of the tighter focus of telephone contacts on dose adjustment and glycaemic control.

Box 6.7 Managing expectations in basal insulin treatment

- Though insulin treatment in some form is likely to be for the long term, this is still type 2 diabetes, and patients are insulin-requiring not insulin-dependent.
- Maintaining lifestyle efforts will maximize benefit; there should be access to specialist dietitians, especially if prandial insulin is needed.
- Although the starting dose is low, repeatedly remind patients that the final daily insulin dose will be much higher, approximately 0.8–1.0 units/kg, i.e. 70–100 units/day; doses will increase for at least the first 3 years, though most of the increase will occur in the first year. To achieve the same HbA_{1c}, the total daily dose of twice-daily detemir is much higher than once-daily glargine (e.g. 77 vs. 44 units).
- These doses should reduce HbA_{1c} by about 1.5% (17 mmol/mol), but post-prandial hyperglycaemia will probably persist.
- Weight will increase by about 4 kg over 3 years, perhaps up to 6 kg over 6 years (UKPDS); in RCTs levemir has weight advantages over NPH and glargine.

Beyond basal insulin: complex regimens

Even when basal insulin treatment has been maximized to achieve good fasting levels, HbA_{1c} remains very poor (e.g. >9%, 75 mmol/mol) in a substantial proportion. Most patients (80% in 4-T) required additional insulin, effectively converting them to MDI, 60% of the total insulin dose being prandial. In general, the more intensive the insulin regimen, the greater the weight gain and risk of significant hypoglycaemia.

Over 6 months, HbA_{1c} fell by about 2% (22 mmol/mol) from 8.9% (74 mmol/mol) using either three times daily prandial insulin added to the basal glargine or conversion to three times daily prandial 50/50 biphasic insulin; in practice, dose titration might not be rigorous enough to achieve this, and an already obese American study population gained a further 4 kg [25]. Several possible strategies are therefore valuable after establishing an optimum basal insulin regimen with oral hypoglycaemic agents (Fig. 6.4). No standard regimen can be stipulated, but consider the following, and individualize the approach.

- Sequentially add prandial insulin to one meal at a time, starting with the most carbohydrate-rich meal, and thereafter to the other main meals. Some patients may not eat breakfast, and long-acting analogue bedtime insulin may maintain satisfactory control until lunch, thereby limiting the number of prandial insulin injections.
- Move to twice-daily prandial biphasic insulin (e.g. Humulin M3, NovoMix 30, Insuman Comb 25); in some short-term studies, this is more effective than basal insulin.
- Move to three times daily prandial biphasic insulin (e.g. Humalog Mix 50), changing the dinner-time dose to a lower mix (e.g. Humalog Mix 25) if more intermediate-acting insulin is needed to achieve good fasting levels. This regimen is as effective as a full basal-bolus regimen.
- Add twice-daily exenatide (unlicensed and no RCTs reported).

However, the durability of these regimens is not assured, and results of long-term outcome studies are badly needed, for example the 2-year DURABLE study.

Beyond complex regimens: the patient poorly controlled on multiple daily insulin doses plus oral hypoglycaemic agents

Regrettably there are no RCTs to help guide practice in this common, difficult and distressing clinical problem, the frequency of which could appear to the sceptical as undermining the concept of the limitless impact of insulin. The syndrome is characterized by:

- glycaemic control that has not improved with insulin, or improved transiently but returned to pre-insulin treatment levels or worse;
- high total daily insulin doses, often greater than 1 unit/kg body weight or more than 100 units;

- increasing weight, with associated worsening insulin resistance features (rising blood pressure, deteriorating lipid profile).

There are no simple explanations or easy solutions, but consider the following (Fig. 6.4).

1 Taking into account the results of the recent glycaemia trials, the duration of diabetes and complications, would focusing on more achievable, non-glycaemic targets be a better use of time and resources?

2 Modifying oral agents, for example:
   (a) Add metformin up to 1 g b.d., though most patients will already be taking it. The results are variable and not as striking in practice as in clinical trials.
   (b) Give a trial of modified-release metformin in patients previously intolerant of immediate-release metformin.
   (c) Some patients may respond to reinstating a discontinued sulphonylurea.
   (d) Add sitagliptin 100 mg daily (licensed) or vildagliptin 50 mg b.d. (unlicensed), which may modestly lower HbA_{1c} (0.5–0.7%, 6–8 mmol/mol) over 6 months when given to patients poorly controlled on high doses of insulin.
   (e) Add pioglitazone 15 mg daily, increasing very gradually up to 45 mg if beneficial and tolerated.

3 Add exenatide or liraglutide (unlicensed).

4 Bariatric surgery in the obese or very obese patient on multiple ineffective medications with or without late complications.

Bariatric surgery

Bariatric surgery (Greek *baros* meaning 'weight') is the term used for all surgical procedures to reduce weight. Restrictive procedures (e.g. laparoscopic adjustable gastric banding) markedly reduce stomach volume and decrease food intake. The most commonly used and most effective routine bariatric procedure, the Roux-en-Y gastric bypass (Fig. 6.5), reduces stomach volume and causes some degree of malabsorption. Roux-en-Y bypass causes greater weight loss than restrictive procedures (around 60% of excess weight, 10–15 BMI units, or 30–50 kg). Following any procedure there is some rebound weight gain over the years, but this is minor in relation to the overall weight loss. Diabetes resolves (i.e. normoglycaemia with no requirement for diabetes medication) in about 80% after Roux-en-Y bypass, dyslipidaemia improves in nearly all patients (though hypercholesterolaemia itself may not improve), and hypertension in about three-quarters. Non-alcoholic fatty liver disease and sleep apnoea often dramatically improve. The diabetes is more likely to resolve in patients on tablets, as opposed to insulin, and those with a shorter duration of diabetes. Diabetes resolves within days of bypass procedures,

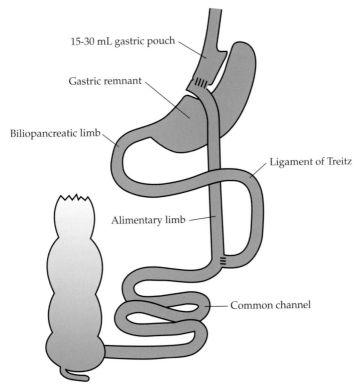

Fig. 6.5 Roux-en-Y gastric bypass, the commonest and most effective standard bariatric procedure

well before weight loss occurs, but takes months to occur after restrictive surgery. GLP-1 levels substantially increase, and remain elevated for years after bypass, but other hormones influencing satiety and appetite (e.g. PYY) are probably involved. Alternatively, bypass of the proximal gut may exclude as yet unknown 'anti-incretin' or 'decretin' hormones.

Roux-en-Y bypass is usually performed laparoscopically, is safe (operative mortality about 0.5%), and NICE suggests considering it in diabetic patients with a BMI of 35–40. Careful postoperative management is important (Box 6.8). Ten years after surgery, the Swedish Obesity Study reported a 30% reduction in mortality, with substantial reductions in myocardial infarction and cancers [26], but as yet there are no systematic studies on microvascular complications. It would be surprising if there were no effects, even if the impact of near-normoglycaemia might not be as dramatic as on resolution of hypertension and its associated features (e.g. sleep apnoea, microalbuminuria). Surgical techniques are continually being refined; for example, laparoscopic sleeve (subtotal) gastrectomy, which leaves a small

---

Box 6.8 Practical aspects of diabetes management after bariatric surgery

- Actively reduce diabetes medication during any preoperative weight loss programme.
- High risk of hypoglycaemia: stop oral hypoglycaemic agents immediately before surgery, and anticipate dramatic and rapid reductions in prandial insulin requirements after surgery.
- Rapid-acting analogues rather than soluble insulin are recommended once the patient is eating again.
- After surgery avoid agents with gastrointestinal effects or side-effects (metformin, α-glucosidase inhibitors, GLP-1 analogues); use insulinotropic agents (sulphonylureas, meglitinides, DPP-4 inhibitors) with care.
- Long-term vitamin and mineral supplementation is required in bypass patients (multivitamins, iron, calcium and vitamin D, vitamin B_{12}).
- Retinopathy can markedly deteriorate if HbA1C falls rapidly in the previously poorly-controlled patient. Ensure ophthalmological follow-up within two months (see Chapter 9).

Source: after Vetter *et al.* [27]

---

tubular gastric remnant, is a relatively new restrictive procedure (with removal of the appetite-regulating ghrelin produced in the gastric fundus being a possible endocrine mechanism for weight loss). Although its place in the bariatric repertoire is not yet clear, it can be used as a single procedure in the moderately obese or as a bridging procedure in the high-risk severely obese patient, converting it later, after initial weight loss, to a Roux-en-Y bypass or a biliopancreatic diversion with duodenal switch.

New developments

While many new drugs are in early development, probably only one novel group of agents will be introduced over the next few years, the type 2 sodium glucose cotransporter (SGLT2) inhibitors. Inhibition of glucose reabsorption in the proximal renal tubules by the prototype clinical compound dapagliflozin is insulin independent and causes mild glycosuria and diuresis without hypoglycaemia. In short-term studies, HbA_{1c} reduction is moderate, up to 0.9% (10 mmol/mol), dose-dependent (2.5, 5 and 10 mg daily), and associated with weight loss up to 4 kg. Dapagliflozin is effective in poorly controlled patients taking combination insulin and oral hypoglycaemic treatments. Similar results are seen in monotherapy, and patients in very poor control (HbA1c >9%, 75 mmol/mol) already with glycosuria had HbA1C reductions of nearly 2% (22 mmol/mol).

Genital infections are more common with high-dose treatment (20 mg vs. 10 mg). Several other SGLT2 inhibitors, for example sergliflozin, are in late-stage development. High-ratio biphasic insulins (e.g. containing up to 70% rapid-acting analogue) may be introduced and have a place in intensified insulin regimens, though long-term benefits may be limited. Insulin degludec, a very long-acting soluble insulin basal analogue, may be of value. Further down the line are G protein-coupled receptor 119 (GPR119) agonists, which seem to have a dual action on intestinal L cells to promote GLP-1 secretion and on the β-cell. Experimentally, combination with DPP-4 inhibitor treatment increases their therapeutic effect.

References

1. Tattersall R. *Diabetes: The Biography*, pp. 131–5. Oxford: Oxford University Press, 2009. Robert Tattersall brilliantly summarizes this most contentious of diabetes studies.
2. Wu RR, Zhao JP, Jin H *et al.* Lifestyle intervention and metformin for treatment of antipsychotic-induced weight gain: a randomized controlled trial. *JAMA* 2008;299:185–93. PMID: 18182600.
3. Kooy A, de Jager J, Lehert P *et al.* Long-term effects of metformin on metabolism and microvascular and macrovascular disease in patients with type 2 diabetes mellitus. *Arch Intern Med* 2009;169:616–25. PMID: 19307526.
4. Salpeter S, Greyber E, Pasternak G, Salpeter E. Risk of fatal and nonfatal lactic acidosis with metformin use in type 2 diabetes mellitus. *Cochrane Database Syst Rev* 2006;(1):CD002967. PMID: 16437448.
5. de Jager J, Kooy A, Lehert P *et al.* Long term treatment with metformin in patients with type 2 diabetes and risk of vitamin B-12 deficiency: randomised placebo controlled trial. *Br Med J* 2010;340:c2181. PMID: 20488910.
6. Brown JB, Conner C, Nichols GA. Secondary failure of metformin monotherapy in clinical practice. *Diabetes Care* 2010;33:501–6. PMID: 20040656.
7. Esposito K, Giugliano D, Nappo F, Marfella R. Regression of carotid atherosclerosis by control of postprandial hyperglycemia in type 2 diabetes mellitus. Campanian Postprandial Hyperglycemia Study Group. *Circulation* 2004;110:214–19. PMID: 15197140.
8. Fasano CJ, O'Malley G, Dominici P, Aguilera E, Latta DR. Comparison of octreotide and standard therapy versus standard therapy alone for the treatment of sulfonylurea-induced hypoglycemia. *Ann Emerg Med* 2008;51:400–6. PMID: 17764782.
9. Charbonnel B, Defronzo R, Davidson R *et al.* Pioglitazone use in combination with insulin in the prospective pioglitazone clinical trial in macrovascular events study (PROactive 19). *J Clin Endocrinol Metab* 2010;95:2163–71. PMID: 20237169.
10. Sanyal AJ, Chalasani N, Kowdley KV *et al.* Pioglitazone, vitamin E, or placebo for non-alcoholic steatohepatitis. *N Engl J Med* 2010;362:1675–85. PMID: 20427778.
11. Ambrosius WT, Danis RP, Goff DV Jr *et al.* Lack of association between thiazolidinediones and macular edema in type 2 diabetes: the ACCORD eye substudy. *Arch Ophthalmol* 2010;128:312–18. PMID: 20212201.

12. Zinman B, Hoogwerf BJ, Durán Garcia S *et al.* The effect of adding exenatide to a thiazolidinedione in suboptimally controlled type 2 diabetes: a randomized trial. *Ann Intern Med* 2007;146:477–85. PMID: 17404349.

13. Pan C, Yang W, Barona JP *et al.* Comparison of vildagliptin and acarbose monotherapy in patients with Type 2 diabetes: a 24-week, double-blind, randomized trial. *Diabetic Med* 2008;25:435–41. PMID: 18341596.

14. Meier JJ. The contribution of incretin hormones to the pathogenesis of type 2 diabetes. *Best Pract Res Clin Endocrinol Metab* 2009;23:433–41. PMID: 19748061.

15. Gribble FM. RD Lawrence Lecture 2008: Targeting GLP-1 release as a potential strategy for the therapy of Type 2 diabetes. *Diabetic Med* 2008;25:889–94. PMID:18959599.

16. Rosenstock J, Fonseca V. Missing the point: substituting exenatide for non-optimized insulin: going from bad to worse! *Diabetes Care* 2007;30:2972–3. Comment on *Diabetes Care* 2007;30:2767–72. PMID: 17965313.

17. Yoon NM, Cavaghan MK, Brunelle RL, Roach P. Exenatide added to insulin therapy: a retrospective review of clinical practice over two years in an academic endocrinology outpatient setting. *Clin Ther* 2009;31:1511–23. PMID: 19695400.

18. Leahy JL. What is the role for insulin therapy in type 2 diabetes? *Curr Opin Endocrinol Diabetes* 2003;10:99–103.

19. Davies M, Storms F, Shutler S, Bianchi-Biscay M, Gomis R. Improvement of glycemic control in subjects with poorly controlled type 2 diabetes: comparison of two treatment algorithms using insulin glargine. ATLANTUS Study Group. *Diabetes Care* 2005;28:1282–8. PMID: 15920040.

20. Russell-Jones D, Vaag A, Schmitz O *et al.* Liraglutide vs insulin glargine and placebo in combination with metformin and sulfonylurea therapy in type 2 diabetes mellitus (LEAD-5 met+SU): a randomised controlled trial. *Diabetologia* 2009;52:2046–55. PMID: 19688338.

21. Pradhan AD, Everett BM, Cook NR, Rifai N, Ridker PM. Effects of initiating insulin and metformin on glycemic control and inflammatory biomarkers among patients with type 2 diabetes; the LANCET randomized trial. *JAMA* 2009;302:1186–94. PMID: 19755697.

22. Holman RR, Farmer AJ, Davies MJ *et al.* for the 4-T Study Group. Three-year efficacy of complex insulin regimens in type 2 diabetes. *N Engl J Med* 2009;361:1736–47. PMID: 19850703.

23. Bretzel RG, Nuber U, Landgraf W, Owens DR, Bradley C, Linn T. Once-daily basal insulin glargine versus thrice-daily prandial insulin lispro in people with type 2 diabetes on oral hypoglycaemic agents (APOLLO): an open randomised controlled trial. *Lancet* 2008;371:1073–84. PMID: 18374840.

24. Swinnen SG, DeVries JH. Contact frequency determines outcome of basal insulin initiation trials in type 2 diabetes. *Diabetologia.* 2009;52:2324–7. PMID: 19756479.

25. Rosenstock J, Ahmann AJ, Colon G, Scism-Bacon J, Jiang H, Martin S. Advancing insulin therapy in type 2 diabetes previously treated with glargine plus oral agents: prandial premixed (insulin lispro protamine suspension/lispro) versus basal/bolus (glargine/lispro) therapy. *Diabetes Care* 2008;31:20–5. PMID: 17934150.

26. Sjöström L, Narbro K, Sjöström CD *et al.* Effects of bariatric surgery on mortality on Swedish obese subjects. *N Engl J Med* 2007;357:741–52. PMID: 17715408.

27. Vetter ML, Cardillo S, Rickets MR, Iqbal N. Narrative review: effect of bariatric surgery on type 2 diabetes mellitus. *Ann Intern Med* 2009;150:94–103. PMID: 19153412.

Further reading

Kaul S, Bolger AF, Herrington D, Giugliano RP, Eckel RH. Thiazolidinedione drugs and cardiovascular risks: a science advisory from the American Heart Association and American College of Cardiology Foundation. *J Am Coll Cardiol* 2010;55:1885–94. PMID: 20413044.

Krentz AJ, Bailey CJ. *Type 2 Diabetes in Practice*, 2nd edn. London: Royal Society of Medicine Press, 2005.

Nathan DM, Buse JB, Davidson MB *et al*. Medical management of hyperglycemia in type 2 diabetes: a consensus algorithm for the initiation and adjustment of therapy. A consensus statement of the American Diabetes Association and the European Association for the Study of Diabetes. *Diabetes Care* 2009;32:193–203. PMID: 18945920.

National Institute for Health and Clinical Excellence. Type 2 diabetes: newer agents (partial update of CG66), CG87, May 2009. Available at www.nice.org.uk/CG87shortguideline

National Institute for Health and Clinical Excellence. Obesity, CG43, December 2006 (expected review November 2011). Available at www.nice.org.uk

Websites

Electronic Medicines Compendium (eMC). Searchable site for summaries of product characteristics (SPCs) of all drugs available in the UK. Available at www.emc.medicines.org.uk

Infections in diabetes

CHAPTER 7

Key points

- Consider infection in any sick diabetic patient.
- Clinical and laboratory features of serious infection in diabetes are often undramatic, in part because of the impaired inflammatory responses that occur especially in patients with advanced neuropathy.
- Postoperative infections are frequent and are associated with increased morbidity and mortality, particularly in poorly controlled patients.
- Simple urinary tract and skin infections may become complicated and dangerous (e.g. renal abscess, emphysematous pyelonephritis and necrotizing fasciitis).
- Admit to hospital when there is doubt, do not undertreat, and give antimicrobial treatment for longer than you would in a non-diabetic person.
- Work closely with radiologists, microbiologists and surgeons.

Introduction

Infections in patients with diabetes are a persistent trap for both the inexperienced and world-wise physician. Whenever someone with diabetes presents unwell, always consider the possibility of infection. High blood glucose levels predispose to some acute infections, especially postoperatively, but other mechanisms are involved, for example the effects of long-standing hyperglycaemia on small and large blood vessels and on the nervous and immune systems. However, among common infections,

Practical Diabetes Care, 3rd edition. © David Levy.
Published 2011 by Blackwell Publishing Ltd.

only candidal and staphylococcal infections of the skin and mucosae seem to be 'specific' to poorly controlled diabetes.

There are countless case reports of unusual infections in diabetes, but few well-controlled prospective studies or RCTs. While there is a reasonable evidence base for treatment of diabetic foot infections, infections elsewhere remain a real diagnostic and treatment challenge.

Diabetes and the chronic low-grade infection of periodontal disease are linked in both directions: diabetes has an adverse effect on periodontal health, and periodontal disease seems to be associated with poor glycaemic control and diabetes complications, especially macrovascular disease. Demonstrating the latter link and establishing improved glucose control and a lower risk of complications with improved dental hygiene is difficult.

Types of infections

- Common infections are also common in diabetes, though it is still controversial whether chest and urinary tract infections are in fact more common in people with well-controlled diabetes compared with non-diabetic individuals.
- Common infections occurring in unusual sites, especially staphylococcal infections (see below).
- Unusual infections occurring in unusual sites: some serious but rare infections seem mostly to occur in people with diabetes (e.g. rhinocerebral mucormycosis, 'malignant' otitis externa and Fournier's gangrene); the whole urinary tract and the limbs are susceptible to invasive gas-forming organisms. Pyrexia of unknown origin in someone with diabetes is a real challenge. Fortunately, new imaging techniques, especially fluorodeoxyglucose positron emission tomography (FDG-PET) and PET/computed tomography (CT), will be of great diagnostic help in these cases (though hyperglycaemia requires correction for efficient PET scanning results).

Methicillin-resistant *Staphylococcus aureus* and *Clostridium difficile* infections

These two organisms are responsible for serious, usually hospital-acquired, infections. MRSA is present in about 30–40% of diabetic foot ulcers in the UK, higher than the reported prevalence in South Asia (10%) but lower than that in other European countries, for example Greece (80%) [1]. Nasal MRSA carriage predisposes to foot infections, and community-acquired MRSA infections in patients not previously treated with antibiotics is probably increasing. The role of MRSA in ulcers that are not clinically infected is not known, but in animal studies the organism itself has increased procoagulant and proinflammatory properties compared with sensitive MRSA, and these characteristics are compatible with the clinical course of serious MRSA infections.

Diabetes itself does not seem to be associated with an increased risk of either antibiotic-associated diarrhoea or *C. difficile* infections, but foot ulcer patients are more likely to be treated for prolonged periods with antibiotics associated with *C. difficile* infections (cephalosporins, quinolones and clindamycin).

The high incidence of these infections has led to more restrictive hospital antibiotic guidelines for acute infections. In general, penicillins, vancomycin and gentamicin are emphasized over the broader-spectrum quinolones and cephalosporins. Clindamycin, while being associated with a higher risk of *C. difficile*, is nevertheless a narrow-spectrum antibiotic and on balance its use is encouraged. Follow local hospital policies for inpatient treatment, but wherever care is given to these threatened patients, antibiotic therapy must always be appropriate for the severity of the infection; in particular bear in mind the high risk of limb loss in severe diabetic foot infections.

Chest infections

Advanced autonomic neuropathy may impair the perception of pleuritic pain. Most surveys do not indicate a higher mortality for people with diabetes from general community-acquired pneumonias, but these studies may conceal a worse out-of-hospital mortality rate. Specifically, pneumococcal and influenzal infections are not more common (though bacteraemic pneumococcal infection may be), but carry a greater morbidity and mortality, highlighting the need for widespread immunization in diabetic patients. Infections with some organisms are more common in diabetes, for example:

- *Staphylococcus aureus*;
- *Mycobacterium tuberculosis* (increasingly recognized link between both type 1 and type 2 diabetes and tuberculosis in high-prevalence areas, but even in developed countries diabetes seems to carry a greater risk of treatment resistance and death);
- Gram-negative organisms, especially *Klebsiella pneumoniae*, particularly associated with empyema.

Infections after surgery

Coronary bypass surgery
Because this is a common and standard procedure, much of the epidemiological work on postoperative infections has been carried out in bypass patients. Lessons are probably generalizable to other forms of surgery.

Poorly controlled diabetes (e.g. HbA_{1c} > 8.5%, 69 mmol/mol, or admission glucose > 9.2 mmol.L, 166 mg/dL) predicts increased risk of major superficial and deep infections (including mediastinitis, thoracotomy site, septicaemia and vein harvest site) after coronary bypass surgery. Diabetes, renal failure and obesity (BMI 30–40) each carry a similar risk; the cumulative risk may therefore be very high in some patients. Bilateral internal thoracic artery grafts and associated ischaemia may contribute to chronic sternal wound infections in people with diabetes or chronic heart failure. Negative-pressure dressings and possibly hyperbaric oxygen therapy (see below) may be of value in treating these uncommon but very severe infections. Diabetes does not appear to be a risk factor for infections of implanted pacemakers or cardioverter-defibrillators. Although there is strong epidemiological evidence for a close relationship between glycaemic control and surgical outcomes, there are no large-scale trial data, nor are there likely to be.

Lower limb total joint replacement surgery
Poor preoperative glycaemic control in patients having total hip and knee replacement is associated with urinary tract and wound infections. Associated postoperative risks (ileus, stroke, postoperative haemorrhage and transfusion) contribute to delayed discharge and increased risk of death [2]. Patients with diabetes more frequently require hip replacement revision surgery as a result of deep infection, especially if they have cardiovascular complications.

Urinary tract infections (*British National Formulary, section 5.1.13*)
Type 1 patients in the long-term EDIC study were no more likely to have cystitis than non-diabetic women. Poor glycaemic control and vascular complications were not associated with increased risk of cystitis and pyelonephritis, but cystitis was strongly associated with sexual activity. Few of these patients had advanced neuropathy: bladder dysfunction caused by autonomic neuropathy is generally thought to be an important factor contributing to urinary tract infections (UTIs). Patients with heavy proteinuria are more likely to have asymptomatic bacteriuria, and the two may be linked via endothelial dysfunction.

Asymptomatic bacteriuria
In males asymptomatic bacteriuria does not occur more commonly in diabetes, but it is twice as common in women with diabetes compared

with non-diabetic women. Evidence is contradictory on the benefits of treatment, one study suggesting there was no difference in the rate of development of subsequent definite UTI, the other the opposite. The preferred approach following a positive urine culture is vigilance but no immediate treatment, except in pregnancy.

Management of symptomatic UTI (Table 7.1)

In diabetic patients, 80% of UTIs involve the upper tract, and bilateral involvement is more frequent. Other complications are more frequent. *Escherichia coli* remains the usual organism, but *Proteus* spp., *Enterobacter* spp., *Enterococcus faecalis*, *Klebsiella pneumoniae* and group B streptococci are also common.

Treat bacterial cystitis for at least 7 days, possibly 14 days, longer than in a non-diabetic patient, because of the tendency to involve the upper renal tract. Treat pyelonephritis as in non-diabetic patients, but always admit for blood and urine culture, intravenous antibiotic treatment and to intensify diabetes treatment where possible, as bacteraemia is about four times more likely to occur. Be vigilant for the development of a perinephric abscess (occasionally caused by haematogenous spread of *Staphylococcus aureus*) and the rare but possibly fatal emphysematous pyelonephritis.

Choice of antibiotic

- Uncomplicated cystitis: trimethoprim 200 mg b.d.
- Pyelonephritis: gentamicin, followed by trimethoprim or amoxicillin.
- In the very sick patient: ceftazidime 0.5–1 g every 12 hours, or cefuroxime 0.75–1.5 g every 6–8 hours.
- Once fever and systemic symptoms have resolved, transfer to oral antibiotics and maintain for 14 days.

In practice all patients with symptomatic UTIs more severe than simple cystitis should have a renal tract ultrasound scan. Recurrent UTIs require urological involvement, but low-dose prophylaxis can be started with trimethoprim 100 mg daily. Unfortunately, cranberry products do not seem to be effective (and may be high in glucose).

Emphysematous pyelonephritis (and emphysematous cystitis) is almost specific to people with diabetes. The organism is either *E. coli* or another Gram-negative organism generating gas (carbon dioxide) through unclear mechanisms. Unilateral nephrectomy used to be the only option, but intensive medical treatment (including hyperbaric oxygen therapy where available) has improved the very poor prognosis. Emphysematous pyelonephritis and renal abscesses are best seen on CT; manage closely with the urologists. Consider them in patients slow to respond to standard intensive treatment for UTI.

Table 7.1 Urinary tract infections in diabetes

Infection	Clinical features	Diagnostic procedures	Microbiology and suggested treatment	Comments
Cystitis	Frequency, dysuria, suprapubic pain	Urine culture Ultrasound of renal tract to exclude upper tract involvement	*E. coli, Proteus* spp. Trimethoprim (Ciprofloxacin)	Less common organisms include *Klebsiella* spp., group B streptococci, enterococci, *Pseudomonas*
Pyelonephritis	Fever, loin pain	Urine culture Ultrasound of renal tract	*E. coli, Proteus* spp. Gentamicin followed by trimethoprim Third-generation cephalosporins (e.g. cefotaxime, ceftriaxone, ceftazidime) Piperacillin/tazobactam	Consider bilateral involvement
Emphysematous pyelonephritis	Fever, loin pain, poor response to antibiotics	Plain X-ray, ultrasound, CT scan	*E. coli*, other Gram-negative bacilli (e.g. *Klebsiella* spp.) Treatment as above	ITU, percutaneous drainage, emergency nephrectomy sometimes needed, hyperbaric oxygen may help

Perinephric abscess	Fever, loin pain, poor response to antibiotics (fever persisting for > 4 days after start of antibiotic treatment)	Ultrasound, CT scan	E. coli, other Gram-negative bacilli, Staph. aureus from haematogenous spread	Consider surgical drainage
Papillary necrosis	Fever, loin and abdominal pain	Ultrasound, intravenous urography		
Fungal	All the above can occur, depending on site of infection	Difficult to diagnose, especially difficult to distinguish from colonization; urine culture	Candida spp.	Oral fluconazole

Source: after Hakeem et al. [3].

Abdominal infections

Signs and symptoms may be subtle and undramatic. Patients with auto-nomic neuropathy have reduced abdominal visceral sensitivity. The most common specific abdominal infection is peritonitis in patients undergoing peritoneal dialysis. Gram-positive organisms, especially *Staphylococcus aureus*, are usually responsible, but Gram-negative infections occur; those caused by *Pseudomonas* spp. and *Serratia marcescens* carry a poorer prog-nosis. Other abdominal infections include:
- emphysematous cholecystitis, usually polymicrobial infections (Gram-negative organisms and anaerobes);
- gynaecological infections (remember small occult pelvic abscesses);
- hepatic abscess (most commonly *Klebsiella* spp.), uncommon in the UK;
- retroperitoneal abscess;
- psoas abscess (see below, musculoskeletal infections).

Soft-tissue infections

Cellulitis

A spreading infection of the epidermis, dermis and subcutaneous fat, common in diabetes, frequently recurrent and associated with infected foot ulcers. Where there is no coexisting foot ulceration (always check carefully for minor skin breaks and interdigital fungal infection), treat as in a person without diabetes, covering the most likely organisms (*Staphylococus aureus* and β-haemolytic streptococci, usually group A). Blood cultures are usually negative, but culture any fluid from unrup-tured blisters. Exclude coexisting deep venous thrombosis, and give pro-phylactic anticoagulation in immobilized patients.

Treatment

Oral antibiotics are suitable if there is limited or no involvement of the legs and no foot ulceration. A 7- day course of co-amoxiclav (or ciprofloxacin where available) are suitable, but review frequently, as infections can spread rapidly. Oral macrolides (erythromycin, clarithromycin) are probably not potent enough in this situation, and metronidazole is not necessary. Always err on the side of caution: an initial course of 24–48 hours of intravenous antibiotics (if possible ambulatory) is often valuable. High-dose intravenous benzylpenicillin and flucloxacillin are currently recommended, clindamycin in the penicillin-allergic, vancomycin where MRSA is known or suspected. Systemically unwell patients who have had previous antibiotic treatment should be started on a third-generation cephalosporin (e.g. ceftazidime) until more specific advice and culture results are available. Where there is a large volume of infected tissue, especially in the presence of ischaemia or oedema, 2–4 weeks of treatment is sometimes necessary; diuretics and elevating the feet reduce leg oedema and the risk of skin breaks. Widespread desquamation during recovery is characteristic of streptococcal infection.

Necrotizing fasciitis

This is fulminating gangrene of the skin caused by rapidly spreading microvascular thrombosis affecting subcutaneous fat, dermis and muscle. Diabetes is a risk factor in up to 30% of cases (other factors include chronic alcoholism, immunosuppression and recent surgery). It usually occurs in the limbs, but any skin surface can be involved, including the feet, face and neck (where it is often of dental origin). Mortality is 20–40% from sepsis and multiorgan failure. At the onset, cutaneous signs are usually unimpressive, but irregular dusky blue and black patches appear and extend rapidly. It is a surgical emergency requiring intensive medical support. Think of necrotizing fasciitis in any diabetic patient with severe cellulitis; confirm with immediate ultrasound or CT.

Microbiology
- Predominantly Lancefield group A β-haemolytic streptococci.
- Less severe infections are seen with group C and G β-haemolytic streptococci.
- Fournier's gangrene is a specific form of necrotizing fasciitis, involving the perineum, genitalia and perianal area: multiple organisms can be involved, for example *Staphylococcus aureus*, *E. coli*, anaerobes (clostridia, *Bacteroides* or anaerobic streptococci). It is also described in the feet, face and neck (often of dental origin).
- Community-acquired MRSA-associated necrotizing fasciitis has been described and is usually associated with other underlying medical conditions, diabetes included.
- *Vibrio vulnificans*, found in warm coastal waters of the southern hemisphere, is increasing.

Management
Obtain immediate surgical advice. High-dose intravenous benzylpenicillin (e.g. > 14 g/day) and clindamycin (900 mg t.d.s.) should be given for streptococcal infection, metronidazole and cephalosporin for suspected Fournier's gangrene. Hyperbaric oxygen treatment probably reduces tissue loss, but is not usually available quickly enough.

Diabetic foot infections (see also Chapter 10)

Multidisciplinary teamwork with specialist podiatrists is crucial. Patients in primary care must be referred for specialist wound débridement and dressing, which are as important as antibiotic treatment. Worsening

Table 7.2 Simple clinical classification of diabetic foot ulcers (IDSA-IWGDF) [4]

Clinical classification according to degree of infection	Description	Hospitalization rate (%)	Amputation rate (%)
Uninfected	No purulence or evidence of inflammation	0	3
Mild infection	Two signs of inflammation, e.g. pain/induration, < 2 cm cellulitis around ulcer, infection limited to skin and subcutaneous tissue	4	3
Moderate infection	More than one of the following: > 2 cm cellulitis around ulcer, lymphangitis, spread beneath fascia, abscess, gangrene, involvement of muscle, tendon or bone	52	46
Severe infection	Local infection with systemic toxicity (e.g. fever, hypotension, leucocytosis, impaired renal function)	89 (15% required multiple hospitalization)	88

clinical features of infection are associated with increasing rates of hospitalization and eventual amputation (Table 7.2).

Clinically uninfected ulcers do not benefit from 'prophylactic' antibiotic treatment. Distinguishing non-infected ulcers from mild infections is therefore important, and a CRP of 17 mg/L has been suggested as a cutoff [5]. Where there is a clinical infection, antibiotic treatment (Table 7.3) should be guided by the following factors.

- Chronicity: the more chronic, the less likely treatment for Gram-positive pathogens alone will be sufficient.

Table 7.3 Antibiotics frequently used in diabetic foot infections and their spectrum of activity

Antibiotic	Formulation		Relative activity against specific pathogens				Comments
	Oral	IV	S. aureus	Streptococcus	Enterobacteriaceae	Anaerobes	
Penicillins (BNF section 5.1.1)							
Benzylpenicillin	–	Y	+	++++	+	++	Do not use penicillin V
Flucloxacillin	Y	Y	++++	+++	0	++	Avoid long courses; can cause delayed cholestatic jaundice
Co-amoxiclav	Y	Y	++++	++++	++	+++	Important broad-spectrum antibiotic; currently less approved (C. *difficile* risk)
Amoxicillin/ ampicillin	Y	Y	+	++++	++	++	Less used
Piperacillin/ tazobactam	N	Y	++++	++++	+++	++++	Very broad spectrum, including *Pseudomonas* spp.
Cephalosporins (BNF section 5.1.2.1)							
Cefuroxime	Y	Y	++++	++++	++	++	Less approved (C. *difficile*)

(Continued)

Table 7.3 (*Continued*)

Antibiotic	Formulation		Relative activity against specific pathogens				Comments
	Oral	IV	S. aureus	Streptococcus	Enterobacteriaceae	Anaerobes	
Ceftriaxone/ ceftazidime	N	Y	+++	+++	++++	++	Useful agent in severe infections in penicillin-sensitive patients or when mixed organisms are suspected
Fluoroquinolones (BNF section 5.1.12)							
Ciprofloxacin	Y	Y	+++	++	++++	0	Good bone penetration; well tolerated in long courses in ambulatory care; generally less approved (*C. difficile*)
Levofloxacin	Y	Y	+++	+++	++++	+	
Anaerobic agents							
Clindamycin (*BNF section 5.1.6*)	Y	Y	++++	+++	0	++++	Good bone penetration. Important anti-staphylococcal agent. Narrow spectrum but associated with diarrhoea

Metronidazole (BNF section 5.1.11)	Y	Y	0	0	0	++++	Anti-anaerobic only. Do not use routinely
Others							
Vancomycin/teicoplanin (BNF section 5.1.7)	Y*	Y	++++	+++	0	++	MRSA or penicillin-allergic patients
Imipenem/cilastatin (BNF section 5.1.2.2)	N	Y	++++	++++	++++	+++	Similar spectrum to piperacillin/tazobactam
Rifampicin (BNF section 5.1.9)	Y	N	++++	0	+++	++++	In combination for anti-staphylococcal regimen (MRSA active)

* Vancomycin only.
BNF, British National Formulary.
Source: after Lipsky [4].

- Depth: superficial, deep, bone involvement.
- Community or hospital-acquired infection, and associated probability of specific organisms, for example MRSA in hospitalized patients, sensitive streptococci in first community-acquired infection, mixed organisms in chronic infection, presence of anaerobic/gas-forming organisms.
- Presence of ischaemia (anaerobes) and osteomyelitis (staphylococci).
- Recent antibiotic treatment and antibiotic sensitivities.

Deep cultures, especially of tissue, are important in guiding treatment and limiting the use of broad-spectrum antibiotics, but results will not be available for several days. *Staphylococcus aureus* and streptococci should always be covered. It is difficult to give guidance for individual cases, but consider the following.

- Do not undertreat: symptoms and signs of infection can be attenuated or obscured in diabetic neuropathy, which always accompanies foot ulceration. If in doubt about the severity of the infection or whether it can be managed in the community, admit the patient for intravenous treatment.
- Abscesses are difficult to detect clinically in oedematous feet, and often become evident only when surgical or podiatrist débridement has been performed, or on magnetic resonance imaging (MRI).
- Infections can spread with alarming speed.
- Surgical liaison is often needed, especially when there is peripheral vascular disease, and frequent discussion with the microbiology team is important.
- No topical antibiotic preparation is currently licensed for ulcers.

Osteomyelitis

Osteomyelitis in the foot usually occurs adjacent to a neuropathic ulcer; it rarely occurs with completely intact skin, though small puncture wounds, especially in flexures of the toes and at their tips, can sometimes heal up after infection has entered. Clinically therefore it is difficult to exclude osteomyelitis, but an ulcer in excess of $2\,cm^2$ and a positive 'probe-to-bone' test are the best clinical indicators of its presence (though there is continuing doubt about the reliability of the 'probe-to-bone' test; see Chapter 10) [6]. When there is radiological suspicion of osteomyelitis, especially of midfoot bones, but without clinical ulceration, then consider Charcot neuroarthropathy (see Chapter 10). The painless 'sausage toe' – with characteristic swelling and dusky skin, probably caused by local ischaemia – usually conceals underlying distal osteomyelitis, though radiologically it can be difficult to detect, because normal distal phalanges vary in appearance. Heel osteomyelitis is also difficult to spot radiologically.

Osteomyelitis can progress very rapidly, and if it is suspected, repeat films every month to detect subtle cortical changes. MRI may show marrow oedema, but Charcot neuroarthropathy gives the same appearance.

Bone infection in diabetes is nearly always caused by *Staphylococcus aureus*. Open biopsy and culture will confirm, but this is rarely needed except when there is high suspicion of another organism, or failure to respond to prolonged high-dose anti-staphylococcal antibiotics.

Treatment
Surgery is often needed when there is infection proximal to the phalanges, especially in the presence of peripheral vascular disease. However, the common situation of distal infection involving the phalanges in a well-perfused neuropathic foot can often be managed with long (3–6 month) courses of anti-staphylococcal bone-penetrating antibiotics (flucloxacillin, quinolones and clindamycin), and up to 75% of cases of forefoot osteomyelitis complicating ulceration can be eradicated in the medium to long term with 3-monthly cycles of antibiotics guided by repeated MRI scans [7]. In the outpatient setting, the quinolones are often well tolerated, and can be given twice daily. Flucloxacillin is sometimes poorly tolerated, requires dosing four times daily, and can cause hepatitis. In the otherwise well patient, clindamycin is also a good choice, though there is a higher risk of antibiotic-associated diarrhoea and *C. difficile* infection. During treatment small pieces of bone (sequestra) are often spontaneously discharged through the tip of the toe, or can be picked out by the podiatrist. Ultimately sclerosis or resorption occurs. Closure of any local ulceration usually (but not always) signals healing.

Uncommon infections characteristic of diabetes

Malignant otitis externa
'Malignant' otitis externa is usually caused by *Pseudomonas aeruginosa*. Disproportionate pain, discharge and hearing loss are the warning features, but diagnosis is often delayed. Involvement of the skull through osteomyelitis with secondary cerebral venous thrombosis are late manifestations. Joint surgical management with the ENT and microbiology/infectious disease teams and prolonged systemic and topical anti-pseudomonal antibiotics are required.

Rhinocerebral mucormycosis
Extremely uncommon (I have never seen a case), though frequently quoted in the literature, and said to be associated with DKA. Beginning with face or eye pain, there is progressive ocular involvement: proptosis,

ophthalmoplegia and severe constitutional upset. Venous and arterial thromboses of the head and neck are described.

Ophthalmic infections
Staphylococcal endophthalmitis after cataract surgery, though rare, is more common in diabetes. There are also sporadic reports of endogenous endophthalmitis resulting from septicaemia originating from an infection elsewhere, especially diabetic foot lesions (*Staphylococcus*), liver abscess (*Klebsiella*) and UTI (*E. coli*). Always consider a potentially serious eye infection whenever a diabetic patient presents with a red eye.

Cardiac infections
Mitral annular calcification is more frequent in diabetes, and affected valves can become infected. Staphylococcal valve infection is more common than viridans streptococcal infection in diabetic patients, who are more likely to be on dialysis; mortality is much higher in diabetes.

Musculoskeletal infections
Many have been described, and they often present as pyrexia of unknown origin, as do many other infections in diabetes. They include:
• septic arthritis (including the sternoclavicular joint)
• epidural abscess
• discitis
• psoas abscess
• vertebral osteomyelitis.
   Staphylococcus is the most common organism, but *Streptococcus* and the pneumococcus are also encountered. These are often indolent infections resistant to early diagnosis, but should be considered in poorly controlled, complicated diabetic patients with focal, especially lower back pain. Always be alert to the possibility of 'metastatic' infection in patients with infected foot ulceration or osteomyelitis. MRI is valuable in delineating the anatomical extent of a known infection, but combined FDG-PET/CT scanning is becoming the investigation of choice in localizing obscure infections and in the investigation of pyrexia of unknown origin, common scenarios in people with diabetes.

References
1. Bowling FL, Salgami EV, Boulton AJM. Larval therapy: a novel treatment in eliminating methicillin-resistant *Staphylococcus aureus* from diabetic foot ulcers. *Diabetes Care* 2007;30:370–1. PMID: 17259512.
2. Marchant MH Jr, Viens NA, Cook C, Vail TP, Bolognesi MP. The impact of glycaemic control and diabetes mellitus on perioperative outcomes after total joint arthroplasty. *J Bone Joint Surg Am* 2009;91:1621–9. PMID: 19571084.

3. Hakeem LM, Bhattacharyya DN, Lafong C, Janjua KS, Serhan JT, Campbell IW. Diversity and complexity of urinary tract infection in diabetes mellitus. *Br J Diabetes Vasc Dis* 2009;9:119–25. PMID: not available.
4. Lipsky BA. A report from the international consensus on diagnosing and treating the infected diabetic foot. *Diabetes Metab Res Rev* 2004;20(Suppl. 1):S68–S77. PMID: not available.
5. Jeandrot A, Richard JL, Combescure C *et al*. Serum procalcitonin and C-reactive protein concentrations to distinguish mildly infected from non-infected diabetic foot ulcers: a pilot study. *Diabetologia* 2008;51:347–52. PMID: 19571084.
6. Butalia S, Palda VA, Sargeant RJ, Detsky AS, Mourad O. Does this patient with diabetes have osteomyelitis of the lower extremity? *JAMA* 2008;299:806–13. PMID: 18285592.
7. Valabhji J, Oliver N, Samarasinghe D, Mali T, Gibbs RG, Gedroyc WM. Conservative management of diabetic forefoot ulceration complicated by underlying osteomyelitis: the benefits of magnetic resonance imaging. *Diabetic Med* 2009;26:1127–34. PMID: 19929991.

Further reading

Edmonds ME, Foster AVM. *Managing the Diabetic Foot*. Oxford: Wiley-Blackwell, 2005.

Foster AVM, Edmonds ME. *Diabetic Foot Care: Case Studies in Clinical Management*. Oxford: Wiley-Blackwell, 2010.

Diabetic renal disease

CHAPTER 8

Key points

- Increasing albuminuria and falling eGFR are independent predictors of renal and cardiovascular outcomes; patients with macroalbuminuria and low eGFR require the most intensive management. This requires careful interpretation of trends as well as one-off measurements.
- Serious cardiovascular events are much more common than end-stage renal disease in patients with diabetic nephropathy.
- Urinary albumin measurements have large variability, but the albumin/creatinine ratio (ACR) is probably the most stable measurement.
- Regression of microalbuminuria to normoalbuminuria is frequent in both type 1 and type 2 diabetes.
- Angiotensin blockade does not reduce the risk of developing microalbuminuria in type 1 diabetes; there is no clear evidence in type 2, but many patients will require angiotensin blockade for other reasons.
- Management of microalbuminuria: glycaemic control in type 1, multimodal treatment (Steno-2) in type 2.
- Management of macroalbuminuria: full angiotensin blockade, primarily with ACE-i; intensive cardiovascular risk factor management. Be alert for anaemia and early renal bone disease.
- Refer judiciously to nephrologists, taking into account all circumstances, especially the likelihood of macrovascular events versus renal end points.
- Always consider type 1 patients in end-stage renal disease for pancreas as well as renal transplantation.

Practical Diabetes Care, 3rd edition. © David Levy.
Published 2011 by Blackwell Publishing Ltd.

Overview of diabetic kidney disease

End-stage renal disease (ESRD) is a common and terrible outcome of diabetes. However, recent data in both type 1 and type 2 diabetes are encouraging. In type 1 diabetes, where not long ago diabetic nephropathy was almost inevitable after 20–30 years, fewer than 1% of patients diagnosed in Sweden between 1977 and 1985 developed ESRD, and rates of dialysis take-on throughout Europe were stable during the 1990s, despite rising prevalence and longer survival in type 1 diabetes. Even in type 2 diabetes, at least in the USA, the rising incidence of ESRD between 1990 and 1996 in people over 45 years has now been replaced by a consistent decrease up to 2006 in all age groups, amounting to 2–4% per year. This must reflect improved multimodal management of type 2 diabetes [1]. However, the challenge remains formidable, and reducing this costly end-stage complication requires widespread action at primary-care level to diagnose and intercept increasing albuminuria and falling eGFR as early as possible and to treat them vigorously with the best evidence-based means.

Renal disease in type 1 diabetes

Any degree of albuminuria caused by diabetes is very unusual within 5 years of diagnosis, and should be thoroughly investigated (for example, I have seen a teenage type 1 patient with early-onset microalbuminuria and hypertension who turned out to have Cushing's disease). Nevertheless, functional renal changes do occur shortly after diagnosis, including renal hypertrophy (increased kidney volume) and hyperfiltration, associated with elevated GFR (> 135–150 mL/min). Early renal hypertrophy may increase the risk of developing microalbuminuria, though hyperfiltration does not. Changes on renal biopsy occur within a decade of diagnosis in young people and are associated with lack of nocturnal dipping on ambulatory blood pressure testing. Microalbuminuria may appear or temporarily worsen during periods of very poor glycaemic control, but this may be due to the hyperglycaemia or to the medical problems, especially systemic infection, that precipitated the poor control.

In a typical population of type 1 patients, about 15% will have microalbuminuria, 5% macroalbuminuria, and 3% will be in renal failure. Prepubertal duration of type 1 diabetes may contribute less than postpubertal duration to the development of renal disease, and onset under the age of 5 years seems to delay the development of nephropathy. Regression from microalbuminuria to normoalbuminuria is very common (up to one-third of cases), but annually about 2% of microalbuminuric patients progress to macroalbuminuria, cumulatively significant in this young population.

Non-modifiable risks for progression of diabetic renal disease
- Diabetes duration
- Initial albumin excretion rate (AER).

Modifiable or partly modifiable risks
- Blood pressure
- Smoking
- Insulin resistance characteristics (e.g. low HDL-cholesterol, elevated triglycerides, degree of abdominal obesity, inflammatory markers such as white blood count and fibrinogen)
- Total cholesterol.

Renal disease in type 2 diabetes

In contrast with type 1 diabetes, at diagnosis up to 10% of type 2 patients already have microalbuminuria and a small proportion overt proteinuria. A global study found microalbuminuria in 40% and macroalbuminuria in 10%. As in type 1 diabetes, hyperfiltration is common, occurring in 10–20%, depending on the measurement method used, and can occur even in patients with IGT. In UKPDS, progression from microalbuminuria to macroalbuminuria was only slightly more frequent in type 2 diabetes than type 1, about 3% annually, though other estimates are a little higher, around 5%; another 2% progress annually from microalbuminuria to macroalbuminuria, and from macroalbuminuria to significant renal impairment or renal replacement therapy. Dyslipidaemia (low HDL, elevated apolipoprotein B) and other factors associated with the metabolic syndrome (e.g. elevated fibrinogen) predict progression to overt nephropathy, again as in type 1 diabetes. The dyslipidaemia (and worse hypertension) may partly account for the higher rate of diabetic nephropathy found in ethnic minority African, African-Caribbean and South Asian patients, in the UK and elsewhere. While the fear of renal failure is always present, the reality is that the likelihood of death from cardiovascular disease, is greater than the risk of progressing nephropathy, especially when there is renal impairment (serum creatinine $> 175\,\mu mol/L$, $2\,mg/dL$), at which level the annual mortality is about 12% [2].

Other (non-diabetic) nephropathies

The reported frequency of non-diabetic nephropathy in patients with proteinuria varies with the criteria used to justify renal biopsy. Perhaps up to one-third of proteinuric type 1 patients have non-diabetic glomerular disease, but in type 2 patients, selected on the basis of absent retinopathy, the rate is lower, around 10%. Many renal units screen for non-diabetic renal diseases using standard serological tests (e.g. ANF, ANCA, complement), but renal biopsy is very rarely performed these days unless these tests are strongly indicative or there are unusual clinical features, for example:

- rapid deterioration in renal function;
- suspicious urinary sediment, red cell casts;
- sudden development of nephrotic syndrome (see below);
- short duration (e.g. less than 5 years) of otherwise uncomplicated type 1 diabetes.

Even when these features occur, biopsy usually shows typical diabetic renal disease. The clinical benefit of identifying alternative or additional renal parenchymal disease has not been established, but these are subtle matters and patients with any of these unusual features need a nephrology opinion. The full range of non-diabetic renal disease can be encountered on biopsy, but a large retrospective study in the USA [3] found, in decreasing order of prevalence, focal segmental glomerulosclerosis, minimal-change disease, IgA nephropathy, and membranous glomerulonephritis.

Do not forget renal stone disease, which is more common in people with the metabolic syndrome (increasing risk with increasing numbers of defined components) and type 2 diabetes, and which is associated with chronic kidney disease (CKD).

ESR and CRP in diabetic nephropathy

A high erythrocyte sedimentation rate (ESR) due to elevated fibrinogen synthesis is a non-specific indicator of CKD, and values between 25 and 55 mm/hour would be expected, with a weak upward trend with advancing stage of CKD. In contrast, CRP is normal or only slightly elevated (e.g. about 12 mg/L in CKD stage 5), and barely increases even in haemodialysis patients (about 7 mg/L). CRP is therefore a reliable marker of infection in patients with CKD [4].

Microscopic haematuria, sometimes heavy, occurs in about 70% of patients with macroalbuminuria, and is not a reliable indicator of non-diabetic renal disease; however, all patients with macroalbuminuria need a renal tract ultrasound scan.

Stages of CKD: estimated glomerular filtration rate

Serum creatinine is no longer regarded as a sufficiently accurate estimate of renal function, since a normal or near-normal serum creatinine may mask markedly impaired renal function, especially in the elderly. eGFR is now routinely reported, nearly always using the MDRD equation, which takes into account age, gender, serum creatinine and ethnic origin (black vs. other ethnicities). Since serum creatinine is a term in the calculation, its variability and effect on the resulting eGFR must be taken into account, especially with eGFR values above 60 mL/min, where precision is particularly poor. The resulting stages of CKD should be used

Table 8.1 Stages of chronic kidney disease (CKD) and diabetes

CKD stage	eGFR range (mL/min)	Description	Cardiovascular risk (odds ratio, univariate, non-diabetic subjects)	Comments
Normal	≥ 90		–	Only normal if no other evidence of renal disease (in which case stage 1)
				Possibility of 'elevated' eGFR during periods of hyperfiltration (poor glycaemic control)
				Cardiovascular risk depends on level of proteinuria
Stage 1	≥ 90	Kidney damage with normal or increased eGFR	–	Evidence of other renal disease (e.g. APCKD), proteinuria, haematuria, structural abnormalities (e.g. reflux nephropathy, renal artery stenosis)
				Cardiovascular risk dependent on level of proteinuria
Stage 2	60–89	Kidney damage with mild decreased eGFR	1.5	With other evidence of renal disease
				Risk of cardiovascular disease greater than that of requiring renal replacement therapy

Stage 3	30–59	Moderate decreased eGFR	2–4	Use metformin with caution and stop if any other contraindication Anaemia and bone disease common (FBC, B_{12}, folate, ferritin, bone screen, including PTH) Most patients in this stage will die of cardiovascular disease, rather than ESRD
Stage 4	15–29	Severe decreased eGFR	4–10	Specialist advice needed for treatment and planning for renal replacement therapy Stop metformin. Sulphonylureas, insulin and possibly glitazones suitable
Stage 5	< 25 or dialysis	Kidney failure	10 to > 50	

APCKD, adult polycystic kidney disease; FBC, full blood count.

as a broad guide only, and rate of change of eGFR, as well as its absolute value, is very important (Table 8.1). There is concern about the rigid use of referral criteria based on CKD stage. Most people, even those with diabetes, who have CKD stage 3 are elderly and may not have risk factors for progression to ESRD, compared with risk factors for a moderately increased cardiovascular risk. The benefit of nephrology referral in many of these patients, as opposed to careful control of vascular risk factors, which could be more efficiently done in primary care, is questionable.

Diabetic nephropathy

An important term for a syndrome comprising macroalbuminuria, hypertension, and reduced eGFR (i.e. CKD stage 2 or worse, and deteriorating). It should be used precisely, because it defines a group with a very high risk of cardiorenal events. Data from ADVANCE show that in patients with type 2 diabetes (the same probably applies to type 1 diabetes) with macroalbuminuria (ACR > 34 mg/mmol, 300 mg/g) and eGFR below 60 mL/min, cardiovascular events are increased threefold and renal events 22-fold.

Quantification of urinary albumin excretion

The following methods are in current use:
- spot early-morning urine specimen expressed as ACR (mg/mmol or mg/g): albumin excretion corrected for urine output;
- 24-hour urinary albumin excretion (mg per 24 hours);
- timed (usually overnight) AER (μg/min);
- urinary albumin concentration *uncorrected* for creatinine (i.e. mg/L).

ACR is widely used as a screening test, and increasingly to monitor response to treatment, on account of its simplicity for both the patient and the laboratory. Reliable point-of-care methods for measuring ACR are now available (e.g. DCA Vantage). Urinary albumin concentration in a spot specimen (point-of-care HemoCue Albumin 201) has its advocates, but so far has not been widely adopted. Although ACR correlates well with 24-hour urinary albumin excretion, there are difficulties with its universal adoption [5].
- Its definition is not agreed worldwide (see below): the original definitions of microalbuminuria and macroalbuminuria were based on 24-hour collections.
- The lower limits for microalbuminuria defined by ACR are higher in females than males (24-hour urinary creatinine excretion is lower in females).
- 24-Hour urinary creatinine measurement falls with age, especially in females. ACR increases with age, and for precision age- and sex-adjusted values should be used.
- Early-morning (first pass) specimens should always be analysed.

Factors that may falsely increase urinary albumin excretion include the following.
- Strenuous exercise can increase ACR in normal people to 6–8 mg/mmol (53–70 mg/g), but it settles to baseline within 24 hours.
- Fever/systemic infection.
- Very poor glycaemic control leading to hyperfiltration.
- Contrary to widespread belief, asymptomatic UTI (see Chapter 7) does not cause proteinuria or microalbuminuria. Management of albuminuria should not be delayed on account of bacteriuria.

Urinary albumin versus protein measurements
Because of the significance of microalbuminuria in diabetes practice it is usual to measure urinary albumin; once patients transfer to the renal team, the degree of proteinuria is less of a concern, and in any case gram, rather than milligram, protein leakages are the rule. Renal units therefore often use protein/creatinine ratios. Albumin constitutes about 70% of total urinary protein; the distinction is of importance in the microalbuminuric range.

Reference ranges for albumin excretion (Table 8.2)
Normoalbuminuria
The normal range for AER is usually quoted as 1.5–20 μg/min, with a geometric mean of 6.5 μg/min, approximately equivalent to 10 mg per 24 hours (AER is logarithmically, not normally distributed). This value is similar to the detection limit of most laboratory assays. ACR in healthy volunteers and in non-microalbuminuric type 2 patients is about 0.4 mg/mmol (males) and 0.5 mg/mmol (females).

Microalbuminuria
Microalbuminuria is defined as:
- urinary albumin excretion 30–299 mg per 24 hours;
- AER 20–199 μg/min;
- ACR 2.5/3.5 to 20 mg/mmol (USA 30–299 mg/g);
- there may be intermittent stick-positive proteinuria.

The threshold for microalbuminuria using ACR is higher in females than males. In the UK threshold values are usually quoted as 2.5 mg/mmol (22 mg/g) or more in males, and 3.5 mg/mmol (31 mg/g) or more in females, though 2.0 and 2.8, respectively, are also used, for example in Canada. Using a factor of 8.8 for conversion of SI to traditional units, the range defining microalbuminuria is not the same in the UK and in the USA; agreement is needed. The classic clinical trials used different definitions for microalbuminuria (e.g. DCCT > 40 mg per 24 hours; UKPDS > 50 mg/L).

Table 8.2 Definitions of albuminuria

Screening method	Normoalbuminuria	Microalbuminuria	Macroalbuminuria
Albumin/ creatinine ratio	Male: < 2.5 mg/ mmol (22 mg/g) Female: < 3.5 mg/ mmol (31 mg/g)	2.5/3.5 to 20 mg/ mmol (USA 30–299 mg/g)	> 20 mg/mmol (USA ≥ 300 mg/g)
Timed (usually overnight) albumin excretion rate (μg/min)	< 20 (some studies < 25)	20–199	≥ 200
24-hour urinary albumin excretion (mg per 24 hours)	< 30	30–299	≥ 300

Macroalbuminuria

Macroalbuminuria is defined as:

- urinary albumin excretion ≥ 300 mg per 24 hours;
- AER ≥ 200 μg/min;
- ACR > 20 mg/mmol (USA ≥ 300 mg/g);
- persistent stick-positive proteinuria (1 to 3+) is invariable.

Nephrotic syndrome

In the IDNT study of irbesartan in diabetic nephropathy (2001), more than 40% of patients had the nephrotic syndrome, defined as:

- total urinary protein > 3.5 g/day;
- urinary albumin > 2.2 g/day;
- ACR > 2.2 g/g (250 mg/mol).

Traditionally, the syndrome also includes:

- hypoalbuminaemia (serum albumin < 35 g/L);
- hypercholesterolaemia (total cholesterol > 6.7 mmol/L, 260 mg/dL) or statin use;
- peripheral oedema, or use of a loop diuretic [6].

Definitional minutiae apart, proteinuria of this degree carries a poor prognosis, both renal and cardiovascular, with a risk of rapid deterioration in GFR and high mortality, as in non-diabetic renal disease. Because of the high cardiorenal risk, and because with vigorous treatment a certain proportion can be brought into remission (see below), it is important to identify these patients as early as possible, and to establish joint management with the renal team.

Thyroid function in nephrotic syndrome
Protein-bound thyroid hormone loss can be massive in heavy proteinuria. TSH secretion is stimulated, and although patients are clinically euthyroid, thyroid function tests may suggest early hypothyroidism, i.e. TSH 5–10 mU/L, low-normal free T_4 (10–15 pmol/L). This phenomenon is well known in children, but less recognized in adults [7]. It does not respond to L-thyroxine treatment. The converse is important: if this thyroid profile emerges, then check urinary protein levels before embarking on further thyroid investigations.

Diagnosis of microalbuminuria

Urinary albumin measurements have high biological variability, but ACR is less variable than 24-hour urinary albumin measurements (13% vs. 27%). Nevertheless, for diagnostic purposes the recommendation remains that a positive screening test for microalbuminuria (usually ACR) should be followed up with three timed urine samples over the next 6 weeks. If two or three samples are positive, then the diagnosis is confirmed. If a timed urine sample is used for screening, then only two confirmatory tests are required. This difficult procedure is particularly important in younger normotensive type 1 patients, who may be committed unnecessarily to long-term angiotensin blockade treatment. Common sense must be used here: stick-positive proteinuria with a single macroalbuminuric timed sample is sufficient. Albumin in urine is stable at room temperature for 7 days (and up to 30 days at 4°C), so multiple specimens can be stored for a single delivery to the laboratory.

'Renoprotection' in normotensive non-microalbuminuric patients

There is a widespread belief that because of the benefits of angiotensin blockade treatment in microalbuminuria and macroalbuminuria, 'renoprotection' with these agents might reduce the risk of normotensive normoalbuminuric patients developing microalbuminuria. This situation frequently occurs in type 1 diabetes, but the DIRECT-Renal study (2008) in which patients were treated with high-dose candesartan for 5 years did not prevent microalbuminuria [8]. Good glycaemic control (HbA_{1c} 7.0%, 53 mmol/mol or lower) is the only reliably effective preventive measure in type 1 patients, reducing the incidence of microalbuminuria in DCCT by 30–40%.

In type 2 diabetes, RCTs are less clear. In the BENEDICT study, treating hypertensive patients (mean BP 150/87 mmHg) with the ACE-i trandolapril 2 mg daily reduced the risk of progressing from normoalbuminuria to microalbuminuria by about 50% over 4 years [9]. This benefit was not seen with high-dose candesartan (32 mg daily) in the DIRECT-Renal study, either in normotensive patients (mean BP 123/75 mmHg) or those with relatively well-controlled hypertension (mean BP 140/80 mmHg). However, normotensive type 2 patients with persistently negative microalbuminuria are unusual (and may have late-onset type 1 diabetes), and many type 2 patients will have other indications for angiotensin blockade (hypertension, established macrovascular disease or risk factors for it).

Management of microalbuminuria

Type 1 diabetes: the glycaemic approach

Microalbuminuric type 1 patients are hypertensive relative to normoalbuminuric patients, though many will not have blood pressure that reaches the criterion level for either hypertension (BP > 140/90 mmHg) or even pre-hypertension (120–140/80–90 mmHg; see Chapter 11). Glycaemic control is still very important, and CSII should be offered where available to motivated individuals not achieving HbA_{1c} below 7.0% (53 mmol/mol) on an intensified insulin regimen. Smoking is an independent risk factor for microalbuminuria (as in type 2 diabetes) and should be actively targeted. Aspirin or lipid-lowering treatment is of no value. Angiotensin blockade treatment is usually considered essential, but spontaneous regression of microalbuminuria is frequent, particularly if:

- HbA_{1c} is reasonable (e.g. < 8%, 64 mmol/mol);
- systolic blood pressure is below 115 mmHg;
- total cholesterol under 5.1 mmol/L (198 mg/dL) and triglycerides under 1.64 mmol/l (145 mg/dL), which they are likely to be in most type 1 patients;
- microalbuminuria is of short duration [10].

In patients with low-grade microalbuminuria (e.g. ACR 3–5 mg/mmol, 26–44 mg/g) it is therefore reasonable to intensify glycaemic control, target cessation of smoking and monitor ACR every 3–6 months to assess trends in AER before starting angiotensin blockade, particularly in women of childbearing age. Treatment, if started, must be titrated to the highest recommended dose, postural symptoms permitting (but, intriguingly, ACE-i treatment is not consistently associated with regression of microalbuminuria, another reason to consider improving glycaemic control as primary management).

Type 2 diabetes: the multimodal approach

In a typical general practice population of type 2 patients, about one-quarter will have microalbuminuria. It is a strong independent risk factor for cardiovascular mortality (at least twofold increased risk), and even minor degrees of microalbuminuria within the reference range show a strong consistently graded cardiovascular risk. Other cardiovascular risk factors, traditional and otherwise, are highly prevalent in people with microalbuminuria, in particular hypertension: nearly all patients have blood pressure in excess of 140/90 mmHg. Renal tract ultrasound scan, especially in people with established microalbuminuria, is necessary to exclude unrelated structural abnormalities. Resting ECG should probably be done annually; although there are no clear guidelines on this, the cardiovascular risk at this stage remains the major concern.

Smoking increases the risk of progression from microalbuminuria to macroalbuminuria and is independently associated with a more rapid fall in eGFR. Quitting markedly reduces the risk of albuminuria progression, and is a priority target (in general as well, of course). However, intervention in all other risk factors is critical. Steno-2 (2008) in type 2 patients with mid-range microalbuminuria found that with intensive targeting of several factors for 8 years, cardiovascular deaths and events (and the need for laser treatment of retinopathy) were reduced by about 50% over the following 6 years, even after allocation to intensive or conventional treatment had stopped. End-stage renal failure, autonomic neuropathy, coronary interventions and amputations were all markedly reduced, though not all targets, especially glycaemia, were achieved (Table 8.3 and Box 8.1) [11]. The intensive targets of Steno-2 are now routinely achieved, and show that mortality and complications can be substantially reduced in high-risk type 2 patients, though these are not short-term gains.

Glycaemic control and microalbuminuria

Nephropathy seems to be the most responsive of the microvascular complications to glycaemic intervention. In the UKPDS tighter glycaemic control (average HbA_{1c} 7%, 53 mmol/mol) decreased risk of progression to microalbuminuria and to clinical albuminuria by about one-third, albeit over a very long period (9–12 years), and there was also an impressive risk reduction in doubling of serum creatinine. In the ADVANCE study very tight glycaemic control (mean HbA_{1c} 6.3%, 45 mmol/mol) reduced the risk of developing microalbuminuria by about 10% compared with less tight glycaemic control (7.0%, 53 mmol/mol), and of new or worsening nephropathy by 20%, but neither glycaemic target is realistic in the long term. Nevertheless, in a comprehensive management regimen it should be possible to emphasize glycaemic control where there are renal complications. High-dose B-vitamin therapy (folic acid, B_6 and B_{12})

Table 8.3 Steno-2 study: stringent targets, modest achievements, remarkable outcomes (values for the intensive group)

Variable	Target	Baseline (mean or median)	End of follow-up (13.3 years)
Urinary albumin excretion (mg per 24 hours)		78	69
Systolic blood pressure*	<130–140	146	140
Diastolic blood pressure	<80	85	74
HbA$_{1c}$, % (mmol/mol)	<6.5 (48)	8.4 (68)	7.7 (61)
Fasting plasma glucose, mmol/L (mg/dL)		10.1 (182)	8.9 (160)
Total cholesterol, mmol/L (mg/dL)*	<4.5 to 4.9 mmol/L	5.4 (210)	3.8 (147)
LDL cholesterol, mmol/L (mg/dL)		3.4 (133)	1.8 (71)
Triglycerides. mmol/L (mg/dL)	<1.7	1.8 (159)	1.1 (99)

* Blood pressure and cholesterol targets fell as this long trial progressed.

Box 8.1 Summary of targets in microalbuminuric type 2 patients (achieved levels at the end of the randomization period in Steno-2)

- Blood pressure < 130/75 mmHg
- HbA$_{1c}$ < 8.0% (possibly ~6.5%: ADVANCE)
- Total cholesterol < 4.1 mmol/L (160 mg/dL)
- Triglycerides < 1.3 mmol/L (116 mg/dL)
- Full dose ACE-i or ARB treatment
- Aspirin in patients with known cardiovascular disease
- Smoking cessation

hastens the decline in GFR and increases vascular events in patients with nephropathy; ensure that microalbuminuric patients are not taking these vitamins. This is another reminder always to take a comprehensive medication history, and to actively discourage vitamin supplements in diabetes [12].

Angiotensin blockade treatment
There are relatively few large-scale studies of angiotensin blockade treatment in microalbuminuric type 2 patients. ACE inhibitors and ARBs are equally effective in reducing albuminuria and slowing the decline in eGFR; trialled agents include enalapril 20 mg daily and telmisartan 80 mg daily. IRMA-2 (2001) found that full-dose irbesartan (300 mg daily) was more likely to prevent progression to macroalbuminuria over 2 years than 150 mg daily. Full doses of any agents should be used in this situation.

Management of diabetic nephropathy

Investigations
1 Mid-stream urine if leucocytes on routine urinalysis.
2 Renal tract ultrasound scan:
  (a) Normal renal length is about 11 cm, correlating weakly with height and BMI; it is about 10 cm in South Asian and oriental subjects. Kidneys are large in the poorly controlled, hyperfiltering patient (see above) and the level of proteinuria is related to kidney size. Even in advanced diabetic renal disease the kidneys are not particularly small (~10 cm), compared with the typically shrunken kidneys (~8 cm) of advanced chronic non-diabetic renal disease. Adult polycystic kidney disease may coexist with diabetes, though the two conditions are not associated.
  (b) Obstruction (stones, tumour, prostatic enlargement, papilla).
  (c) Discrepancy in kidney size: if marked (i.e. > 1 cm), suggests renal artery stenosis (see below).
  (d) Bladder size and residual volume (neuropathic bladder).
3 Full blood count, CRP, ferritin, vitamin B_{12}, folate, prostate-specific antigen.
4 Fasting lipids.
5 Bone screen, including parathyroid hormone (PTH) when eGFR <60 mL/min, or when serum creatinine > 150 μmol/L (1.7 mg/dL).
6 12-lead ECG. Any hint of ischaemia should be investigated early, though standard treadmill tests may be unhelpful because of the extensive diffuse coronary artery disease that occurs in diabetes, and poor exercise tolerance. The best non-invasive investigations in this

group of patients are not known, and stress echocardiography, radio-nuclide scanning and CT scan for coronary artery calcium score all have their advocates.

7 Regular measurement of albuminuria. An increase may herald nephrotic syndrome; a decrease may signify response to treatment.

Specialist referral

Most guidelines suggest referral to a renal physician when eGFR is 40–50 mL/min or serum creatinine reaches about 150 μmol/L (2 mg/dL). Whether all these patients should remain under nephrology care, as opposed to only those with major risk factors for progression of renal impairment, is debated (see above). Younger or ethnic minority patients with heavy proteinuria or uncontrolled blood pressure should be prioritized. The greater problem is patients with rapidly progressing renal impairment, and many patients are referred far too late, with 30–40% of diabetic patients fulfilling the criterion for 'late referral', i.e. requiring renal replacement therapy within 4 months of referral. Many first attend the renal clinic with poorly controlled glycaemia and blood pressure, and taking suboptimal angiotensin blockade treatment and lipid-lowering treatment. Anaemia and renal bone disease are common.

Renal artery stenosis

Atherosclerotic renal artery stenosis affecting the ostium or proximal renal artery is common in type 2 diabetes. It is usually asymptomatic and considered where there is widespread macrovascular disease, hypertension, renal impairment and renal asymmetry on ultrasound. 'Flash' pulmonary oedema is characteristic, related to activation of the renin–angiontensin–aldosterone pathway. Duplex ultrasound (including assessment of intrarenal resistive index) and magnetic resonance arteriography are definitive investigations.

Longitudinal studies and historical fashion hinted that revascularization could slow the rate of decline in renal function (though there was no long-term benefit on blood pressure). However, the ASTRAL trial (2009) found that well-defined outcomes after revascularization (renal function or event(s), blood pressure, cardiovascular outcomes or death) were no different from a group given optimum medical treatment [13]. The similar CORAL study has not yet reported, but the era of invasive management of atherosclerotic renal artery stenosis is probably coming to an end.

Proteinuria reduction and management of hypertension (Table 8.4)

Trial data in proteinuric type 1 patients is limited and quite old. Reducing blood pressure to less than 130/75 mmHg should result in remission

Table 8.4 Summary of angiotensin blockade treatment of albuminuria

	Type 1 diabetes	Type 2 diabetes
Reducing progression of normoalbuminuria to microalbuminuria	No evidence	If hypertensive, use full-dose ACE-i If treated hypertension or normotensive, no clear evidence
Reducing progression of microalbuminuria to macroalbuminuria	If persistent, use full-dose ACE-i Strict glycaemic control (HbA$_{1c}$ <7.0%)	Target BP < 140/80 mmHg, preferably lower Use full-dose ACE-i or ARB; both equally effective for albuminuria reduction Full-dose ACE-i may reduce macrovascular events (HOPE)
Reducing progression of macroalbuminuria to serious renal end points	Target BP < 130/75 mmHg Full-dose ACE-i	Target BP < 135/85, achieve < 140/75 mmHg Full-dose ARB (irbesartan 300 mg daily, losartan 100 mg daily, telmisartan 80 mg daily)
Nephrotic-range proteinuria		Full-dose ACE-i. Consider ACE-i/ARB combination or direct renin inhibitor/ARB treatment if ACE-i side-effects; alternatively ARB or ACE-i with spironolactone Unlicensed: monitor renal function 2–3 monthly and be alert for hyperkalaemia

or regression of proteinuria in 20–30% of patients, so long as full-dose ACE-i treatment is used.

In type 2 diabetes, two large-scale trials reporting in 2001 give clearer guidance. Full-dose ARB treatment (irbesartan in the IDNT study; losartan in the RENAAL study) significantly reduced progression from proteinuria to ESRD, with relatively modest achieved blood pressure (140/75, target $< 135/85$ mmHg), using on average three to four antihypertensive agents. In IDNT, the renal benefits of irbesartan were not matched by a group treated with amlodipine, despite similar blood pressure levels; amlodipine is an effective antihypertensive agent but does not reduce proteinuria. ACE inhibitors and ARBs have not been directly compared, though they are probably equally effective in reducing renal and cardiovascular end points, but there is some uncertainty over dose equivalents. In the AMADEO trial (2007), telmisartan 80 mg daily was slightly more effective and had a longer-lasting effect in reducing proteinuria than losartan 100 mg daily, but these differences are unlikely to be important in the individual.

However, patients in the IDNT and RENAAL studies had severe diabetic renal disease. Each year about 10% died, progressed to ESRD or doubled their serum creatinine. At baseline, they had moderate renal impairment (serum creatinine 150–170 μmol/L, 1.7–1.9 mg/dL), heavy proteinuria (ACR 140 mg/mmol, 1.25 g/g; or 2 g albumin per 24 hours). Lipids, blood pressure and glycaemia were all poorly controlled. In IDNT, there was a clear relationship between the degree of albuminuria above 1 g per 24 hours and the rate of decline in renal function. Conversely, the greater the fall in proteinuria, the better the renal outcome. Unfortunately, these remain observations, and the factors influencing the response to angiotensin blockade are not known.

In addition to blood pressure control and angiotensin blockade with a single agent, more complex drug strategies have been used, but so far not in major RCTs. They are worth considering when responses to conventional management are not sufficiently effective, but they are not yet licensed.

High-dose ARB treatment
Proteinuria continues to fall more than blood pressure at very high ARB doses, three or four times the standard doses (e.g. irbesartan 900 mg daily, valsartan 640 mg daily). They appear to be safe and without increased risks of hyperkalaemia or hypotension, but currently would be prohibitively expensive.

High-dose lisinopril
Lisinopril 40 mg daily has additional proteinuria- and blood pressure-reducing effects compared with 20 mg daily in proteinuric type 1 patients,

and without increased adverse effects [14]. This regimen is likely to be safer than combined ARB and ACE-i treatment (see below).

Low-dose spironolactone

Low-dose spironolactone (25 mg daily) in addition to angiotensin blockade reduces proteinuria by about a further 30% in heavy proteinuria, but some of the effect may be related to blood pressure reduction. Hyperkalaemia is a problem, but carefully monitored this may be a valuable agent in some patients. The selective aldosterone blocker eplerenone 50–100 mg daily also additionally reduces proteinuria, but is not licensed in diabetes, because of the high risk of hyperkalaemia.

Combined ACE-i and ARB treatment

This combination was fashionable a few years ago in the management of both hypertension and proteinuria, based on a small study in diabetes that was not confirmed. A major clinical trial (VA NEPHRON-D) is studying the effects of losartan plus lisinopril versus losartan alone on the progression of diabetic nephropathy to hard renal end points. The ONTARGET study (2008) found that telmisartan and ramipril together reduced proteinuria more than ramipril alone, but hard renal end points (dialysis, doubling of serum creatinine and death) were increased on dual therapy and eGFR fell quicker. However, this was in a mixed population, albeit huge, and not primarily proteinuric diabetic patients. Although a cautious trial of combination treatment is worthwhile in heavy proteinuria that has not responded to maximum treatment with a single agent, it should not be used routinely and should be initiated and supervised by a specialist team. Near-complete blockade of the renin–angiotensin–aldosterone system may compromise physiological responses to acute hypovolaemia, for example bleeding, vomiting or diarrhoea, with a risk of acute kidney injury. Advise patients taking combination therapy to stop both if there is vomiting or diarrhoea, and present to the emergency department.

Combined ARB and direct renin inhibitor (aliskiren) treatment

In the AVOID study (2008), aliskiren 300 mg and losartan 100 mg daily reduced ACR by 20% more than placebo, for a similar decrease in blood pressure (to 135/78 mmHg) [15]. This is an encouraging combination, as is aliskiren and irbesartan 300 mg each daily, but the cardiorenal end point ALTITUDE study is not expected to report until 2012. Like combined ACE-i and ARB treatment, it may be worth a trial in individuals with heavy proteinuria, especially those who suffer ACE-i side-effects.

Other management problems in diabetic nephropathy

Glycaemic control

Once nephropathy is established, good control of blood pressure and lipids is probably more important than glycaemic control. Observational studies abound and show that, for example, patients with advanced renal failure entering renal replacement programmes survive longer with a low HbA_{1c}, or that haemodialysis patients with HbA_{1c} above 8% (64 mmol/mol) have an increased risk of sudden death but not myocardial infarction compared with those with HbA_{1c} of 6% (42 mmol/mol) or less [16]. Since nearly all patients with diabetic nephropathy will have advanced macrovascular disease, the cautions of ACCORD should probably be heeded more than observations, and reasonable control (e.g. HbA_{1c} 7.5–8.5%, 59–69 mmol/mol), avoiding hypoglycaemia, will probable serve patients well until formal RCTs of glycaemic control in advanced diabetic renal disease are reported. Regardless, glycaemic control is often difficult to achieve in renal impairment because of:

- other diabetic complications associated with long-duration diabetes (e.g. hypoglycaemia unawareness, gastroparesis);
- decreasing insulin requirements with progressing renal impairment (due to decreased renal insulin clearance and degradation, though it is not a sufficiently reliable factor that insulin doses can be prophylactically reduced as renal impairment progresses, partly because renal failure is itself an insulin-resistant state);
- changes in insulin requirements during and after dialysis sessions;
- the need to discontinue or change doses of non-insulin drugs, and increasing reliance on insulin;
- long-term poor control, partly responsible for the renal impairment itself.

In some, poor nutrition and appetite, decreased muscle and fat mass, and belated awareness of the need for good glucose control conspire to cause very low HbA_{1c} levels. These cannot now be considered safe, but neither can double-figure HbA_{1c} values.

Blood pressure

The benefits of blood pressure treatment in advanced CKD are not established, but home systolic blood pressure readings between dialysis sessions probably give better prognostic information than readings taken in the dialysis unit. Optimum systolic blood pressure is probably 120–130 mmHg, with increased cardiovascular mortality occurring with systolic blood pressure measurements above 180 or below 110–120 mmHg [17]. Antihypertensive treatment is surprisingly well tolerated in these patients. Angiotensin-blocking agents, beta-blockers and calcium channel blockers are all suitable; many patients will be taking loop diuretics.

Cardiac disease

Coronary artery disease is common but dyspnoea or atypical chest symptoms are more common than classical angina in these patients with very limited exercise tolerance. At the onset of dialysis, about 30% of patients have ischaemic heart disease, and heart failure and concentric left ventricular hypertrophy (LVH) are very common. Events are distressingly frequent: type 2 haemodialysis patients have an 8% annual rate of myocardial infarction or coronary death, higher than the 6.6% rate reported in the placebo group of the pioneering 4S study. There is concern that repeated episodes of myocardial stunning during haemodialysis sessions may contribute to heart failure and poor survival. Heavy coronary artery and cardiac valvular calcification is very common, and nearly all type 1 patients have significant coronary artery disease, often with heavy calcification. As in patients with normal renal function, the best algorithm for investigation and management is not known. Resting ECG remains important, but few patients can do standard exercise tolerance tests. Routine two-dimensional echocardiography is limited but certain measurements (e.g. height-indexed left atrial volume) may be of prognostic value. Dobutamine stress echo is not currently recommended for patients with advanced CKD, but stress myocardial perfusion imaging and eventually cardiac MRI may be valuable. Pretransplantation coronary angiography is now routine, as is carotid Doppler scanning.

Lipids (see Chapter 12)

Any patient with any degree of albuminuria or renal impairment must take a statin in the long term. The cardiovascular benefits are at least as great as in patients with normal renal function. Early vigorous treatment, aiming for LDL 1.7–1.8 mmol/L (65–70 mg/dL) and probably lower, is needed. Delaying statin treatment until dialysis does not reduce the very high cardiovascular event rates (4D study, atorvastatin 20 mg daily, 2005; AURORA, rosuvastatin 10 mg daily, 2009), but most patients will have been treated for many years before entering ESRD. There was no excess of serious statin-related muscle side-effects in these studies (i.e. myositis and rhabdomyolysis), and although new proteinuria may occur in a very small proportion, it is tubular proteinuria that does not impact on renal function. In RCTs, statins (especially simvastatin in the HPS, and atorvastatin in CARDS) have a mildly beneficial effect on eGFR, reducing the rate of fall compared with placebo-treated patients. These benefits seem to be particularly great in proteinuric patients, although statins do not reduce new-onset proteinuria or increase regression to normoalbuminuria [18].

However, one study found that in heavily proteinuric non-diabetic patients treated with angiotensin blockers, atorvastatin halved proteinuria from about 2 g per 24 hours to 1 g per 24 hours over a year.

Other agents

Ezetimibe 10 mg daily combined with simvastatin 20 mg daily is safe and effective in pre-dialysis patients, although there are no end-point studies, but avoid fibrates, especially gemfibrozil, and statin–fibrate combinations. Fibrates, much less used now, increase serum creatinine. If increased creatinine synthesis is the reason (one view), then there should be no effect on renal function; another view is that they may decrease production of vasodilatory prostaglandins, and therefore have a real effect on renal function. Serum creatinine may increase by up to 30%, in which case the drug should be withdrawn. Fibrates and angiotensin-blocking agents used together can therefore cause an alarming increase in serum creatinine, especially in patients with impaired renal function; the fibrate should be withdrawn, as it is unlikely to be of prognostic value. High-dose ω-3 fatty acids (e.g. Omacor 4 g daily) improve postprandial lipaemia in the nephrotic syndrome.

Peripheral vascular disease

Peripheral vascular disease and neuro-ischaemic foot lesions are common in patients with nephropathy and ESRD. Medial arterial calcification is widespread and leads to spuriously high systolic blood pressure measurements on Doppler testing (and is responsible for the severe systolic hypertension that is so difficult to manage). Absent foot pulses on clinical examination is the most reliable indicator of peripheral vascular disease in these patients, but the presence of peripheral oedema (stasis, venous disease, heart failure and hypoalbuminaemia) makes evaluation of peripheral vasculature difficult. Assess ischaemic limbs for suitability for angioplasty or vascular bypass. Small and medium arteries can be affected by a specific form of calcification known as calciphylaxis, usually occurring in dialysis patients. Severe skin necrosis and distal limb gangrene can occur. It is very difficult to treat; hyperbaric oxygen might help.

Neuropathy

Most patients with renal impairment will have advanced, though not always symptomatic, peripheral neuropathy. Many will have additional peripheral vascular disease, putting their feet at very high risk of ulceration and gangrene. Regular podiatrist supervision with intensification of input where required and education in foot care can reduce the frequency of serious foot lesions.

Retinopathy

This is extremely common. Type 1 patients may have 'burned out', previously laser-treated, but currently inactive retinopathy. Others suffer recurrent bleeding from proliferative retinopathy, with vitreous and preretinal haemorrhages, frustratingly even in the presence of good glycaemic and blood pressure control. Maculopathy, with or without proliferative changes, with its associated risk of progressive and severe visual loss, is common in type 2 patients.

Renal bone disease

Difficult territory for the non-specialist, but now encompasses disturbed mineral metabolism, abnormalities of bone histology (renal osteodystrophy) and extraskeletal features, such as vascular calcification [19]. These all require specialist management, but significant bone disease can occur relatively early in diabetic CKD and both primary and secondary care teams need to be aware of it, as abnormalities of mineral metabolism and cardiovascular disease may be linked. Secondary hyperparathyroidism may occur as early as stage 2 CKD. Perform bone screen, including PTH, once eGFR is below 60mL/min (i.e. CKD stage 3 or worse), along with routine diabetes blood work. The spectrum of renal bone disease is wide, from adynamic bone disease and osteomalacia, associated with low PTH levels, to severe secondary hyperparathyroidism and classical osteitis fibrosa with high PTH levels, contributing to vascular calcification and increased fracture risk. Both syndromes are common, but adynamic bone disease is very frequent in stage 5 CKD patients, and vitamin D analogues and phosphate binders are partly responsible.

The aims are to reduce the calcium $\times$ phosphate product and to normalize PTH levels. Vitamin D analogues are used where serum calcium is low, but there is much interest in calcimimetics (e.g. cinacalcet) that significantly reduce PTH and the calcium $\times$ phosphate product. The hope is that cinacalcet, now used widely, may have a more consistent long-term effect than vitamin D analogues, and may reduce soft-tissue and vascular calcification.

Anaemia

The normochromic anaemia of erythropoietin deficiency occurs earlier, i.e. at a higher eGFR, in diabetic nephropathy than in non-diabetic renal disease. By CKD stage 3, about 20% of patients have Hb below 11g/dL [20]; anaemia may be more common in men. Prospective non-RCT data strongly linked anaemia with hard end points (e.g. in RENAAL, Hb < 13.8g/dL was associated with progression to ESRD, and Hb < 11.3g/dL with both ESRD and death). Guidelines therefore suggested achieving Hb of 11–13g/dL using one of the erythropoietin-stimulating agents (ESAs).

The most used, recombinant human erythropoietin, is usually given by weekly subcutaneous injection, in the hope that it will improve quality of life, reduce the risk of progression to LVH in pre-dialysis CKD patients, decrease hospitalization in end-stage renal failure, and reduce the incidence of cardiovascular events.

In 2006, two non-placebo-controlled studies (CHOIR and CREATE) that compared achievment of mean Hb of 13 versus 11 g/dL were published. Neither showed the expected major advantages of full anaemia correction, with no decrease in cardiovascular risk but possibly improved quality of life. The definitive placebo-controlled TREAT study (2009) used another ESA, darbepoetin, in type 2 patients with moderate renal impairment and anaemia (eGFR ~30 mL/min, Hb 10.4 g/dL) to raise mean Hb to 12.6 g/dL (placebo 10.6 g/dL). Overall, cardiovascular events were not increased, but the risk of stroke was doubled in the darbepoetin group. Reported hypertension, and both venous and arterial thromboembolic events, were more common. Quality-of-life measures barely changed. Partial correction of anaemia to about 11 g/dL is therefore warranted.

Coexisting iron deficiency is very common and must be fully corrected to maximize the benefit of ESAs. In view of the new lower target level many patients will require only iron treatment (and possibly folate and vitamin B_{12}). Oral and intravenous routes are equally effective in correcting iron deficiency in CKD, but intravenous iron is quicker, is better tolerated and may have a greater effect on quality of life. It can easily be given as a single outpatient infusion, is relatively inexpensive and should be used more than it is [21]. Target ferritin is above 100 μg/L. If an ESA is needed once patients are iron replete, refer to the renal team. ESAs require frequent monitoring, including blood pressure, which can rise. From the diabetes point of view, ESAs increase the number of young red cells, which, less exposed to ambient glycaemia, may cause a factitious fall in HbA_{1c}.

Renal replacement therapy

The decision to start dialysis is often difficult. The clinical decision is based on many factors, including the presence of uraemic symptoms and weight loss, and biochemical measurements including serum creatinine (e.g. serum creatinine 700–800 μmol/L (small mu), eGFR < 12–14 mL/min, falling albumin, hyperkalaemia). For haemodialysis patients, vascular access is usually undertaken when eGFR is about 25 mL/min. Distal vascular calcification often prevents use of the radial artery, and an elbow fistula is often required. Everyone must be made aware of the value of the antecubital fossa vessels, and venous cannulation should be avoided at this site in a pre-dialysis patient.

Until recently peritoneal dialysis was preferred, especially in people with diabetes, as it carried improved medium-term survival and preservation of residual renal function compared with haemodialysis. The emergence of the serious complication of encapsulating peritoneal sclerosis has tempered enthusiasm for the technique of late, and there has been a consistent decline in the use of peritoneal dialysis over the past 10 years.

Renal transplantation is now routine for ESRD patients with diabetes, a transformation over the past 20 years. However, survival is still not as high as in non-diabetic transplant patients. The results of live donor transplantation are consistently better than with deceased donor kidneys. Worse glucose control after transplantation is associated with poorer patient (but not graft) survival, but studies are retrospective and as in other areas hyperglycaemia may be a marker of less measurable but more important factors.

Pancreas, kidney–pancreas and islet transplantation

Renal transplantation is appropriate for both type 1 and type 2 patients, but in type 1 patients always consider whether pancreatic or islet transplantation might also be beneficial, especially in patients with recurrent severe hypoglycaemia, uncontrolled hyperglycaemia despite intensification of insulin treatment, and early potentially reversible microvascular complications (Box 8.2). Pancreas-alone transplants are less often given because of the relatively high rate of graft failure. Simultaneous pancreas–kidney transplants now comprise up to 20% of procedures, as kidney graft survival is at least as high as in kidney-alone transplants, and patient survival higher, probably due to the normoglycaemia achieved after pancreas transplant. Pancreas-after-kidney procedures are also highly successful, whether performed early or late. Long-term restoration of normoglycaemia, defined as non-diabetic HbA_{1c} below 5% (31 mmol/mol) with normal acute insulin response, is now achievable. Microvascular complications, except for autonomic neuropathy, begin to stabilize and improve within a few years, and intermediate measures of cardiovascular risk, for example CIMT, also improve. Despite the formidable surgery, and the need for lifelong immunosuppression, improvement in quality of life in many cases is dramatic.

Islet transplantation
Interest in islet transplantation increased after Shapiro and colleagues in Edmonton reported success in 2000 using a novel islet isolation technique, intra-portal delivery of islets, and steroid-free immunosuppression with

180 | Chapter 8

Box 8.2 Indications for pancreatic transplantation

Simultaneous pancreas–kidney transplant
- Type 1 diabetes with ESRD
- No option for live-related kidney donor
- Patient wishes simultaneous transplant rather than waiting for pancreas after having had a renal transplant

Pancreas-after-kidney transplant transplant
- There is a live kidney donor, and wishes to have a later pancreas transplant
- Patient established with a well-functioning kidney transplant, and wants the additional advantages of stable glucose control

Pancreas alone transplant
- No kidney failure
- Frequent, severe and acute metabolic emergencies (DKA, hypoglycaemia and hyperglycaemia)
- Injected insulin therapy that generated very severe clinical and emotional problems
- Insulin-based management consistently unable to prevent acute complications

Source: after Larsen JL. *Endocr Rev* 2004;25:919–46.

daclizumab, tacrolimus and sirolimus. Around 550 islet transplantations were performed between 2000 and 2006. In an international collaborative study using the Edmonton technique (2006), which permitted up to three islet infusions per patient, nearly half of recipients were insulin independent after a year, about one-quarter had partial graft function (usually requiring some insulin treatment) and the remaining one-quarter had complete graft loss. However, even partial graft function protects against severe hypoglycaemia, one of the major indications for islet transplantation. Further refinements are likely to improve outcome and side-effects, the latter still common even with the slimmed-down immunosuppression regimen [22].

References

1. Burrows NR, Li Y, Geiss LS. Incidence of treatment for end-stage renal disease among individuals with diabetes in the U.S. continues to decline. *Diabetes Care* 2010;33:73–7. PMID: 20040673.
2. Adler AI, Stevens RJ, Manley SE, Bilous RW, Cull CA, Holman RR. Development and progression of nephropathy in type 2 diabetes: the United

Kingdom Prospective Diabetes Study (UKPDS 64). *Kidney Int* 2003;63:225–32. PMID: 12472787.

3. Pham TT, Sim JJ, Kujubu DA, Liu IL, Kumar VA. Prevalence of nondiabetic renal disease in diabetic patients. *Am J Nephrol* 2007;27:322–8. PMID: 17495429.

4. Romão JE, Haiashi AR, Elias RM *et al*. Positive acute-phase inflammatory markers in different stages of chronic kidney disease. *Am J Nephrol* 2006;26: 59–66. PMID: 16508248.

5. Houlihan CA, Tsalamandris C, Akdeniz A, Jerums G. Albumin to creatinine ratio: a screening test with limitations. *Am J Kidney Dis* 2002;39:1183–9. PMID: 12046029.

6. Stoycheff N, Stevens LA, Schmid CH *et al*. Nephrotic syndrome in diabetic kidney disease: an evaluation and update of the definition. *Am J Kidney Dis* 2009;54:840–9. PMID: 19556043.

7. Fonseca V, Thomas M, Katrak A, Sweny P, Moorhead JF. Can urinary thyroid hormone loss cause hypothyroidism? *Lancet* 1991;338:475–6. PMID: 1678446.

8. Bilous R, Chaturvedi N, Sjølie AK *et al*. Effect of candesartan on microalbuminuria and albumin excretion rate in diabetes: three randomized trials. *Ann Intern Med* 2009;151:11–20. PMID: 19451554.

9. Ruggenenti P, Fassi A, Ilieva AP *et al*. Preventing microalbuminuria in type 2 diabetes. Bergamo Nephrologic Diabetes Complications Trial (BENEDICT) investigators. *N Engl J Med* 2004;351:1941–51. PMID: 15516697.

10. Perkins BA, Ficociello LH, Silva KH, Finkelstein DM, Warram JH, Krolewski AS. Regression of microalbuminuria in type 1 diabetes. *N Engl J Med* 2003;348:2285–93. PMID: 12788992.

11. Gæde P, Lund-Andersen H, Parving HH, Pederson O. Effect of a multifactorial intervention on mortality in type 2 diabetes. *N Engl J Med* 2008;358:580–91. PMID: 18256393.

12. House AA, Eliasziw M, Cattran DC *et al*. Effect of B-vitamin therapy on progression of diabetic nephropathy: a randomized controlled trial. *JAMA* 2010;303:1603–9. PMID: 20424250.

13. The ASTRAL Investigators. Revascularization versus medical therapy for renal-artery stenosis. *N Engl J Med* 2009;361:1953–62. PMID: 19907042.

14. Schjoedt KJ, Astrup AS, Persson F *et al*. Optimal dose of lisinopril for renoprotection in type 1 diabetic patients with diabetic nephropathy: a randomised crossover trial. *Diabetologia* 2009;52:46–9. PMID: 18974967.

15. Parving HH, Persson F, Lewis JB, Lewis EJ, Hollenberg NK. Aliskiren combined with losartan in type 2 diabetes and nephropathy. AVOID Study Investigators. *N Engl J Med* 2008;358:2433–46. PMID: 18525041.

16. Drechsler C, Krane V, Ritz E, März W, Wanner C. Glycemic control and cardiovascular events in diabetic hemodialysis patients. *Circulation* 2009;120:2421–8. PMID: 19948978.

17. Agarwal R. Blood pressure and mortality among hemodialysis patients. *Hypertension* 2010;55:762–8. PMID: 20083728.

18. Colhoun HM, Betteridge DJ, Durrington PN *et al*. Effects of atorvastatin on kidney outcomes and cardiovascular disease in patients with diabetes: an

analysis from the Collaborative Atorvastatin Diabetes Study (CARDS). *Am J Kidney Dis* 2009;54:810–19. PMID: 19540640.

19. Gal-Moscovici A, Sprague SM. Bone health in chronic kidney disease–mineral and bone disease. *Adv Chronic Kidney Dis* 2007;14:27–36. PMID: 17200041.
20. New JP, Aung T, Baker PG *et al.* The high prevalence of unrecognized anaemia in patients with diabetes and chronic kidney disease: a population-based study. *Diabetic Med* 2008;25:564–9. PMID: 18445169.
21. Agarwal R, Rizkala AR, Bastani B, Kaskas MO, Leehey DJ, Besarab A. A randomized controlled trial of oral versus intravenous iron in chronic kidney disease. *Am J Nephrol* 2006;26:445–54. PMID 17035697.
22. Shapiro AMJ, Ricordi C, Hering BJ *et al.* International trial of the Edmonton protocol for islet transplantation. *N Engl J Med* 2006;355:1318–30. PMID: 17005949.

Further reading

Larsen JL. Pancreas transplantation: indications and consequences. *Endocr Rev* 2004;25:919–46. PMID: 15583023.
Mehdi U, Toto RD. Anemia, diabetes, and chronic kidney disease. *Diabetes Care* 2009;32:1320–6. PMID: 19564475. Review published a short time before TREAT reported.

Websites
Web-based eGFR calculation (MDRD equation): http://nephron.com/mdrd/default.html and www.kidney.org/professionals/kdoqi/gfr_page.cfm
National Kidney Disease Education Program: www.nkdep.nih.gov

Diabetes and the eye

CHAPTER 9

Key points

- In type 1 diabetes, visual loss resulting from the complications of proliferative retinopathy is now uncommon.
- In type 2 diabetes, visual loss is usually caused by macular oedema that is often resistant to laser treatment and also to improvement with intensive glycaemic control.
- Laser photocoagulation and advanced vitreoretinal techniques have improved the visual prognosis in individual patients.
- Good glycaemic control markedly decreases the emergence and progression of retinopathy in type 1 diabetes; intensive control in UKPDS and ACCORD Eye (HbA$_{1c}$ about 6.5–7.0%, 48–53 mmol/mol) also reduces progression of retinopathy (but probably has no effect on visual outcomes) in type 2 diabetes.
- In UKPDS, more intensive blood pressure control reduced progression of retinopathy, but this benefit was not seen in either ACCORD Eye or ADVANCE, where blood pressure differentials were less pronounced than in the earlier study.
- Adjuvant medical treatment with angiotensin blockade and aspirin does not slow the progression of retinopathy, but fenofibrate seems to have an as-yet unexplained beneficial effect in reducing retinopathy progression (ACCORD) and the need for laser treatment (FIELD).
- Multimodal intervention (e.g. Steno-2 study) holds out the best hope for reduction of retinopathy in type 2 diabetes.
- Intravitreal anti-VEGF agents and systemic protein kinase C inhibitors may be of value.

(Continued)

Practical Diabetes Care, 3rd edition. © David Levy.
Published 2011 by Blackwell Publishing Ltd.

> - Rigorous retinal screening programmes can potentially reduce visual loss, but do not forget other eye pathologies in people with diabetes, especially cataract and glaucoma.
> - Patients attending specialist retinopathy clinics have high rates of other complications, and must be referred to the appropriate clinical setting for intensive medical care.

Introduction

Diabetic retinopathy is the most common clinically significant microvascular complication of diabetes, but cataract is the most common ocular complication, with a prevalence of about 60% in those aged 30–54, five times more frequent than in those without diabetes. Diabetes is also associated with raised intraocular pressure and chronic open-angle glaucoma, and retinal venous and arterial occlusions are also more common. Neovascular age-related macular degeneration (AMD) and diabetic retinopathy have pathogenic features in common (and also some treatment options), and macular degeneration is more common in people with vascular disease, such as hypertension or history of myocardial infarction, though there is no clear link with diabetes. Comprehensive eye screening in diabetes should therefore include all these important pathologies as well as others unrelated to diabetes, including simple refraction problems. Fear of visual loss is common, recurrent and pervasive in many people with diabetes, and is independent of objective measures of retinopathy and visual acuity. The fear is rarely articulated spontaneously, but must be recognized by the diabetes team.

The widespread introduction of retinopathy screening programmes has reduced the need for routine retinal examination in both primary and secondary care. Nevertheless, skilled direct ophthalmoscopy is still an important procedure (Box 9.1). While tight glycaemic control may not be as important in the management of retinopathy in type 2 diabetes as was previously believed, DCCT/EDIC confirms that glycaemia is the main, possibly the only, driving force behind early retinopathy in type 1 diabetes, while multimodal management of type 2 diabetes remains critical. The significance of retinopathy therefore varies with the individual, and is much wider than a referral pathway to the ophthalmology service.

Retinopathy in type 1 diabetes

Clinically significant retinopathy is uncommon within 5 years of diagnosis, but in the population screened for the DCCT, two-thirds with duration of less than 5 years had some detectable retinopathy.

> **Box 9.1 Practical points relating to retinal examination in diabetes**
>
> - Check visual acuity before pupil dilatation.
> - Use 1% tropicamide drops, one drop each eye. Apply to the inner lower lid to aid rapid absorption and decrease discomfort (tropicamide stings, so warn patients).
> - Leave at least 20 min before retinal examination or photography.
> - If pupils do not dilate sufficiently (common in people with dark irises), repeat tropicamide 1% one drop in each eye, and add phenylephrine 2.5% one drop in each eye.
> - Advise patients not to drive for at least 2 hours after drops.
> - Treated open-angle glaucoma and modern lens implants are not contraindications to pupil dilatation (though old traditions die hard), but advise patients about the unlikely possibility of developing a painful red eye, in which case they should attend accident and emergency urgently.
> - Most patients, except younger type 1 patients with no other diabetes complications, should also have a comprehensive annual eye examination with an optometrist.
>
> *Source*: adapted from Dodson PM (ed.) *Diabetic Retinopathy: Screening to Treatment*. Oxford: Oxford University Press, 2008

Undoubtedly the natural history has changed. The Wisconsin study, published in the mid-1980s, showed a near-100% prevalence of some degree of retinopathy after 15–20 years of type 1 diabetes, with proliferative retinopathy peaking at about 60% at 20–35 years' duration, and severe visual impairment in 2.4%. By the early 2000s, at least in Oslo, Norway, the prevalence of proliferative retinopathy at the same duration was only 11%, and in the intensively treated DCCT group fewer than 1% were blind [1]. This gratifying reduction must be due to improved long-term glycaemic control, but strangely there is little evidence that this has occurred. Patients with 20–24 years' duration, especially those with onset before age 15 years, are at the greatest risk of developing proliferative retinopathy; ensure this group has regular retinal screening.

Retinopathy in type 2 diabetes

The picture is quite different in type 2 diabetes, where 20–30% have retinopathy at diagnosis, and 10–25% proliferative retinopathy 10 years after diagnosis. Evidence is conflicting whether blindness caused by diabetic retinopathy is decreasing; however, as recently as 2004, diabetes was still the commonest cause of blindness and visual impairment in working-age people in western Scotland. However, do not underestimate the visual impact of less severe retinopathy; for example, patients with macular oedema have impaired quality of life similar in degree to non-diabetic patients with AMD [2].

Classification of retinopathy

The clinical classification of retinopathy remains important to the clinician and the patient, whereas the many and complex grading systems for severity of retinopathy are more relevant to the epidemiologist and clinical triallist. A simple international retinopathy severity scale has been proposed based on the presence of red lesions only, but the following notes use the more traditional classification of:

1 non-proliferative diabetic retinopathy (NPDR)
2 pre-proliferative diabetic retinopathy
3 proliferative diabetic retinopathy
4 maculopathy
5 advanced diabetic eye disease.

Non-proliferative diabetic retinopathy

Background retinopathy
Microaneurysms
Small, red, intraretinal lesions usually found at the posterior pole of the eye, around the disc and macula. They occur in areas of capillary non-perfusion and show leakage of fluorescein. It is worthwhile estimating the number of microaneurysms as it has some prognostic significance; the more there are, the greater the risk of progression to proliferative retinopathy. On their own they do not reduce visual acuity unless at the macula, where even a very small number can significantly affect vision.

Hard exudates
Waxy yellow dots or plaques formed by extravasated plasma proteins. Like microaneurysms, they occur early in the course of retinopathy, and affect vision only if they form at the macula.

Intraretinal haemorrhages
These are caused by ruptured capillaries situated deeper in the retina than those causing microaneurysms. They can occur in non-diabetic conditions (e.g. anaemia, leukaemia or hypertension) unrelated to diabetes. There are different types, not always clearly distinguished, and several forms may occur in the same retina:
• dot and blot;
• flame-shaped haemorrhages in the retinal nerve fibre layer, which often look striated, are common in non-diabetic hypertension and sometimes also occur transiently in well-controlled type 1 diabetes;

- deeper haemorrhages with irregular outlines;
- large, dark, 'cluster' haemorrhages.

Cotton-wool spots (soft exudates)

These white fluffy-edged lesions, unlike the waxy, more yellow hard exudates, represent accumulation of axoplasmic material adjacent to a retinal infarct. An occasional cotton-wool spot is of little significance, but in greater numbers (> 5) they may indicate rapidly advancing retinopathy, associated hypertension, or unrelated conditions (e.g. vasculitis).

Multiple soft exudates frequently accompany pre-proliferative retinopathy, though this view has been challenged. Distinguish between soft exudates and soft drusen, associated with progression to AMD: drusen occur only at the macula, and symmetrically in both eyes.

Management

Patients with either no retinopathy or with NPDR but no maculopathy are invited for rescreening in England every year. No ophthalmological treatment is required for NPDR, but 6-monthly examination may be valuable in patients with multiple lesions of background retinopathy (sometimes aptly described as 'active' retinopathy), especially if there is poor control of glucose and blood pressure, as there is a risk of rapid progression. In addition, there are several important practical points relating to diabetes management and background retinopathy.

Management of background retinopathy (Box 9.2)

Glycaemic control

Maintaining HbA_{1c} at 7% (53 mmol/mol) in the DCCT reduced the rate of progression in those with background changes at baseline (about 10%

Box 9.2 Management of background retinopathy

- Retinal screening every year, more frequently if 'active' retinopathy.
- Retinal examinations every 3 months in patients starting intensive glycaemic control, especially where baseline HbA_{1c} is high and there is background retinopathy.
- $HbA_{1c} < 7.0\%$ (53 mmol/L) without hypoglycaemia.
- Blood pressure $< 140/80$ mmHg, $< 130/75$ mmHg if microalbuminuria.
- Angiotensin blockade is of little value unless there is microalbuminuria (type 2).
- Optimize lipid profiles; consider fenofibrate in type 2 patients if progressing retinopathy.
- Aspirin in type 2 patients to reduce cardiovascular events.
- Smoking is associated with proliferative retinopathy and visual impairment in type 1 patients. Cessation is a priority.

progression at HbA_{1c} 7%, and about half that rate at 6%, 42 mmol/mol). Almost identical results were obtained in type 2 diabetes in the intensive intervention group in UKPDS. More recent studies have not given consistent messages: neither VADT nor ADVANCE (including a detailed retinal substudy, AdRem [3]) found intensive glycaemic control to improve any measure of retinopathy, but ACCORD Eye showed a substantial effect of very intensive glycaemic control (HbA_{1c} ~ 6.5%), though with an attendant risk of hypoglycaemia and possible increased overall mortality [4]. Taking the results of UKPDS and ACCORD Eye together, patients with retinopathy should aim for HbA_{1c} levels between 6.5 and 7.0%, though it is still not clear whether maculopathy responds in the same way.

DCCT/EDIC demonstrated a dramatic 'legacy' effect of tight glycaemic control on retinopathy in type 1 diabetes; the benefits outlasted the relaxation of intensive control by at least 7 years. However, the effect had disappeared by year 10 of EDIC in adolescents who had entered DCCT. Control was worse than in the adults during DCCT (HbA_{1c} 8.9%, 74 mmol/mol vs. 8.1%, 65 mmol/mol), though there was no difference during EDIC. This finding reinforces the need for the best possible glycaemic control from the outset in type 1 diabetes. Intensive multimodal intervention in the Steno-2 study accounts for a similar legacy effect in type 2 diabetes. Even though glycaemic control was indifferent, retinopathy progression, laser treatment and blindness were all markedly reduced in the original intensively managed group; Steno-2-like interventions should be mandatory, regardless of the glycaemia.

Effect of rapid improvement in glycaemic control on retinopathy
Rapidly improving glycaemic control can cause sometimes dramatic but transient deterioration in retinopathy. It was first noted in the 1980s in studies of intensive control in type 1 diabetes, and later in DCCT. The mechanism is not known, but retinal ischaemia is involved, as the hallmark lesion is cotton-wool spots, which develop within 3–6 months but which usually resolve by 1 year. Laser treatment is occasionally needed, but the eventual visual outcomes are consistently better if good control is maintained. Whenever intensive treatment starts, especially where there is poor baseline glycaemic control, close retinal monitoring is important. DCCT suggests 3-monthly monitoring in high-risk groups, for example:
- in the preconception period and early pregnancy;
- in patients starting pump therapy or any intensive therapy when in poor control;
- any patient with known retinopathy where there has been a fall in HbA_{1c} of over 2% (22 mmol/mol), whatever the reason.

The situation in type 2 diabetes, especially the development of macular oedema, is not clear. Massive reductions in HbA_{1c} (e.g. 4–6%,

44–66 mmol/mol) can occur over a short period with any form of intensive intervention, including bariatric surgery (see Chapter 6). In patients with known retinopathy, monitoring every 3–6 months would be wise, but there is no evidence for this approach, and it may be difficult to organize. Glitazone use has been associated with cases of macular oedema, but in large-scale trials does not seem to be overall more common (see Chapter 6).

Blood pressure and angiotensin blocker treatment
As more trials report, evidence for the benefit of intensive blood pressure reduction on retinopathy in type 2 diabetes becomes less clear-cut, perhaps because patients are entering modern clinical trials with better overall control of blood pressure. In the UKPDS, intensive blood pressure control (144/82 from 160/94 mmHg at baseline) over 6–9 years reduced progression of retinopathy and visual deterioration, but maintaining approximately the same levels for 4 years in the ADVANCE trial (baseline 145/81, achieved 138/78 mmHg) had little benefit, and neither did even more intensive control in ACCORD Eye (baseline 139/77, achieved 119/64 mmHg). Nevertheless in microalbuminuric patients, such as those in Steno-2, blood pressure should be maintained at about 130/70 mmHg in order to contribute to lowering the risk of retinopathy.

Specific drugs have been studied. In EUCLID/EURODIAB (1998) the ACE-i lisinopril reduced the risk of retinopathy progression, including progression to proliferative retinopathy in type 1 diabetes, but it was a short study and the treatment groups were unabalanced. In the large DIRECT studies (2008), candesartan 32 mg daily for 5 years slightly reduced the risk of developing new-onset retinopathy, but did not slow progression of pre-existing retinopathy in type 1 diabetes [5]. In type 2 patients with mild-to-moderate retinopathy, the same regimen improved outcomes (modest effect on regression and reducing overall retinopathy) [6]. All patients had negative microalbuminuria (or they would already have been taking angiotensin blockade). Translating these undramatic findings into clinical practice is difficult. In type 1 patients, it would be difficult to justify this length of drug treatment in patients without retinopathy when DCCT showed that good glycaemic control would have a greater effect on retinopathy prevention and progression (and would reduce all other complications as well), though it might be justifiable in the chronically poorly controlled. Very few type 2 patients escape angiotensin blockade treatment for other indications.

Other agents
Aspirin, even at high doses (e.g. 650 mg/day in the ETDRS study in type 1 and 2 patients), does not benefit retinopathy, but it reduces the risk of myocardial infarction. However, it does not increase the risk of

retinal haemorrhage. Aspirin use should therefore be based on assessment of cardiovascular risk without regard to retinopathy status (see Chapter 11). There is no evidence for its benefit in type 1 patients with isolated background retinopathy. Atorvastatin may slightly reduce the need for laser treatment in type 2 diabetes (CARDS) but the effect was not statistically singnificant. Fenofibrate 200 mg daily in the FIELD study (2007) had a more dramatic effect (40% reduction) on the need for laser treatment in mildly dyslipidaemic type 2 patients, but it had no long-term effect on the lipid profile in this study, so another mechanism must be responsible. Very interestingly, fenofibrate reduced the risk of significant progression of retinopathy in ACCORD Eye (see Chapter 12) in patients already taking simvastatin; two major trials have now confirmed that fenofibrate reduces the risk of severe retinopathy. Although the mechanism is not clear, there may be now some justification for the use of this agent in patients with progressing retinopathy, where all other risk factors are under control. Patients, especially type 1, must stop smoking, as current smoking is associated with proliferative changes and visual impairment.

Pre-proliferative retinopathy

An important diagnosis, as there is a very high risk of progression to proliferative retinopathy and significant visual loss. Pre-proliferative changes are characterized by the following.
- Multiple (> 5) cotton-wool spots.
- Multiple large blot haemorrhages.
- Venous abnormalities: irregularities, beading, looping or reduplication.
- Intraretinal microvascular abnormalities: these resemble new vessels, and branch abnormally (in frequency, number and angulation) but they are intraretinal, so do not cause preretinal or vitreous haemorrhage. It is very difficult for the non-expert to spot them, but like true proliferative retinopathy they are unlikely to occur in isolation, without apparent background changes.

Prompt ophthalmological referral is needed for careful follow-up and possible laser treatment. Despite the dramatic retinal appearances, most patients do not have visual symptoms; discuss the importance of attending appointments.

Proliferative retinopathy

Retinal neovascularization
This comprises NVE (retinal new vessels; new vessels elsewhere), arising from veins, usually at a bifurcation, and NVD (new vessels at the

optic disc). Growth factors, especially vascular endothelial growth factor (VEGF), released from ischaemic retina, lead to proliferation. Proliferating vessels lie in the preretinal space, between the retina and the posterior surface of the vitreous, and may bleed into the preretinal space or the vitreous. Although proliferative retinopathy is characteristic of type 1 diabetes, it frequently occurs in type 2, just as maculopathy is not restricted to type 2 diabetes. Proliferative changes in type 2 patients are associated with advanced coronary artery disease. In the VADT baseline cohort (mean age 62 years, very long duration of 21 years), median Agatston coronary artery calcification score in these patients was about 1000, where a score over 400 suggests a high risk of occlusive coronary artery disease [7]. At the very least, simple cardiac screening tests should be carried out in these high-risk patients, but this requires a high level of integrated diabetes care that is just as important as a retinal screening and referral service. Paradoxically, as retinal screening becomes more efficient, patients may be less likely to be known to their specialist diabetes teams: patients attending retinopathy clinics have a very high rate of associated complications, especially microalbuminuria (about 70% in those with proliferative retinopathy), and there is a high smoking rate (16%) [8]. This is an important message for primary care teams.

Treatment
Treatment of proliferative retinopathy is with panretinal (scatter) laser photocoagulation using green-only lasers. How laser treatment works is still not understood, but it must be applied to areas of capillary non-perfusion and retinal ischaemia. Severe visual loss is reduced by about 50%, but it is destructive treatment and it is important for patients to understand that it stabilizes, but does not improve, visual function. Fortunately, the loss of peripheral and night vision that often occurred with heavy peripheral laser treatment is less common now. Effective treatment, usually requiring 2000 or more retinal burns in each eye over two or more sessions, is demanding for operator and patient alike. Macular oedema can worsen after panretinal laser treatment.

Maculopathy

Maculopathy is retinopathy occurring at or close to the fovea. It is common, occurring in 10% of the VADT cohort, was two to three times more prevalent in Hispanic and African-American groups, and was associated with diastolic hypertension and amputation. Visual impairment is usually caused by macular oedema, macular ischaemia, or a combination of the two. Neither can be diagnosed with direct ophthalmoscopy, though the presence of oedema can be inferred from the frequent finding of a grey patch of retina with central microaneurysms and surrounding (circinate) exudates. Optical coherence tomography is now the most important technique for measuring and monitoring macular oedema. Macular ischaemia can only be definitively diagnosed using fluorescein angiography, though it is not usually needed.

Ophthalmologists use the term 'clinically significant macular oedema' (CSMO; CSME in North America) to describe patterns of macular oedema that if not laser treated will result in significant visual loss. Laser treatment is generally effective where the central macula is involved and visual acuity is 6/9 (20/30) or worse. Other varieties of maculopathy are less responsive, and careful clinical judgement and discussion with the patient is required. Focal laser treatment is used to treat localized retinal thickening; where there is diffuse macular oedema, often associated with circinate exudates, grid laser treatment, avoiding the fovea, is often effective. In long-standing macular oedema, large macular plaques of exudate can occur. While resistant to laser treatment, intensive lipid lowering may help plaque regression. Since these patients usually have other vascular complications, statin treatment is in any case mandatory, but this is one situation where targeting very low LDL levels (e.g. < 1.5 mmol/L, 60 mg/dL) may be helpful, though evidence is sparse. Diabetic maculopathy often does not respond to standard treatment (despite ophthalmologists' frequent requests to diabetes teams, tight glycaemic control of itself does not improve it), and intravitreal and systemic drugs are frequently used off-licence (see below). Maculopathy is strongly associated with obstructive sleep apnoea (OSA) in men.

Advanced diabetic eye disease

Advanced diabetic eye disease is visual loss caused by the complications of proliferative retinopathy or maculopathy. Retinal ischaemia, common to all forms of severe retinopathy, induces a fibrovascular response. The resulting fibrous tissue leads to traction effects, i.e. avulsion of retinal blood vessels, tractional retinal detachment and neovascularization of the iris.

Avulsion of retinal blood vessels causes haemorrhage.

- *Preretinal (subhyaloid) haemorrhage.* Boat-shaped with a horizontal fluid level, and may be precipitated by hypoglycaemia or Valsalva manoeuvre. They often form inferotemporal to the optic disc. If haemorrhage obscures the macula, the presentation is with acute visual loss; elsewhere, there may only be 'floaters'. Preretinal haemorrhage implies proliferative changes, which may be obscured by the haemorrhage. If detected on routine retinal screening, urgent referral is needed, as it may presage a visually catastrophic vitreous haemorrhage.

- *Vitreous haemorrhage.* Again, usually associated with proliferative changes. They are large dense haemorrhages causing acute visual loss. Spontaneous clearing and improvement in vision occurs very slowly, over months, but there is a risk of further bleeds with less chance of resolution. Vitrectomy, usually with endolaser photocoagulation, can achieve impressive results.

Neovascularization of the iris (rubeosis iridis), usually associated with widespread retinal ischaemia or tractional retinal detachment, may lead to rubeotic glaucoma when the canal of Schlemm, draining the aqueous humour, blocks off. Pain is intense, it is difficult to treat, and the visual prognosis is poor. It is fortunately exceedingly rare in modern practice.

Cataract

Diabetes is a strong risk factor for cataract, and it occurs earlier and progresses faster than in the non-diabetic population. Cortical cataract is the most frequent, with its typical radial spoke opacities. Indications for cataract surgery include impairment of vision that reduces quality of life, and suspicion of retinopathy or other retinal or optic nerve pathology obscured by cataract.

Cataract surgery in diabetes is more difficult and carries worse visual outcomes. Complications are more frequent, for example rapid progression of retinopathy, posterior capsule opacification, iris neovascularization and, very rarely, endophthalmitis, but results are continually improving. Systemic α-adrenergic blocking drugs for hypertension, often used in diabetes, are associated with the rare intraoperative floppy iris syndrome. The optimum timing of laser treatment in relation to cataract surgery is still debated [9].

Retinal vascular occlusions

Occlusions of the retinal artery and vein (and their branches) are common. Atherosclerotic risk factors are, naturally, associated with arterial occlusion, and retinal artery occlusions are more common in diabetes, but the association with venous occlusions is less strong. Most patients will present to the ophthalmologist, but diabetes team input is important.

Retinal artery occlusions

Both central and branch retinal artery occlusions frequently result from microemboli from atherosclerotic plaques and calcified cardiac valves. They present with acute unilateral visual impairment. Importantly, the retina may appear normal, but is usually whitened and opacified (segmental if there has been a branch occlusion). The cherry-red spot is characteristic. Investigate a structural source with a carotid Doppler study and an echocardiogram. All vascular risk factors must be carefully managed, especially smoking. There are no specific ophthalmological treatments. Non-arteritic ischaemic optic neuropathy causes painless visual loss through occlusion of the posterior ciliary artery supplying the optic nerve. It has been rarely associated with the phosphodiesterase (PDE)5 inhibitors used in the treatment of erectile dysfunction (see Chapter 10).

Retinal vein occlusions

These are more common than arterial occlusions, and again can be central or branch. They may not be primary events; a thickened atherosclerotic retinal artery overlying a vein at an arteriovenous crossing may disturb blood flow and cause thrombosis. The major risk factor is hypertension, but ocular hypertension and other vascular risk factors are important. The retinal appearance is characteristic and dramatic ('tomato splash'), with widespread haemorrhages, and is sometimes mistaken for advanced retinopathy. Again, management of arterial risk factors is important, but investigate for a prothrombotic cause in patients with previous venous thromboembolic disease. Macular grid treatment is probably the best at present, but anti-VEGF treatments are being trialled, and a 6-month course of intravitreal bevacizumab may improve the visual outcome.

New developments

Several drugs are in development or in clinical trials that may retard progression of pre-proliferative retinopathy or maculopathy. The main interest is in maculopathy, which frequently does not respond to standard treatments. Ruboxistaurin, an orally active protein kinase C β-isoform antagonist, has been in trials for several years. It does not seem to retard progression of retinopathy, but it slows progression of maculopathy and moderately severe to very severe non-proliferative retinopathy. Further trials are in progress. There is increasing interest in agents that bind or antagonize VEGF and which, given by intravitreal injection, are already in widespread use in neovascular AMD. These include the recombinant humanized monoclonal antibodies bevacizumab (Avastin) and its modification ranibizumab (Lucentis); small studies have given inconsistent results but, pending substantive RCTs, they are often used off-licence in macular oedema which is not responding to other treatments, and where the maculopathy is so close to the avascular zone that laser treatment is not possible. There is also interest in their use in proliferative retinopathy, and substantial trials are in progress. Pegaptanib, which binds VEGF, may also prove valuable, as may aflibercept, an inhibitor of VEGF receptor expression. There is concern that systemic absorption of these agents may carry a small risk of thromboembolism. Intravitreal glucocorticoids (e.g. triamcinolone) have been used in macular oedema, but are probably less effective than laser treatment. They tend to cause raised intraocular pressure, and late cataract formation is common.

References

1. Nathan DM, Zinman B, Cleary PA *et al*. Modern-day clinical course of type 1 diabetes mellitus after 30 years' duration: the Diabetes Control and Complications Trial/Epidemiology of Diabetes Interventions and Complications and Pittsburgh epidemiology of diabetes complications experience (1983–2005). *Arch Intern Med* 2009;169:1307–16. PMID: 19636033.
2. Hariprasad SM, Mieler WF, Grassi M, Green JL, Jager RD, Miller L. Vision-related quality of life in patients with diabetic macular oedema. *Br J Ophthalmol* 2008;92:89–92. PMID: 17584999.
3. Beulens JW, Patel A, Vingerling JR *et al*. Effects of blood pressure lowering and intensive glucose control on the incidence and progression of retinopathy in patients with type 2 diabetes mellitus: a randomised controlled trial. *Diabetologia* 2009;52:2027–36. PMID: 19633827.
4. Chew EY, Ambrosius WT, Davis MD *et al*. Effects of medical therapies on retinopathy progression in type 2 diabetes. ACCORD Study Group and ACCORD Eye Study Group. *N Engl J Med* 2010;363:233–44.
5. Chaturvedi N, Porta M, Klein R *et al*. Effect of candesartan on prevention (DIRECT-Prevent 1) and progression (DIRECT-Protect 1) of retinopathy in type 1 diabetes: randomised, placebo-controlled trials. *Lancet* 2008;372:1394–402. PMID: 18823656.
6. Sjølie AK, Klein R, Porta M *et al*. Effect of candesartan on progression and regression of retinopathy in type 2 diabetes (DIRECT-Protect 2): a randomised placebo-controlled trial. *Lancet* 2008;372:1385–93. PMID: 18823658.
7. Reaven PD, Emanuelle N, Moritz T *et al*. Proliferative diabetic retinopathy in type 2 patients is related to coronary artery calcium in the Veterans Affairs Diabetes Trial (VADT). *Diabetes Care* 2008;31:952–7. PMID: 18316393.
8. Al-Ansari SA, Tennant MT, Freve MD, Hinz BJ, Senior PA. Short report: suboptimal diabetes care in high-risk diabetic patients attending a specialist retina clinic. *Diabetic Med* 2009;26:1296–300. PMID: 20002485.
9. Shah AS, Chen SH. Cataract surgery and diabetes. *Curr Opin Ophthalmol* 2010;21:4–9. PMID: 19935423.

Further reading

Dodson PM (ed.) *Diabetic Retinopathy: Screening to Treatment*. Oxford: Oxford University Press, 2008.
Donnelly R (ed.) *Vascular Complications of Diabetes: Current Issues in Pathogenesis and Treatment*. Oxford: Wiley-Blackwell, 2002.
Fong DS, Aiello L, Gardner TS *et al*. Retinopathy in diabetes. *Diabetes Care* 2004;27(Suppl. 1):S84–S87. PMID: 14693935.

Scanlon P, Aldington S, Wilkinson C, Matthews D. *A Practical Manual of Diabetic Retinopathy Management*. Oxford: Wiley-Blackwell, 2009.

Simó R, Hernández C. Advances in the medical treatment of diabetic retinopathy. *Diabetes Care* 2009;32:1556–62.

Websites

Diabetic Retinopathy Candesartan Trials (reported 2008): www.direct-results.org

Royal College of Ophthalmologists. Guidelines for diabetic retinopathy (2005): www.rcophth.ac.uk/about/publications

National Screening Programme for Diabetic Retinopathy (England): retinalscreening.nhs.uk

Diabetic neuropathy

CHAPTER 10

Key points

- Diabetic neuropathy often presents late, frequently with recurrent neuropathic ulceration.
- The 'hot' diabetic foot is a medical emergency.
- Accurate quantification of neuropathy using vibration perception thresholds is prognostic, but rarely systematically performed.
- Good glycaemic control slows progression of neuropathy in type 1 diabetes, but by itself probably has little effect in type 2 diabetes.
- Multimodal treatment (Steno-2) reduces the risk of developing autonomic neuropathy in type 2 diabetes.
- Acute mononeuropathies usually recover spontaneously.
- Continuing education is critical, especially in patients with at-risk feet.

Introduction

The devastating consequences of diabetic neuropathy are seen every day both in hospital – more bed days are taken up with the consequences of diabetic foot ulceration than any other diabetic complication – and in primary care, where sensory symptoms, especially pain, and autonomic neuropathy, especially erectile dysfunction, are common, disabling and depressing symptoms that have a major impact on quality of life. Despite decades of research, increased understanding of the pathogenesis of diabetic neuropathy has not yet translated into useful prophylactic treatment for the common polyneuropathy of diabetes, other than determined glucose control in type 1 diabetes, and Steno-2-type multimodal intervention to reduce autonomic, though not somatic, neuropathy in type 2

Practical Diabetes Care, 3rd edition. © David Levy.
Published 2011 by Blackwell Publishing Ltd.

diabetes. The difficulty of reliably quantifying peripheral neuropathy has limited its inclusion in outcome measurements in the recent type 2 studies, and is partly responsible for the frequent late presentation with ulceration and infection; however, simple tests, for example the monofilament, if widely used, should help identify the highest-risk groups of patients. The evidence base for most aspects of treatment of diabetic neuropathic syndromes is weak, and certainly far less robust than that for other microvascular complications. Finally, it is difficult to estimate even point prevalences of neuropathy because of methodological variability and referral bias. It is certainly common, for example in a contemporary population of adolescents with type 1 diabetes the prevalence, using reliable electrophysiology and autonomic function tests, was 20–25%. Many studies in type 2 diabetes give similar or higher rates.

Enthusiasm for specific drug treatments has waxed and waned. The development of aldose reductase inhibitors in the 1970s and 1980s, initially designed to prevent neuronal accumulation of sorbitol, has been dogged by toxicity or lack of efficacy; supplementation with recombinant nerve growth factor, though logical, was useless. Other treatments have been discredited (evening primrose oil/GLA), despite experimental evidence of efficacy. The protein kinase C inhibitor ruboxistaurin may positively impact on retinopathy (see Chapter 9), but probably does not have a role in other microvascular complications. There is some evidence for the efficacy of the antioxidant α-lipoic (thioctic) acid in alleviating the unpleasant positive symptoms of diabetic neuropathy, and it is available in some countries. The drugs that are relatively specific and effective for neuropathic pain frequently have side-effects that limit their use and titration to optimum analgesic effect.

However, despite general gloom on the pharmaceutical front, much can be done to prevent the most devastating consequences of peripheral neuropathy – recurrent foot ulceration and amputation – through education, high-quality podiatric care and provision of footwear. In addition, symptomatic painful neuropathy is often helped by judicious combinations of medication, and the management of erectile dysfunction, once the subject of many a long and generally unhelpful textbook, has been transformed by the introduction of the PDE5 inhibitors.

Diagnosis of neuropathy

'Neuropathy' is shorthand for 'distal sensorimotor polyneuropathy'.

Symptoms

Though not a symptom of somatic neuropathy, the earliest feature in type 2 diabetes is thought to be erectile dysfunction, which is increasingly recognized as a sensitive indicator of endothelial dysfunction (see below). Somatic neuropathy presents as insidious and often unnoticed numbness with or without paraesthesiae of the toes, progressing proximally to involve the feet and shins. Neuropathic symptoms may be intermittently present for several years before diabetic symptoms. Clinical involvement above the knee is unusual, and the upper limbs are involved late and to a lesser degree – arms have shorter axons than legs. Consider other diagnoses if there are prominent upper limb features, particularly muscle wasting (bilateral carpal tunnel syndromes or ulnar nerve compression, cervical disc disease, syringomyelia). Symptomatic neuropathy can occasionally be a presenting feature of type 2 diabetes. A differential diagnosis, especially when there is pain, must be in the examiner's mind; always attributing pain and other foot symptoms to diabetes can be hazardous, particularly when the clinical features are unusual. By analogy with diabetic nephropathy, there may be other causes of peripheral neuropathy, perhaps in up to 50% of patients (neurotoxic medications, alcohol, vitamin B_{12} deficiency, uraemia, vasculitis, chronic inflammatory demyelinating neuropathy or inherited neuropathy); there is possibly an even wider spectrum of treatable causes [1].

Signs

Stocking distribution sensory loss, starting with the tips of the toes, proceeds proximally eventually, typically to mid-shin. Loss is usually to all sensory modalities, with large and small nerve fibres all affected:

- light touch
- pain (pinprick)
- temperature
- vibration
- proprioception.

However, in some patients, small fibre-mediated modalities (pain and temperature) are preferentially affected, while in others the large-fibre modalities (touch, vibration and proprioception) are primarily involved. In a small proportion, there is severe loss of proprioception, giving rise to a 'pseudo-tabetic' variety, with positive Romberg's sign and instability on standing and walking, especially on uneven surfaces. Wasting of the small muscles of the foot is characteristic, with clawing of the toes and increased exposure of pressure areas on the soles. Clawing is probably due to motor neuropathy with wasting of the intrinsic muscles of the feet, though there may be some contribution from disruption of the plantar fascia.

Feet are often warm and well perfused with bounding pulses and distended veins caused by sympathetic denervation leading to increased blood flow. There is anhidrosis, demonstrated by little or no friction when the back of the examiner's hand is drawn across the sole of the foot. Hair loss on the dorsum of the foot and great toes is usually claimed as an example of trophic neuropathic changes, but it is an unreliable sign, particularly in the elderly; more significant clinically is atrophy of the fibro-fatty tissue of the heel pad. Impressionistically, there is often a smooth, shiny, rather featureless skin (this may be the equivalent in the foot of absent skin wrinkling in the fingers after immersion in water, thought to be due to advanced sympathetic denervation). More prosaically, always examine the skin between the toes for maceration and fungal infections, often sites of bacterial entry, and a risk factor for the development of cellulitis.

If high-risk features are identified on examination, always ask the help of a podiatrist.

- Callus: always precedes neuropathic ulceration, and is not benign in the neuropathic foot, as it increases focal pressure [2]. Callus recurs very quickly, especially in the typically neuropathic foot with its high arches and increased pressure on the balls of the foot. It requires frequent active removal by a podiatrist. Callus at the tip of a toe may conceal underlying abscess or osteomyelitis. Bleeding into callus requires action.
- Blistering at pressure points, sometimes with infection.
- Deeply fissured dry skin, often at the heels, is a possible portal for infection. Hydrating agents such as Flexitol Heel Balm (UK) are available without prescription and should be recommended for regular use.
- Interdigital fungal infection.
- Ingrowing toe-nail, especially if infected; subungual haematoma.
- Cellulitis.

Ankle reflexes are usually absent in established neuropathy. Absent knee reflexes (in the absence of other neuromuscular disorders) suggests advanced neuropathy.

Quantitative and semi-quantitative measurements
For routine clinical examination of the foot, the 2008 ADA/AACE report suggests using one, preferably two, of the following five tests to identify the high-risk foot, as indicators of loss of protective sensation:
- 10 g monofilament
- vibration perception threshold (neurothesiometer)
- 128-Hz tuning fork
- pinprick sensation
- ankle reflexes (use reinforcement if necessary).

10 g monofilament (Fig. 10.1a)
Very simple. Apply the 10 g monofilament perpendicularly to the distal great toe (between the nail fold and the distal interphalangeal joint) until it just buckles; this presents a relatively constant pressure. Formally, 10

(a)

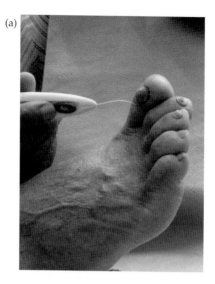

(b)

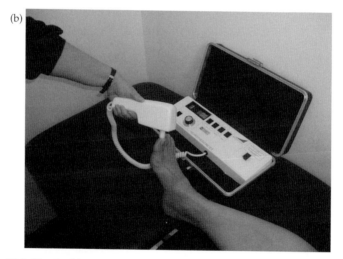

Fig. 10.1 Simple objective measures of peripheral neuropathy. (a) 10 g monofilament. (b) Neurothesiometer: apply perpendicularly to the tip of the pulp of the
great toe, without contacting the nail, having tested the sensation at the sternum.
Increase the voltage slowly until vibration can just be felt. Average three measurements. The feet being tested have typical neuropathic features: high arch,
slight wasting of the small muscles, prominence of the ball of the great and fifth
toes and thickened dystrophic nails

trials are required: eight or more correct responses is normal, while one to seven correct responses indicates reduced sensation; no correct responses indicates absent sensation. Inability to feel the monofilament is a reliable indicator of neuropathy and is associated with a high risk of progression to foot ulceration.

Vibration perception threshold
Vibration is the simplest sensory modality to quantify. The neurothesiometer (Fig. 10.1b) applies an increasing amplitude of vibration to the great toe pulp; inability to feel vibration at above 25 V predicts progression to foot ulceration. Vibration perception threshold (VPT) correlates broadly with other measurements of nerve function (including electrophysiological measurements of nerve conduction), but all neurological functions deteriorate rapidly with age and for more precise diagnosis an age-related measurement should be used (the 25-V threshold underestimates neuropathy in younger people and overestimates it in older people) [3]. Inability to feel vibration of a standard (128 Hz) tuning fork is a reliable but truly insensitive indicator.

Autonomic function tests
These quantify heart rate and blood pressure responses to various standardized manoeuvres, but the full battery of tests described many years ago cannot easily be done in the routine setting. However, measurement of sinus arrhythmia and postural blood pressure drop are simple and useful in the clinical setting (see below).

Nerve conduction studies
Infrequently used, but they can be useful in differentiating diabetic from other neuropathies. Median nerve studies are routinely performed in patients with suspected carpal tunnel syndrome and atypical neuropathies. The neurophysiologist will often do supplementary tests to confirm diffuse polyneuropathy in the upper limb. Ask for a sural nerve sensory action potential amplitude and common peroneal motor nerve conduction velocity in the lower leg, which are simple measurements. An absent sural nerve sensory action potential is a sensitive indicator of diabetic neuropathy.

Education
The strong link between insidious progression of numbness in the feet, lack of protective sensation, and subsequent painless damage is not at all obvious, even to some professionals (Box 10.1). Systematic review of a limited number of non-biased publications concluded, depressingly, that limited patient education alone does not result in meaningful reductions

> **Box 10.1 Key elements of education for patients with neuropathy or previous foot ulceration**
>
> - Formal podiatry review, including peripheral vascular assessment and assessment for orthotic footwear.
> - Regular routine podiatry for nails and callus. Repeatedly advise patients against cutting their own toenails, a depressingly frequent precipitant of ulceration and infection in insensitive feet. In the UK, hospital and community nurses do not cut nails; ask the hospital podiatry team to see inpatients even when there is no acute foot problem.
> - Frequent education: the responsibility of all members of the diabetes team. Emphasize the risk of exposing feet to painless injury:
>   - Always wear footwear (even, perhaps especially, when going to the toilet in the middle of the night).
>   - Pre-test bathwater temperature with the elbow.
>   - Avoid being barefoot at any time, but especially outside on holiday when walking on hot sand, marble floors or temple steps, common causes of severe burns and other injuries to the soles of the foot. Sunbathing with soles exposed to the sun is dangerous.
>   - Feel inside shoes and shake them out before putting them on to avoid penetrating injuries from gravel and other objects.
>   - In severely neuropathic feet, even small irregularities (e.g. a prominent seam in a sock) can cause skin breakdown.
>   - Check feet every day, including between the toes.
> - Ensure secure lines of communication between the patient and specialist podiatry services and that patients with problems, especially early ulceration and injury to neuropathic feet, can have urgent specialist review within 24 hours.

in ulceration and amputation; this finding should steer us towards a more selective and intensive approach to education of high-risk patients [4].

Management of diabetic polyneuropathy

Glycaemic control
In the DCCT, the risk of both peripheral and autonomic neuropathy in type 1 diabetes was reduced by about 50% in the intensively treated group. The EDIC follow-up study used only a standardized questionnaire and clinical examination, but the previously intensively treated group continued to develop symptoms at a greater rate than the previously conventionally treated group [5]. However, clinical signs remained unchanged in both groups, emphasizing the unreliability of clinical examination in detecting

neuropathy, and the importance of symptomatic questioning. Reversing established neuropathy is probably not possible. Even prolonged near-normoglycaemia after pancreas transplantation improved only nerve conduction velocities – significant, but probably not of major concern to most patients. Autonomic function and clinical signs did not improve.

There is no comparably rigorous data for neuropathy outcomes in type 2 diabetes, and it was not studied in the UKPDS. Intensive glycaemic therapy in ACCORD had minor beneficial effects on some measures of peripheral neuropathy, but not VPTs. Multimodal treatment in Steno-2 reduced autonomic, but strangely not peripheral, neuropathy in micro-albuminuric patients, though glycaemia in both intensive and conventional groups was similar, and the other interventions must have been responsible for the improvement.

Pharmacological treatment

No drug is widely licensed in asymptomatic diabetic polyneuropathy. The aldose reductase inhibitors, despite a generally poor efficacy and safety record, continue to be developed and studied, and one, epalrestat, is available in Japan for symptomatic and asymptomatic neuropathy. Some hold the view that previous agents in this class were underdosed on the basis of targeting sorbitol accumulation and osmotic derangement, both theories now discredited. Benfotiamine, a vitamin B_1 derivative, and α-lipoic acid are widely used, and there is experimental and some RCT evidence to support their use in symptomatic neuropathy. Avoid other B vitamins (B_6 and B_{12}) and folate unless there is documented deficiency; they are of no value in routine treatment and may accelerate coexisting diabetic nephropathy (see Chapter 8).

Foot ulceration

The ulcerated, infected and possibly gangrenous foot is a common reason for hospital admission. Anatomically, diabetic foot ulceration is restricted to the region distal to the ankle; proximal lesions are more likely ischaemic, vasculitic, venous, or to have another underlying cause. Most ulcers are predominantly neuropathic, but ischaemia from large-vessel lower limb disease must be carefully excluded. Ulceration always has three components: neuropathy, tissue ischaemia and infection.

Tissue ischaemia is due to large-vessel occlusion or local trauma. 'Large vessel' includes arteries as small as digital vessels, which can become involved in septic thrombophlebitis and lead to gangrene of one or more digits. True microangiopathic (capillary) involvement as seen in the retina and kidney does not occur in the foot, so the common clinical description of 'small-vessel disease', while aptly referring to vessels that are too small in calibre to be amenable to interventional radiology or arterial surgery, suggests a diffuse process that does not occur.

Additional risk factors include deformity, callus and oedema.

Neuropathy

The usual sequence of events leading to ulceration can be summarized as follows:

1 loss of protective sensation (pain and thermal sensation), leading to
2 areas of maximum pressure in the foot exposed to repeated trauma, leading to
3 callus at pressure sites, frequently the ball of the great toe or fifth toe (compare ischaemic ulcers which often occur at acute pressure sites (e.g. tips of the toes, sides of the feet), resulting in
4 ulceration (neuropathic ulcers are usually deep, clean and punched-out, the ulcer margin often being surrounded by callus).

Although any neuropathic patient can develop an ulcer, it characteristically occurs in tall overweight white men with type 2 diabetes. In the UK it is much less frequent in South Asians, the 75% lower risk of amputation partly accounted for by lower rates of smoking, peripheral vascular disease and of neuropathy itself [6]. However, in the USA black and Hispanic patients have notably higher rates of lower-extremity disease, and social deprivation and lack of access to foot care are likely additional factors. Although amputations in type 1 patients have decreased over the past decade, and are very rare in the under thirties, there is a still an 80-fold increased risk compared with the non-diabetic population, and by age 65, men have a cumulative risk of about 20%, women 11%. Foot ulceration carries a 40% increased mortality compared with non-ulcer diabetes patients, and a twofold increased risk compared with non-diabetes, differences that are only partly explained by conventional cardiovascular and other risk factors, including depression [7]. Ulceration requires specialist podiatrist management, but even a superficial wound to a vulnerable foot needs vigilance since infections can spread very rapidly. This is a situation where prophylactic antibiotics are justified. Heel ulceration usually has causes in addition to neuropathy (e.g. ischaemia, prolonged bed rest without adequate heel protection) but is always serious and can lead to rapidly progressing osteomyelitis of the calcaneum (Fig. 10.2).

Ischaemia

If foot pulses are present, there is no significant peripheral vascular disease. However, pulses are often absent or questionably present, especially where there is oedema. Doppler studies are routinely used. If the pulse is monophasic, significant peripheral arterial disease is likely. As with ischaemia generally in diabetes, symptoms are atypical: short proximal

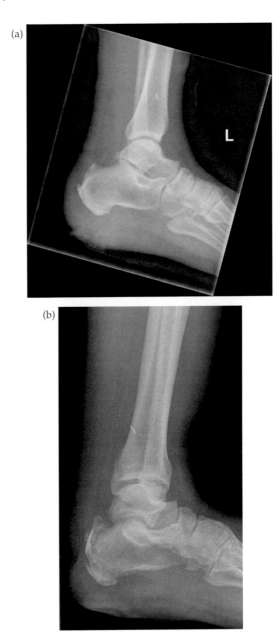

(a)

(b)

Fig. 10.2 Osteomyelitis of the heel: male, aged 67 years, 20 years' duration of type 2 diabetes, HbA$_{1c}$ 12%, proteinuria, mild renal impairment (serum creatinine 111 μmol/L), heel ulcer, feverish. Sensitive *Staphylococcus aureus* on blood culture. (a) Normal foot radiograph. (b) Despite treatment, 1 month later there is osteomyelitis of the heel. Patient died suddenly 2 weeks later, presumed cardiac

iliofemoral stenoses causing classical claudication are uncommon, and multivessel infrapopliteal disease is the usual culprit.

Ankle–brachial pressure index

This is the systolic pressure at the ankle (12-cm sphygmomanometer cuff just above the ankle and inflated until the posterior tibial pulse is obliterated) divided by the systolic pressure in the brachial artery measured conventionally. The ratio is usually over 1.0. Values below 0.6–0.7 signify severe occlusive vascular disease; where there is ulceration, patients should be referred for a vascular opinion, and will require more detailed Doppler studies and magnetic resonance angiography. Medial arterial calcification is widespread in diabetes, occurring in distal vessels of the foot and hand. It commonly leads to falsely elevated systolic foot pressures (though is also associated with systemic systolic hypertension) and an apparently normal ankle–brachial pressure index. A normal index in an ulcerated pulseless foot indicates critical limb ischaemia that requires urgent investigation and treatment.

Infection (see Chapter 7)

Describe carefully what you see and seek permission to take a digital photograph, which will help communication. Although intended for research, the PEDIS system summarizes key elements of diabetic foot ulcers and is useful as a descriptive scheme [8].
- Perfusion (presence of peripheral vascular disease)
- Extent/size
- Depth/tissue loss
- Infection
- Sensation (neuropathy).

Probe-to-bone test

It used to be thought that if a sterile probe hits bone at the base of an ulcer, osteomyelitis was likely. Another view has been proposed: it has low positive predictive value and its main benefit is excluding ostyeomyelitis if the test is negative [9]. The two contrasting views are still held, but positive or negative, it is a useful contributory test in a condition that is difficult to diagnose.

Radiography

Always request a plain foot radiograph for osteomyelitis. Help the radiologists by describing the site of the ulcer. X-ray changes are unlikely within 2 weeks of the onset of osteomyelitis, cortical changes are difficult to distinguish from degenerative joint disease, and abnormalities around the joint spaces can also be found in Charcot neuroarthropathy (see below). Unsuspected fractures, especially involving the metatarsals, are commonly found, and may be precipitants of Charcot joints. MRI (see Chapter 7) is increasingly helpful in detecting the early signs of osteomyelitis and, importantly, its resolution with treatment. Routine blood tests should include CRP, which can help distinguish no infection from mild infection (see Chapter 7); however, where there is no systemic upset, CRP may be quite low, and it is not clear whether antibiotic treatment can be guided by it more reliably than using radiography and clinical examination.

Management
Podiatrists with a special interest in diabetes are the key professionals, and should always be involved. Deep infections, abscesses and spreading infection associated with tissue necrosis require early liaison with surgeons.

The mainstay of treatment is relieving pressure from the ulcer, and complete bed rest will heal most ulcers in 6–12 weeks. In practice this is rarely possible, and total contact casting, where available, allows patients to remain mobile. The technique is simple, but requires fully trained personnel who understand that the methods, precautions and aims differ from those used in fracture management. Poorly applied casts can themselves cause ulceration in these insensitive feet. Casts require changing at least weekly. Off-the-shelf removable casts (e.g. Aircast) are useful where individual casting is not available, or if precautionary immobilization pending further tests or specialist evaluation is required.

Ulcers require meticulous care, including frequent débridement. Adherent fibrinous material at the base of ulcers can delay healing and needs sharp removal with a scalpel. Dressings are important, but should be kept simple where possible. Ulcers should be dressed daily after thorough cleaning with sterile saline. Practice varies widely, but a simple technique uses (i) an antimicrobial dressing such as povidone iodine (Inadine) or nanocrystalline silver (Acticoat), or a simple non-adherent dressing, covered by (ii) a thick protective layer of non-adherent foam (e.g. Allevyn), with (iii) a firmly but not tightly applied conforming stretch bandage. Use minimal amounts of tape, and wherever possible avoid applying it to skin. Many patients have thin skin, and heavily applied tape left for several days can cause skin damage if not carefully removed.

Special dressings designed to liquefy or absorb exudate are widely used and each has their advocates, but the liquefied products are sometimes not easy to remove and can obscure the appearance of the ulcer base. Trial evidence is woefully inadequate here, but it seems that regular simple cleaning and dressing of ulcers is more important than the type of dressing used.

Vascular interventions
Proximal iliofemoral lesions can easily be managed with angioplasty, and bypass surgery is almost never required. Distal disease is more difficult,

because of involvement of multiple smaller-calibre vessels, especially those below the knee and and in the ankle and foot. Improving techniques in endoluminal angioplasty and subintimal angioplasty (for total occlusions) may also be improving the outcome in critical limb ischaemia, but RCTs are needed. Outcomes for distal reconstructive surgery in diabetes are worse than in non-diabetic subjects, with a 50% increased risk at 2 years of death or amputation, even when adjusted for factors such as renal and cardiac disease. Intensive multidisciplinary input is likely to improve outcomes in patients where, by definition, risk factors have not been addressed in the past [10].

Adjunctive treatments for non-healing ulcers
Larval treatment
Where there is a lot of adherent exudate, sterile larval (maggot) treatment can give impressive results, especially when there is MRSA infection [11]. This treatment is more readily accepted by patients than clinical staff.

Growth factors
In vogue a few years ago, recombinant human platelet-derived growth factor (becaplermin 0.01% gel) may accelerate healing of chronic ulcers not responding to standard treatment. Extended use may increase risk of malignancy.

Tissue-engineered skin
Preparations of dermis/epidermis are available, for example Apligraf, living bilayered cell therapy secreting growth factors found in normal skin, and Dermagraft, a fibroblast-derived dermal substitute. As with all studies in diabetic foot ulcers, sufficiently powerful trials are difficult to carry out, but both these agents may help heal full-thickness diabetic foot ulcers more quickly than standard treatment alone.

Hyperbaric oxygen treatment
Systemic hyperbaric oxygen (HBO) is widely used in the USA and Europe, but is available in only a few centres in the UK. HBO promotes wound healing through several mechanisms, including improved oxidative killing of bacteria, and it is speculated that it may increase production of bone marrow-derived endothelial progenitor cells. HBO significantly reduces the risk of major (though not minor) amputations and in an RCT (using hyperbaric air as placebo), over 50% of ulcers remained healed at a year, compared with 30% treated with air [12]. There is reasonable evidence for the use of HBO in refractory osteomyelitis, and arterial ulcers and those associated with calciphylaxis may also benefit. The level of hyperoxygenation achieved at the wound or ulcer site detected by

transcutaneous oximetry correlates reasonably well with positive outcomes of HBO. Case selection is continually improving, and where available the advice of a hyperbaric team is valuable.

**Negative-pressure wound therapy (e.g. vacuum-assisted closure
therapy system)**
Widely used in general surgery, negative-pressure wound therapy
increases the likelihood of wound healing, but is designed for large ulcers
and large soft-tissue deficits, especially after partial foot amputations.

Charcot neuroarthropathy

Charcot neuroarthropathy is a serious and poorly understood condition
associated with rapid destruction of bones and joints and resulting in
bone fragmentation. It occurs only in patients with advanced sensory
and autonomic neuropathy, and is characteristic of long-duration type
1 diabetes with other microvascular complications, especially nephropathy and laser-treated retinopathy, but it is also seen in type 2 diabetes.
Mid-foot bones are characteristically involved, but the metatarsophalan-
geal joints and even the ankle can be affected. A common presentation is
with a tarsometatarsal fracture/dislocation. 'Silent' stress bone injuries
in the foot, detectable on MRI but not plain radiography, may precipitate the acute joint disorganization. When presented with an acute diabetic foot, especially if there is no ulceration, always consider a Charcot
process; diagnosis is often delayed many weeks, by which time considerable joint destruction may already have occurred [13]. Clinically,
they present with painless inflammatory swelling – the affected foot is
usually several degrees warmer than the contralateral foot – but some
patients complain of a poorly localized dull ache, another reason for routinely requesting and carefully scrutinizing radiographs of the foot in all
patients, and repeating at weekly or 2-weekly intervals if clinicial suspicion is high. The difficult differentiation from osteomyelitis is another
reason for taking frequent radiographs; both processes can progress rapidly. Infection usually involves phalanges, metatarsals or calcaneum,
rather than the mid-foot. FDG-PET scanning may differentiate osteomyelitis and Charcot neuroarthropathy more reliably than MRI, but there are
few studies [14]. Coexisting acute Charcot neuroarthropathy and osteomyelitis from an adjacent ulcer is uncommon, but poses a very difficult
diagnostic and therapeutic problem. If there is no recent history of ulceration, a Charcot foot is more likely than osteomyelitis. The more common
problem is the reverse: the severely disorganized bony anatomy of a
chronic Charcot foot leading to ulceration at a bony prominence, often
the medial arch (Fig. 10.3).

Management

Immobilize the foot with total contact casting or Aircast boot as soon as the diagnosis is suspected. Specialist input from podiatrist, orthopaedic surgeon and radiologist is needed. Bisphosphonate treatment with a single intravenous infusion of pamidronate 90 mg should be given, though higher doses have been used, for example 30 mg, 60 mg, and 60 mg at 2-weekly intervals. Bisphosphonates reduce symptoms and markers of bone turnover and destruction, though the long-term benefits are not known, and the fall in bone alkaline phosphatase is not prognostic. The Charcot foot is not osteoporotic after the acute episode, and though long-term oral bisphosphonates are often given, no trials have been performed. However, think of bone health in all patients with diabetes, measure vitamin D levels and supplement appropriately, and request DEXA scans in patients with other risk factor for osteoporosis, foe example type 1 patients with eating disorders.

After the acute phase, custom footwear is vitally important. Seek expert advice on surgical correction of deformity, especially plantar and medial bony protuberances, which predispose to ulceration. The role of more extensive surgery, involving internal fixation, is contentious and requires highly specialized orthopaedic input.

Painful diabetic neuropathy

A distressing syndrome of distal leg and foot pain that occurs in 5–7.5% of a clinic population, though some studies report much higher prevalence rates, up to 15%. The impression is that painful neuropathy is now less common than 10–20 years ago, and this may be due to improving multimodal management of type 2 diabetes. However, it is still probably under-recognized. The pathophysiology is unknown, but the defect may lie in the spinal cord. Poor glycaemic control is common, but by no means invariable. Pain resolves in a minority, and about three-quarters have chronic symptoms lasting several years. Acute pain in the feet and legs ('insulin neuritis') occurs shortly after the start of insulin treatment. Although uncommon now, it is still occasionally seen in people with very high starting HbA_{1c} levels. It resolves spontaneously after a few months. Chronic painful neuropathy seems to be most common in older type 2 patients, but is well described in young women with type 1 diabetes with eating disorders, especially anorexia nervosa [15]. Clinical features are outlined in Box 10.2. These, together with the numbness of coexisting polyneuropathy, give the particularly distressing combination of lancinating pains apparently emanating from an insensitive foot. Making the diagnosis is not always easy, as it is purely clinical, so remember other painful syndromes in diabetes. Patients often hang feet

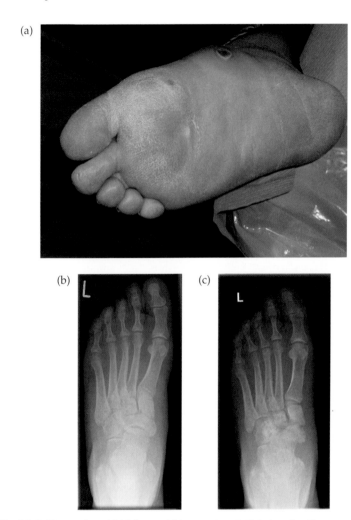

Fig. 10.3 Charcot foot. (a) Male, aged 36 years, type 1 diabetes, duration 15 years. Previous below-knee amputation of the other leg. Short history: he twisted his ankle, and because of profound sensory neuropathy continued to walk on it for the next 2 weeks. Rapidly progressing Charcot neuroarthropathy with disorganization of the mid-foot and secondary ulceration of the medially displaced navicular bone. (b) Female, aged 40 years, long-standing diabetes with very poor control. Minor trauma with apparently normal foot radiograph. (c) Presented with a swollen foot 1 year later, and characteristic appearances of mid-foot Charcot. Lost to follow-up. (d) Nomenclature of foot bones.

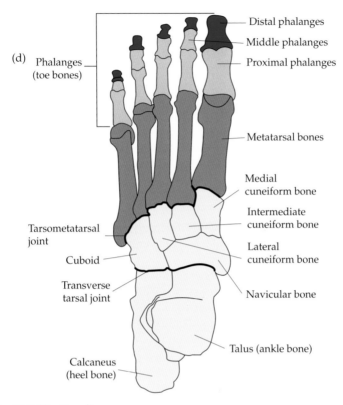

(d) Phalanges (toe bones)

Distal phalanges
Middle phalanges
Proximal phalanges

Metatarsal bones

Medial cuneiform bone
Intermediate cuneiform bone
Lateral cuneiform bone

Tarsometatarsal joint
Cuboid
Transverse tarsal joint

Navicular bone

Talus (ankle bone)

Calcaneus (heel bone)

Fig. 10.3 (Continued)

Box 10.2 Clinical features of painful diabetic neuropathy

Symptoms
- Confined to both lower legs and are symmetrical (compare sciatica)
- Not worsened by exercise (compare ischaemic symptoms)
- Much worse at night

Positive symptoms
- Stabbing/shooting/burning pains, often described in dramatic terms, e.g. red-hot pokers or needles, electric shocks
- Contact hypersensitivity, especially to bedclothes
- Altered sensation (allodynia): stimuli that are not normally painful elicit pain
- Heightened awareness of sensation (hyperaesthesiae)
- Cold feet (not always objectively supported by partners)
- 'Tight skin'

out of bed, out of contact with bedclothes, and find ways of providing counter-irritants, for example soaking their feet in cold water or having their legs massaged.

Other painful neuromyopathic syndromes in diabetes

These include proximal motor neuropathy (syn. diabetic amyotrophy, diabetic neuropathic cachexia), meralgia paraesthetica, diabetic myonecrosis, truncal neuropathy, and 'insulin neuritis'.

Management
Podiatric supervision and foot education where there is distal polyneuropathy. Improving glycaemic control in chronic painful neuropathy has no proven value, but it should be attempted nonetheless.

Medication and other strategies (Table 10.1)
Studies with many drugs have shown statistically significant pain relief beyond the large placebo effect, but this is not always translated into useful therapeutic benefit in the individual patient. Considerable patience is required from the diabetes team and patient while attempting to optimize pain relief. Painful neuropathy is undertreated.

Vitamins and other dietary supplements do not help unless there is documented vitamin deficiency or alcoholism. The efficacy of simple analgesics such as paracetamol and non-steroidal anti-inflammatory drugs (NSAIDs) is not supported by meta-analysis, but it would be remiss not to suggest them. Use the second-line analgesics with care, but they are almost as effective as tricyclic antidepressants. Tramadol can be started at 50 mg b.d., increasing to 200 mg b.d., but it has opiate side-effects, including dependency and tolerance. Oxycodone is similar; use a modified-release preparation (e.g. OxyContin) starting at 10 mg daily [16].

Antidepressants are used for their analgesic effects. Selective serotonin reuptake inhibitors (SSRIs) and selective noradrenaline reuptake inhibitors (SNRIs), often preferred because of their better side-effect profile and simpler dosage titration, are less effective than tricyclics [number needed to treat (NNT) 2 vs. 6]. Sub-antidepressant doses of amitriptyline are effective in neuropathic pain; start at 10 mg nocte, increasing to a maximum of about 100 mg. They are not well tolerated at high doses, with prominent anticholinergic symptoms. See Table 10.1 for doses of other antidepressant analgesics. They can cause ECG changes, particularly at high doses (heart block, ventricular premature beats, prolonged QT interval); request periodic ECGs.

Table 10.1 Stepped therapies for management of neuropathic pain

	Monotherapy	Combinations	Additional measures
First line	Tricyclic antidepressant (TCA), e.g. amitriptyline (*BNF*, section 4.3.1) Antiepileptic (AE), e.g. gabapentin or pregabalin (*BNF*, section 4.8.1)	Low-dose TCA + AE	Paracetamol or paracetamol-based compound analgesic, e.g. co-dydramol
Second line	Lignocaine patch (Capsaicin cream) (*BNF*, section 10.3.2) Alternative antidepressant, e.g. duloxetine 60 mg daily (BNF section 4.3.4), or other SNRI/SSRI, e.g. venlafaxine 15–150 mg daily (*BNF*, section 4.3.4), fluoxetine 20 mg daily (*BNF*, section 4.3.3) Opioids, e.g. tramadol, morphine, oxycodone	Opioid with TCA or AE	TENS Acupuncture Physiotherapy Occupational therapy
Third line (refer to specialized pain management service)	Alternative opioids Neuromodulation		Above together with psychological assessment and support

BNF, British National Formulary.
Source: adapted from Bennett (2010).

Conventional anticonvulsants (carbamazepine, phenytoin) are effective, but require dose titration and do not seem to be very well tolerated. The centrally acting γ-aminobutyric acid (GABA) antagonists gabapentin, and its derivative pregabalin, have NNTs of about 4, between those of the tricyclic antidepressants and the SSRIs. Gabapentin has a wide dose range, and should be started at a low dose (e.g. 300 mg daily), increasing slowly up to 2.4 g daily. Side-effects (dizziness, somnolence, headache and diarrhoea) occur in 10–20% of patients, and frequently limit its use, despite its efficacy. Pregabalin is also licensed for use in neuropathic pain, and is usually effective at a dose of 150–300 mg daily, though it can be used up to 600 mg daily. Because of their side-effect profile, slow titration is better than rapid dose escalation over a few days.

Combination therapies may be valuable (see Table 10.1), but at this stage ask the pain team for advice.

Topical treatments
The evidence base for topical treatments in painful neuropathy is weak, but because they do not have systemic effects they are valuable as additional treatments, especially when systemic agents are limited by side-effects (even generous use of capsaicin cream gives systemic exposure that is much less than found in chilli-eaters worldwide).

- OpSite dressing (Flexigrid) or spray is non-pharmacological and is free from side-effects, and is worthwhile trying on this basis alone. It presumably acts by reducing contact discomfort and allodynia.
- Isosorbide dinitrate spray (Isocard 30 mg/dose, one spray to each leg at bedtime) may act by local vasodilatation or nitric oxide donation.
- Topical 0.075% capsaicin cream (Axsain) is pharmacologically sound (it depletes sensory nerve endings of substance P, which may account for exacerbation of pain at the start of treatment). However, it requires three or four applications a day for maximum efficacy (and to reduce the initial pain), which is difficult to sustain.
- Lignocaine 5% in large patches (e.g. Versatis, UK) is useful in postherpetic neuralgia, and though currently unlicensed may also be valuable in painful neuropathy. Up to three patches, applied to the point of maxmum pain, can be used for up to 12 hours a day.

Mononeuropathies and other focal syndromes

Peripheral mononeuropathies
Upper limb
Carpal tunnel syndrome (median nerve)
Carpal tunnel syndrome is very common (remember the association with primary hypothyroidism, especially in type 1 diabetes) and may present

with atypical symptoms, as it is often superimposed on diabetic polyneu-ropathy. Consider it in any patient presenting with pain or ache in the forearm or hand, especially at night; classical presentation with pain and numbness in the thumb, index and middle fingers is relatively uncom-mon. Request median nerve conduction studies and refer for decompres-sion. The surgical outcomes are either as good as or rather worse than in non-diabetic individuals. The clinical impression is that symptom relief is often less satisfactory; this may reflect other components in the dia-betic hand as well as coexistent polyneuropathy. Ulnar neuropathy is also associated with diabetes, entrapment occurring at the elbow or in the forearm; pain and numbness may occur in the ring and little fingers.

The diabetic hand
In long-standing (usually type 1) diabetes the hands are affected not only by polyneuropathy and median/ulnar mononeuropathies, but by three significant connective tissue complications.
• *Cheiroarthropathy* (generalized connective tissue thickening/limited joint mobility) affecting the small joints of the hand, resulting in minor reduction in mobility and inability to closely oppose the palms of the hands (prayer sign).
• *Dupuytren's contracture*: up to four times more common in diabetes.
• *Tenosynovitis/trigger fingers*: increased about 10-fold in diabetes [17].
   In its advanced state, the hand is stiff, slightly painful, immobile and weak. All but the cheiroarthropathy can be managed, but an expert hand surgeon is needed to identify the most usefully treatable components. It is worth mentioning the threefold increased risk of adhesive capsulitis of the shoulder in diabetes, again particularly in type 1 diabetes. It also per-sists longer, can be bilateral and is more resistant to standard treatments.

Lower limb
Foot drop, caused by a common peroneal nerve mononeuropathy, is uncommon. Meralgia paraesthetica (lateral femoral cutaneous nerve, L2–L3) presents with sensory symptoms, usually burning or numbness in the anterolateral thigh, sometimes aggravated by standing or walking, with a variable hypoaesthetic area on examination. It may be due to com-pression at the inguinal ligament, and is probably more common in peo-ple with diabetes. Nerve conduction studies can help, and local steroid injection preceded by confirmatory nerve block has been reported to be useful. Usually no specific treatment is needed, and reassurance about the self-limiting nature of the condition is sufficient; however, there is an important distinction to be made from proximal motor neuropathy. The current fashion for wearing jeans low-slung over the hips may be contributory.

Proximal motor neuropathy
Also known as diabetic amyotrophy or diabetic neuropathic cachexia, it is uncommon, and the impression is that it is becoming less frequent. It is probably a lumbosacral plexopathy, rather than a femoral mono-neuropathy. It usually occurs in men in their fifties or sixties, often with long-standing type 2 diabetes, taking oral hypoglycaemic agents. It has a subacute onset with symmetrical thigh weakness and wasting, and there is always pain that is deep, burning and aching and, like other neuro-pathic pain, worse at night. Profound weight loss of more than 20 kg and anorexia are common, usually leading to a presumptive malignant diag-nosis, which must be excluded with routine laboratory tests including prostate-specific antigen plus chest and lumbar and thoracic spine radio-graphs. Blood glucose and HbA$_{1c}$ may be unexpectedly low, on account of the anorexia. Insulin treatment aborts the weight loss. The natural his-tory is of slow spontaneous improvement over about 18 months.

Focal diabetic muscle infarction
Focal myonecrosis usually occurs in the vastus muscles of the thigh, very rarely in the abdominal and upper limb muscles, and presents with acute thigh pain not associated with trauma. There is sometimes a palpable and tender mass and erythema; consider infection first. It usually occurs in poorly controlled diabetes with advanced microvascular complications. MRI will demonstrate the infarction and associated muscle oedema. It resolves with conservative treatment and analgesia.

Truncal neuropathy
An unusual mononeuropathy involving one or more intercostal nerves that presents with acute onset of pain in a dermatomal distribution. Cutaneous hyperaesthesia is characteristic. It is very occasionally associ-ated with herniation of the intercostal or abdominal muscles. Osteoporotic or malignant spinal collapse would be the usual primary diagnoses; shin-gles would become obvious. Spontaneous recovery occurs over several months.

Cranial mononeuropathies
About 40% of oculomotor nerve palsies (cranial nerves III, IV and VI) occur in people with diabetes. Lateral rectus (VI) palsy and painful III nerve palsy with pupillary sparing are common, especially in type 1 diabetes. They are probably due to focal microvascular thrombosis in a capillary supplying the peripheral course of the nerve. They do not require brain MRI unless there are atypical features, for example pupil-lary involvement, other neurological symptoms or signs, or more than one episode.

Autonomic neuropathy

Asymptomatic autonomic neuropathy is very common, especially if sensitive diagnostic methods are used to detect it, but only a small proportion of patients develop significant symptoms beyond erectile dysfunction. Impairment of cardiovascular reflexes is probably irreversible, but requires vigilance during anaesthesia (see Chapter 3), and in long-term follow-up in ACCORD was associated with a 1.5- to 2.0-fold increased risk of all-cause and cardiovascular death. Gastrointestinal symptoms and postural hypotension are rare but can be debilitating. Treatment options for advanced autonomic neuropathy are limited, but the associated unstable blood glucose control in type 1 diabetes is an indication for considering pancreas or islet transplantation. Intensive multimodal intervention in microalbuminuric type 2 patients (glycaemia, blood pressure, lipids and lifestyle) significantly reduced the risk of progression to autonomic neuropathy in the Steno-2 study. Glycaemic control alone is not the important factor here: intensive glycaemic control in ACCORD did not reduce mortality [18].

Diagnosis
Cardiovascular autonomic reflexes (Table 10.2)

These are the only tests routinely available for the diagnosis of early autonomic neuropathy. Because there are no clear treatment options, they are required only when there is a clinical problem, for example establishing the cause of gastrointestinal symptoms or in preoperative assessment. The simplest test of vagal function is heart rate variation (sinus arrhythmia) with standardized deep breathing (5s inspiration, 5s expiration). It requires only a single-lead ECG rhythm strip. Decrease in systolic blood pressure after standing will detect orthostatic hypotension and is presumptive evidence of sympathetic neuropathy (other causes having been excluded). The other tests of vagal function (heart rate response to Valsalva manoeuvre and the lying/standing ratio) are too complicated for occasional use.

Management of autonomic neuropathy syndromes
Symptomatic postural hypotension

Uncommon, and correlates poorly with measured blood pressure fall, but can be disabling. It is usually worse in the morning. As a late complication it is often associated with nephropathy, posing the difficult balance of valuable renal protection with angiotensin blockade and the resulting postural symptoms, especially with ACE inhibitors. These patients also often have recumbent hypertension, demonstrable on ambulatory blood pressure testing, adding to the difficulties of management. Very careful

Table 10.2 Autonomic function tests

	Normal	Borderline	Abnormal
Heart rate variation to deep breathing (beats/min)	⩾15	11–14	⩽10
Systolic blood pressure fall 2 min after standing (mmHg)	⩽10	11–29	⩾30

Source: after Ewing and Clarke [25].

adjustment of antihypertensive agents is needed, minimizing the use of diuretics, vasodilators and tricyclics. Short-acting agents (e.g. captopril) can be valuable for use during the night. Mechanical devices and graduated compression stockings and similar aids are of little practical value. Other, unlicensed, treatments can be considered, but use with great care and with specialist input.

- Fludrocortisone (*British National Formulary*, section 6.3.1): valuable, but hypertension, especially nocturnal, is a major problem. Start at a low dose (e.g. 50 μg daily) with frequent monitoring of blood pressure and electrolytes.
- DDAVP (desmopressin) (*British National Formulary*, section 6.5.2) is of anecdotal value, for example 0.1 mL of nasal solution or one dose of nasal spray (each 10 μg) at bedtime. Hyponatraemia is a risk; monitor electrolytes frequently.
- ESAs have been occasionally used in people with very severe postural symptoms (there seems to be a link between autonomic neuropathy and anaemia, even in the absence of nephropathy). Discuss in detail with the nephrology team.

Erectile dysfunction

This is the commonest neuropathic complication: 20% of men have erectile dysfunction (ED) at diagnosis, increasing to 34% at 12 years (UKPDS). The prevalence in a newly diagnosed Kuwaiti population was 30%, and nearly 50% in a large survey of Canadians attending their primary-care physicians [19]. The relationship between potency and peripheral neurological function is weak, but there is a large evidence base strongly relating ED to cardiovascular risk factors and the metabolic syndrome, the effects probably mediated through increasing impairment of endothelial function. This association is of less immediate interest to the patient than to his physician. However, diabetes carries an independent and disproportionate risk

of ED (around threefold), and there is a very important link between ED
and silent myocardial ischaemia, and between ED and all-cause and cardiovascular death, the risk increasing with worsening degrees of ED [20].

Vigorous correction of cardiovascular risk factors is crucial, but apart
from the 1-year data from the Look AHEAD study of intensive lifestyle
intervention (see Chapter 5) there is little evidence that this translates
into improved erectile function. In the ONTARGET/TRANSCEND studies, angiotensin blockade treatment over 5 years did not improve ED; neither do statins. Fortunately, practice has been revolutionized by the PDE5
inhibitors, first introduced in 1998. Successful outcome of PDE5 inhibitor
treatment improves compliance with other treatments, for example antihypertensive medication, resulting in better blood pressure control, and
very importantly is independent of glycaemic control [21].

History
Distinguish between ED and loss of libido; the latter may be psychogenic
or, more rarely, endocrine in origin. Pain (e.g. Peyronie's disease), significantly more common in diabetes, or balanitis, may be another factor. The
duration of ED is not a reliable indicator of aetiology.

Drug history
A detailed medication history is important:
- antihypertensives (thiazides more likely to cause ED than beta-blockers);
- psychotropics of all kinds (SSRIs are associated with ED, reduced libido
  and delayed ejaculation, and with reduced gonadotrophin and testosterone and elevated prolactin levels);
- alcohol, tobacco, cannabis.

Examination
- Peripheral pulses, abdominal aortic aneurysm, and arterial bruits.
- Knee and ankle jerks, vibration sense at feet (though normal VPT does
  not exclude autonomic dysfunction).
- Genitalia: testicular size, penile abnormalities.
- Features of hypopituitarism.

Investigations
There is increasing interest in the hypogonadism associated with type
2 diabetes, and it is much more recognized than before, but the field is
complicated by difficulties with definitions and continuing problems
with the standardization of laboratory measurements of serum testosterone. However, there is reasonable agreement that total testosterone below 11 nmol/L (3.2 ng/mL) in the presence of sexual symptoms
(absence of early morning erections, ED and lower frequency of sexual

thoughts) identifies hypogonadism [22]. It is associated with increased visceral adiposity and the metabolic syndrome. Around one-quarter of type 2 males may be hypogonadal, about twice the rate in non-diabetic men [23]. However, the aetiology is not clear, with no consistent patterns of gonadotrophins – various studies report low, normal or high values. Perform a physical examination and check baseline endocrine tests (luteinizing hormone, testosterone, prolactin). Remember the association between genetic haemochromatosis, hypogonadism and type 2 diabetes. Diabetes does not confer protection against prolactinomas, other pituitary tumours or Kallmann's syndrome, or other causes of primary hypogonadism (mumps orchitis, Klinefelter's syndrome, itself associated with truncal obesity and insulin resistance, even when treated). A trial of testosterone replacement therapy is often warranted (*British National Formulary*, section 6.4.2), with appropriate monitoring, but is best done by an andrologist or a practitioner with experience of using the multiple products for testosterone replacement therapy now available.

PDE5 inhibitors (British National Formulary, section 7.4.5)
These drugs, of which three are currently available, increase the availability of vasodilatory nitric oxide by inhibiting cyclic AMP. The prototype drug, sildenafil, has been joined by vardenafil and the long-acting tadalafil. Sildenafil should be taken about an hour before intercourse; the others are effective within about 30 min. The only absolute contraindication is concomitant nitrate therapy (including nicorandil), which carries a risk of severe hypotension. They should not be taken at the same time as potent CYP3A4 inhibitors (erythromycin, ketoconazole, various antiretroviral agents, large quantities of grapefruit juice). There is some evidence that regular, as opposed to on-demand, use of these drugs is not only effective (especially with the long-acting tadalafil) but may improve outcomes through some form of 'conditioning'. There is no clinically significant difference in the clinical outcomes with any agent; all are less effective in diabetes than in non-diabetic subjects (overall about 50% response rate, compared with 70–80%). Most patients will require the maximum recommended doses. If one agent is ineffective, it is worth trying another.

Adverse effects common to all three include headache, dyspepsia, nausea, visual disturbances, flushing, nasal congestion, back pain and myalgia. Non-arteritic ischaemic optic neuropathy, usually unilateral, has been rarely reported with sildenafil and tadalafil (see Chapter 9). It presents with blurred vision or visual field loss within hours of taking the drug; recovery is variable. Vascular risk factors including diabetes and a history of myocardial infarction and hypertension are associated with this form of optic neuropathy, so the causal association is not clear.

Other approaches
Sublingual apomorphine is less effective than the PDE5 inhibitors, but can be used in patients taking nitrates. It is no longer available in the UK. Intracavernosal injections, intraurethral alprostadil, vacuum tumescence devices and surgical implants have a limited place, but all require specialist andrologist referral after documented failure of PDE5 inhibitors used properly at the maximum recommended (or tolerated) doses. Combination therapy may be helpful. There is a hint that successful treatment of OSA improves erectile function.

Gatrointestinal dysfunction
Gastroparesis is failure of stomach emptying, through a combination of vagal neuropathy, reduction in gastric pacemaker cells and neurohormonal changes. Acute elevations in blood glucose levels also delay gastric emptying. Early on there may be only slight fullness or early satiety after meals; more advanced symptoms are episodic nausea and vomiting, leading to ketoacidosis (sometimes recurrent and frequent), weight loss and malnutrition. Vomiting on an empty stomach first thing in the morning suggests a non-neuropathic cause [24]. In longstanding type 1 diabetes, consider gastroparesis if glycaemic control worsens abruptly, especially if there is unexpected hypoglycaemia (mismatch of food absorption and mealtime insulin) or recurrent ketoacidosis precipitated by vomiting. Bear in mind the association between significant eating disorders, advanced microvascular complications and gastroparesis. In type 2 diabetes, enquire carefully about symptoms of gastroparesis before starting GLP-1 analogues, which act in part through delaying gastric emptying, and use with caution in patients with advanced peripheral neuropathy – GLP-1 analogues may uncover advanced but asymptomatic autonomic dysfunction (see Chapter 6).

Management of gastroparesis
Upper gastrointestinal endoscopy may show concurrent pathologies, or retained food residue. Quantify the delayed gastric emptying with a nuclear medicine study (the percentage of a standard radiolabelled solid meal retained after 4 hours should be less than 10%). Drug treatment is often unsatisfactory, but try metoclopramide 5–10 mg t.d.s. (not in patients under 20 years old), or preferably domperidone 10–20 mg t.d.s. before meals. Erythromycin (a motilin agonist) increases gastric emptying but itself can cause nausea. Low-dose erythromycin suspension (e.g. 125 mg t.d.s.) before meals has been reported to be effective and well tolerated for several months. Inpatients can be given intravenous erythromycin (e.g. 3 mg/kg body weight 8-hourly).

Promptly admit patients with episodic vomiting for intravenous fluids and insulin. Detailed dietary advice is needed. Because liquid emptying is less affected than solid, suitable liquid enteral supplements may be helpful during exacerbations not requiring hospitalization. For intractable cases, an implantable gastric pacemaker is available. While it does not decrease overall symptoms, it reduces the frequency of vomiting.

Large bowel involvement
Constipation is common, as a result of large bowel atony. Diarrhoea is episodic, lasting a few days, then remitting. It characteristically occurs at night, when it may be associated with faecal incontinence. Weight loss and malabsorption do not occur. Episodic severe diarrhoea, like gastroparesis, is more common in middle-aged type 1 patients with very long duration of diabetes and other evidence of microvascular complications. Bacterial overgrowth is said to be common, and a 7–10 day course of oxytetracycline or erythromycin (each 250 mg q.d.s.) relieves symptoms in about 50%. Patients should keep a supply in reserve at home. Intractable diabetic diarrhoea may respond to treatment with somatostatin analogues.

References

1. Freeman R. Not all neuropathy in diabetes is of diabetic etiology: differential diagnosis of diabetic neuropathy. *Curr Diab Rep* 2009;9:423–31. PMID: 19954686.
2. Boulton AJ, Meneses P, Ennis WJ. Diabetic foot ulcers: a framework for prevention and care. *Wound Repair Regen* 1999;7:7–16. PMID: 10231501.
3. Bloom S, Till S, Sonksen P, Smith S. Use of a biothesiometer to measure individual vibration thresholds and their variation in 519 non-diabetic subjects. *Br Med J* 1984;288:1793–5. PMID: 6428547.
4. Dorresteijn JA, Kriegsman DM, Assendelft WJ, Valk GD. Patient education for preventing diabetic foot ulceration. *Cochrane Database Syst Rev* 2010;(5): CD001488. PMID: 20464718.
5. Martin CL, Albers J, Herman WH *et al.* Neuropathy among the Diabetes Control and Complications Trial cohort 8 years after trial completion. *Diabetes Care* 2006;29:340–4. PMID: 16443884.
6. Chaturvedi N, Abbott CA, Whalley A, Widdows P, Leggetter SY, Boulton AJ. Risk of diabetes-related amputation in South Asian vs. Europeans in the UK. *Diabetic Med* 2002;19:99–104. PMID: 11874424.
7. Iversen MM, Tell GS, Riise T *et al.* History of foot ulcer increases mortality among individuals with diabetes: ten-year follow-up of the Nord-Trondelag Health Study, Norway. *Diabetes Care* 2009;32:2193–9. PMID: 19729524.
8. Schaper NC. Diabetic foot ulcer classification system for research purposes: a progress report on criteria for including patients in research studies. *Diabetes Metab Res Rev* 2004;20(Suppl. 1):S90–S95. PMID:15150820.
9. Lavery LA, Armstrong DG, Peters EJ, Lipsky BA. Probe-to-bone test for diagnosing diabetic foot osteomyelitis. Reliable or relic? *Diabetes Care* 2007;30: 270–4. PMID: 17259493.

10. Malmstedt J, Leander K, Wahlberg E, Karlström L, Alfredsson L, Swedenborg J. Outcome after leg bypass surgery for critical limb ischemia is poor in patients with diabetes: a population-based cohort study. *Diabetes Care* 2008;31:887–92. PMID: 18268064.

11. Bowling FL, Salgami EV, Boulton AJ. Larval therapy: a novel treatment in eliminating methicillin-resistant *Staphylococcus aureus* from diabetic foot ulcers. *Diabetes Care* 2007;30:370–1. PMID: 17259512,

12. Löndahl M, Katzman P, Nilsson A, Hammarlund C. Hyperbaric oxygen therapy facilitates healing of chronic foot ulcers in patients with diabetes. *Diabetes Care* 2010;33:998–1003. PMID: 15106239. The results of this study support the findings of a Cochrane systematic review of 2004.

13. Chantelau E. The perils of procrastination: effects of early vs. delayed detection and treatment of incipient Charcot fracture. *Diabetic Med* 2005;22:1707–12. PMID: 16401316.

14. Basu S, Chryssikos T, Houseni M *et al.* Potential role of FDG PET in the setting of diabetic neuroosteoarthropathy: can it differentiate uncomplicated Charcot's neuroarthropathy from osteomyelitis and soft-tissue infection? *Nucl Med Commun* 2007;28:465–72. PMID: 17460537.

15. Steel JM, Young RJ, Lloyd GG, Clarke BF. Clinically apparent eating disorders in young diabetic women: associations with painful neuropathy and other complications. *Br Med J* 1987;294:859–62. PMID: 3105777.

16. Gimbel JS, Richards P, Portenoy RK. Controlled-release oxycodone for pain in diabetic neuropathy: a randomized controlled trial. *Neurology* 2003;60:927–34. PMID: 12654955.

17. Smith LL, Burnet SP, McNeil JD. Musculoskeletal manifestations of diabetes mellitus. *Br J Sports Med* 2003;37:30–5. PMID: 12547740.

18. Pop-Busui R, Evans GW, Gerstein HC *et al.* Effects of cardiac autonomic dysfunction on mortality risk in the Action to Control Cardiovascular Risk in Diabetes (ACCORD) Trial. *Diabetes Care* 2010;33:1578–84. PMID: 20215456.

19. Grover SA, Lowensteyn I, Kaouache M *et al.* The prevalence of erectile dysfunction in the primary care setting: importance of risk factors for diabetes and vascular disease. *Arch Intern Med* 2006;166:213–19. PMID: 16432091.

20. Gazzaruso C, Giordanetti S, DeAmici E *et al.* Relationship between erectile dysfunction and silent myocardial ischemia in apparently uncomplicated type 2 diabetic patients. *Circulation* 2004;110:22–6. PMID: 15210604.

21. Scranton RE, Lawler E, Botteman M *et al.* Effect of treating erectile dysfunction on management of systolic hypertension. *Am J Cardiol* 2007;100:459–63. PMID: 17659929.

22. Wu FC, Tajar A, Beynon JM *et al.* Identification of late-onset hypogonadism in middle-aged and elderly men. *N Engl J Med* 2010;363:123–35. PMID: 20554979.

23. Corona G, Mannucci E, Petrone L *et al.* Association of hypogonadism and type II diabetes in men attending an outpatient erectile dysfunction clinic. *Int J Impot Res* 2006;18:190–7. PMID: 16136189.

24. Camilleri M. Diabetic gastroparesis. *N Engl J Med* 2007;356:820–9. PMID: 17314341.

25. Ewing DJ et al. *Diabetes Care.* 1985;8:491–8.

Further reading

NICE Guidelines
Type 2 diabetes: footcare. CG10 (January 2004, expected review May 2011).
Neuropathic pain: the pharmacological management of neuropathic pain in adults in non-specialist settings. CG96.

Foot examination and risk assessment
Boulton AJ, Armstrong DG, Albert SF *et al.* Comprehensive foot examination and risk assessment: a report of the task force of the foot care interest group of the American Diabetes Association, with endorsement by the American Association of Clinical Endocrinologists. *Diabetes Care* 2008;31:1679–85. PMID: 18663232.

The diabetic foot
Bennett MI (ed.) *Neuropathic Pain*, 2nd edn. Oxford: Oxford University Press, 2010.
Cheer K, Shearman C, Jude EB. Clinical Review: managing complications of the diabetic foot. *Br Med J* 2009;339:b4905. PMID: 19955124.
Edmonds ME, Foster AVM. *Managing the Diabetic Foot*. Oxford: Wiley-Blackwell, 2005.
Foster AVM, Edmonds ME. *Diabetic Foot Care: Case Studies in Clinical Management*. Oxford: Wiley-Blackwell, 2010.
Jones TH (ed.) *Testosterone Deficiency in Men*. Oxford: Oxford University Press, 2008.
Tesfaye S, Boulton A (eds.) *Diabetic Neuropathy*. Oxford: Oxford University Press, 2009.

Websites
International Working Group on the Diabetic Foot (International Diabetes Federation): www.iwgdf.org
Patient information: National Diabetes Information Clearinghouse (NIH): www.diabetes.niddk.nih/gov/DM/pubs/neuropathies
Horwell neurothesiometer, Scientific Laboratory Supplies: www.scientificlabs.co.uk

Hypertension

CHAPTER 11

Key points

- Successful treatment of hypertension in diabetes has more widespread benefits than any other risk-factor intervention, but there is limited evidence for benefit on eye and peripheral nerve complications.
- Accelerated arterial stiffening, associated with increased systolic blood pressure, occurs early in type 1 diabetes, even when there is no microalbuminuria.
- Start treatment if blood pressure exceeds 140/90 mmHg.
- Generally, a systolic blood pressure target of less than 140 mmHg (ACCORD); values under 130 mmHg are not evidence-based, yet widespread in guidelines; apart from ACCORD no important clinical trials have achieved this target.
- Early combined pharmacological treatment is logical.
- Fixed-dose combinations are valuable.
- Apart from the use of angiotensin-blocking agents being used early, and probably as first-line treatment in all type 2 patients, there is little evidence for the superiority of one group over another, and all are valuable.
- Ambulatory blood pressure monitoring is important in diagnosis and management, especially resistant hypertension.
- Resistant hypertension is very common in type 2 patients. The rational use of diuretics is often the key to successful management.

Introduction

Despite more clinical trials than any other aspect of diabetes, many questions still remain about hypertension. Treatment targets continued to fall

Practical Diabetes Care, 3rd edition. © David Levy.
Published 2011 by Blackwell Publishing Ltd.

after UKPDS (1998), but even in contemporary trials with the most stringent treat-to-target protocols they are rarely achieved (see Chapter 8). Because antihypertensive agents, like statins, have log-linear dose–response characteristics, progressive blood pressure lowering requires increasing intensity of treatment, with attendant risks of side-effects, expense and most importantly the possibility of limited improvement in long-term outcomes. Establishing an evidence-based target was therefore important. The hypertension arm of ACCORD (2010) established in the early 2000s was still able to justify randomizing type 2 patients to systolic targets of 140 or 120 mmHg [1]. The to some surprising outcome was that in patients with established diabetes and risk factors for, or evidence of, macrovascular disease, maintaining systolic blood pressure (SBP) at about 120 mmHg conferred no macrovascular advantage compared with a less intensive achieved level of about 133 mmHg, apart from the expected reduction in stroke outcome. Even more counter-intuitive was the finding that intensive lowering of blood pressure did not reduce progression of retinopathy [2]. However, the baseline blood pressure (139/76 mmHg) was already relatively well-controlled hypertension, not far from existing treatment targets, and lower than the achieved level in the intensively controlled group of UKPDS (144/82 mmHg). Similar to the ACCORD glycaemic study, it appears we have reached the practical limits to significant improvements in outcomes using conventional treatments especially in patients with established vascular disease, contrasting with the epidemiological evidence in mostly healthy populations. The striking exception remains proteinuric patients and as in the glycaemic studies and the UKPDS findings, compared with the studies in longer-duration diabetes, we are left with the question of whether patients with more recent onset type 2 diabetes and presumably less vascular disease might benefit from more stringent blood pressure control.

Nevertheless, intensive lowering of blood pressure from UKPDS-like levels (baseline 160/94 mmHg) has consistently dramatic beneficial effects in diabetes. In the UKPDS, microvascular complications and stroke were both reduced by about 40%, and heart failure by more than 50%, though there was no significant effect on myocardial infarction. However, in contrast to the well-established legacy effects of glycaemia (and multimodal treatment in Steno-2), the 10-year UKPDS follow-up found that the vascular benefit of intensive blood pressure lowering was abolished as soon as control was relaxed. Despite the continuing controversies, there is agreement on several major areas (Box 11.1).

Pathophysiologically, hypertension comprises elements of vasoconstriction (probably mediated by renin) and volume (salt) overload, or in many cases both. The rediscovery of this basic concept is important for the treatment of hypertension, in particular resistant hypertension, a common

> **Box 11.1 Areas of agreement in the management of hypertension in type 2 diabetes**
>
> - Hypertension treatment confers more widespread benefit than treatment of any other cardiovascular risk factors.
> - Hypertension is often easier to control in the long term than glycaemia.
> - Treatment thresholds.
> - Treatment priorities in terms of antihypertensive drug classes.
> - The need for two or more agents for adequate blood pressure control in most hypertensive diabetic people (ACCORD), three or more in other studies.
> - Systolic blood pressure (or possibly pulse pressure), as indicator of arterial stiffness, should be the main target of treatment.

problem in diabetes. Most patients therefore require a drug or combination of drugs that address salt overload (i.e. a diuretic), which increase renin, and a drug or drugs that block the renin–angiotensin–aldosterone system. Low-renin hypertension is common in diabetes (renin levels decrease with age, and are characteristically low in black subjects). In future, measurement of plasma renin levels may help diagnose and guide treatment of resistant hypertension [3].

Type 1 diabetes

At diagnosis, blood pressure is no higher than that of non-diabetic people. In the absence of microalbuminuria, blood pressure changes with time in a similar fashion to that of non-diabetic people, but anticipating it by some 15–20 years. SBP is higher at all ages, while diastolic blood pressure (DBP) starts to fall earlier than in non-diabetic subjects; the result is a strikingly higher pulse pressure at all ages and durations of diabetes, indicating accelerated arterial ageing and stiffening. For example, about 15% of 18–24 year old Finns were hypertensive ($\geq 140 / \geq 90$ mmHg), increasing to about 20–25% in the 25–40 year old group (Fig. 11.1). Similar rates are found across Europe (EURODIAB study). By their early thirties, type 1 subjects have higher pulse pressures at any level of albuminuria than young people without diabetes [4]. Actively look for hypertension, especially if there is no microalbuminuria: blood pressure, especially during the night, starts to rise at the same time, or even before, microalbuminuria occurs. Blood pressure can also rise in intensively treated patients who gain weight, together with some other features of the insulin resistance syndrome. The concept of pre-hypertension (SBP 120–139 mmHg, DBP 80–89 mmHg) is especially useful here as an indicator of likely progression to true hypertension, with emphasis on lifestyle interventions, as there is no evidence yet for the benefit of pharmacological treatment.

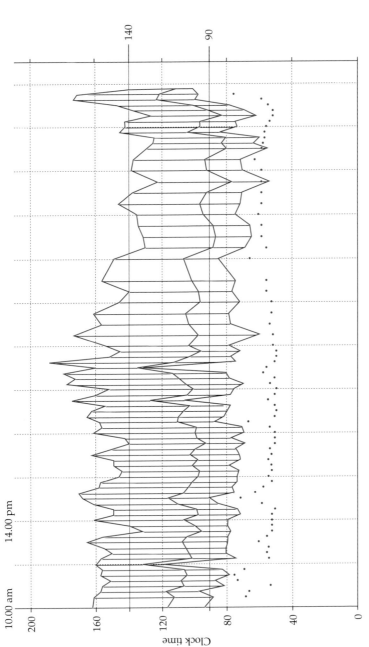

Fig. 11.1 Ambulatory blood pressure record showing systolic hypertension in long-standing type 1 diabetes. Male, aged 50 years, type 1 diabetes, duration 24 years. No retinopathy ever, negative microalbuminuria, normal age-related vibration perception threshold; lifelong non-smoker, BMI 24. Lipids normal on no treatment. Casual clinic blood pressure readings about 150/90 mmHg over past 1–2 years. Striking systolic hypertension with adequate nocturnal dip. Probably increased vascular stiffness. Since no microalbuminuria, treated initially with calcium-channel blocker, not angiotensin-blocking agent, but will probably need another agent, for example a thiazide diuretic. Upper continuous line, systolic blood pressure; middle continuous line, mean arterial pressure; lower continuous line diastolic blood pressure. Dotted line, pulse rate

Once microalbuminuria is established, then angiotensin blocker treatment is mandatory, regardless of blood pressure (see Chapter 8).

Blood pressure should be monitored carefully in young people under 18 with diabetes, most of whom will currently have type 1 diabetes, though this is likely to change. However, it is important to use age-, gender- and height-related measurements (see Numbers, Conversions and Tables). Prehypertension is defined as a blood pressure between the 90th and 95th percentile, which should be managed with intensive lifestyle input; in patients with persistent measurements above the 95th percentile medication can be considered, especially if there is microalbuminuria, but this requires detailed and careful discussion.

Type 2 diabetes

In striking contrast with type 1 diabetes, about three-quarters of type 2 patients are definitely hypertensive ($\geq 140/\geq 90$ mmHg) at diagnosis, and nearly all macroalbuminuric patients are hypertensive. Black patients have an especially high prevalence of hypertension, hypertensive nephrosclerosis and LVH, an independent predictor of coronary death (Fig. 11.2). Isolated systolic hypertension (SBP > 140, DBP < 90 mmHg), again with a major contribution from increased arterial stiffness, is common, as is atherosclerotic renal artery stenosis (see Chapter 8).

Thresholds and targets for treatment

Type 2 diabetes

Thresholds and targets for treatment are shown in Table 11.1. There is general agreement that treatment should start once blood pressure is persistently greater than 140/90 mmHg. Targets for treatment have in some cases run ahead of the evidence; until ACCORD (Box 11.2), only one large clinical trial had achieved an SBP of less than 130 mmHg. While event rates were lower than anticipated in ACCORD, reducing its power, there are no clear benefits of intensive blood pressure lowering in high-risk hypertensive type 2 patients, and targeting SBP less than 140 mmHg is sufficient except in proteinuric patients.

Management

Assess end-organ damage

Current microalbuminuria levels and retinopathy status should be known.

Macrovascular

- Assess for peripheral vascular disease (foot pulses, carotid, renal and femoral bruits, abdominal palpation for aortic aneurysm). A bruit in the left flank is more likely to be splenic than renal.

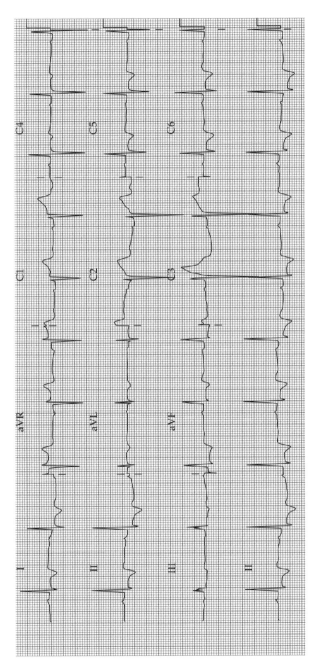

Fig. 11.2 Left ventricular hypertrophy (LVH) in diabetic hypertension. South Asian male, aged 59 years, presenting with accelerated hypertension and a left branch retinal vein thrombosis. No secondary cause found. Poor glycaemic control, very poor medication adherence. Clear 'strain' pattern across left ventricular leads, but voltage criteria for LVH not fulfilled. Even with optimum treatment, including mandatory angiotensin blockade, annual cardiovascular mortality is about 2% (LIFE, 2002), four times higher than in the high-risk patients (LVH an inclusion criterion for those aged 55 or older) in ACCORD (2010)

Table 11.1 Blood pressure management standards in type 2 diabetes

Standard	Blood pressure (mmHg)	Recommending organizations
Treatment threshold	≥140/≥90	BHS-IV
	>140/80	NICE
Treatment target	<140/80	BHS-IV, NICE (if no end-organ damage), ACCORD (implied)
	<130/80	NICE, BHS-IV, JNC 7 (if end-organ damage is present)
Proteinuria ≥ 1 g per 24 hours	<125/75	BHS-IV

BHS, British Hypertension Society (2004); NICE (2009); JNC, Joint National Committee (USA, 2003).

Box 11.2 Outline of ACCORD blood pressure study

- Hypothesis/target: intensive group, target SBP < 120 mmHg; standard group, target SBP < 140 mmHg
- Mean follow-up 4.7 years
- Treat-to-target: any routine blood pressure treatment strategy permitted. Mean number of agents: intensive, 3.4; standard, 2.1
- Baseline blood pressure 139/76 mmHg
- Mean achieved blood pressure: intensive, 119/64 mmHg; less intensive, 134/71 mmHg
- Outcomes
  - No difference in major cardiovascular outcomes
  - Stroke (small numbers) and macroalbuminuria: significantly reduced in intensive group
  - No difference in microalbuminuria or progression of retinopathy
- Adverse effects
  - Hypotension more frequent in intensive group, but still < 1%
  - eGFR lower (80 vs. 75 mL/min) and serum creatinine higher (97 vs. 88 μmol/L) in intensive group

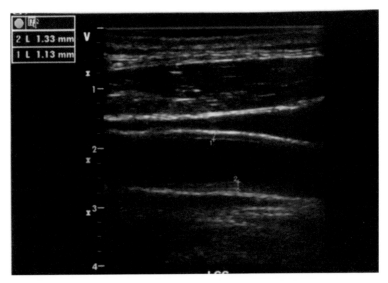

Fig. 11.3 Carotid intima–media thickness as a cardiovascular risk factor.
Increased common carotid intima–media thickness (CIMT). Male, aged 75 years,
diet-controlled diabetes. No other significant risk factors. Normal CIMT
values are age-related, between 0.4 and 0.9 mm. Values over 1 mm are reliably
associated with increased cardiovascular events. Left common carotid artery
(CCA) intima–media thickness is 1.13 mm (1). Focal thickening (1.3 mm) on the
posterior wall of the CCA, just below the bifurcation, but no plaque (2). Intensive
risk factor intervention is required, but it is not yet clear whether interventions,
especially LDL lowering, that may reduce CIMT are associated with reduced
event rates. The PROG-IMT project may help resolve this important question.
Courtesy of Caroline Westgate, London Medical

- LVH cannot be assessed clinically. Standard ECG criteria (SV1 + RV6 >
  35 mm; RV5 or RV6 > 25 mm; or SV1 or SV2 > 25 mm; ± 'strain' pattern)
  correlate poorly with echocardiography, which should be requested
  whenever there is ECG evidence of LVH. It is sometimes difficult to
  distinguish between LVH and ischaemia on ECG (see Fig. 11.2).
- Ultrasound scan of the common carotid artery for CIMT and the presence of atherosclerotic plaque. CIMT over 1 mm is a reliable indicator
  of cardiovascular risk, but the presence of plaque may be even more
  significant. In type 2 diabetes, increased CIMT is strongly associated
  with abnormal SPECT myocardial perfusion (Fig. 11.3).

Blood pressure measurement

Automated digital blood pressure devices are accurate and in widespread use, but manual measurements are still important, as an initial

---

Box 11.3 Practical aspects of blood pressure measurement

- Blood pressure measurements taken by doctors in clinics are substantially higher (9/7 mmHg) than those taken by non-medical staff. In the ambulatory care setting, doctors should therefore no longer be permitted access to blood pressure equipment.
- Ensure sufficient length of the upper arm is exposed to allow proper cuff use; cuffs must not be applied over clothing, especially if sleeves are rolled up and constricting the upper arm.
- Support the arm at heart level.
- Measure blood pressure sitting; standing blood pressure should be measured in patients with complications. Orthostatic hypotension is common, and may not reach a maximum until 1–2 min after standing up. Be patient.
- Decrease cuff pressure slowly (2 mm/s) and take measurements to the nearest 2 mmHg.
- Korotkoff phase V (disappearance) is used for DBP; where sounds can be heard to zero, use phase IV (muffling).
- Remember that blood pressure is one of the most important measurements in diabetic patients; never rush measurements.
- Dipstick urine test (preferably automated) for proteinuria; resting 12-lead ECG.

---

clinic reading may be misleading. Practical advice for blood pressure measurement, adapted from the British Hypertension Society guidelines (2004), is shown in Box 11.3.

Home blood pressure monitoring

Affordable automated equipment is now widely available (recommended validated equipment only; the British Hypertension Society website has details of currently approved devices). Wrist monitors, while more convenient than upper arm monitors, are more difficult to use reliably because of the need to keep the wrist at heart level while the measurement is being taken. Home blood pressure measurements, like ambulatory blood pressure monitoring (ABPM), are lower than casual clinic readings by about 10/5 mmHg, but still correlate reasonably with echocardiographic estimations of left ventricular mass [5]. Home devices cannot be used for diagnosing hypertension, but they are of value in monitoring response to treatment when supported by clinic or office blood pressure measurements. Studies have shown significant reduction in medication and costs, and in some cases permanent discontinuation of treatment, with no significant worsening of blood pressure, though ambulatory pressures may be slightly higher [6]. Some patients will become anxious through measuring their blood pressure too frequently, the same problem posed by home blood glucose monitoring. Time spent explaining the physiological importance of minute-to-minute adjustment of blood pressure is worthwhile, and this can be shown more graphically using ABPM print-outs. Self-measurement of blood pressure opens up real possibilities for innovative programmes to improve blood pressure control, in combination with traditional and more time-consuming methods.

Ambulatory blood pressure monitoring

Mean 24-hour ABPM correlates better with cardiovascular risk and target organ damage than casual blood pressure readings. 'Non-dipping' (failure of nocturnal blood pressure to fall about 10%) is associated with increased left ventricular mass, and increased blood pressure variability is also associated with increased target organ damage independent of mean blood pressure. Box 11.4 lists some uses of ABPM.

Diagnostic thresholds for ABPM in non-diabetic subjects have been updated in the light of important long-term prospective cardiovascular outcome studies [8] (Table 11.2). Though fewer than 10% of the subjects in the studies had diabetes, because of the higher cardiovascular risk in diabetes at any given blood pressure, they are worthwhile clinical targets; in patients with nephropathy, at the highest cardiovascular risk, optimal values, though daunting to achieve, should nevertheless probably be targeted.

Sustained lifestyle interventions

While most hypertensive patients will need some pharmacological treatments, introducing a portfolio of lifestyle changes will enhance the benefits of existing medication (e.g. thiazide diuretics with dietary salt reduction), and possibly also reduce the need for additional medication. Individual responses vary, and there are few large interventional trials. Discuss and reinforce all the following [9].

- *Reducing salt intake.* Average sodium intake in the USA is about 180 mmol/day, up to half consuming more than 300 mmol/day. Given these huge intakes, the recommendation to reduce intake to less than 6 g NaCl (< 2.4 g sodium or < 100 mmol/day) should have clinically important effects on blood pressure. Advise patients not to add salt to food at mealtimes, though prepackaged foods and salty snacks are major culprits, as well as monosodium glutamate. Response can be monitored, with valuable feedback to patients, by requesting urinary sodium with ACRs or 24-hour urinary albumin measurements. Reducing urinary sodium excretion by 30–45 mmol per 24 hours only modestly reduces blood pressure, but reduced cardiovascular events by 25% in a long-term follow-up, even though the original interventions

---

Box 11.4 Situations where ambulatory blood pressure measurements may be helpful

- Where variable clinic measurements hinder decision-making on further management.
- In suspected white-coat hypertension (persistent elevated clinic measurements, but normal measurements outside the clinic setting); the white-coat effect is the same phenomenon in patients with treated hypertension. However, white-coat hypertension is important as blood pressure rises may be frequent and caused by minor daily stresses that normally would not cause a hypertensive surge. The cardiovascular prognosis may not be substantially different from that of sustained hypertension. White-coat hypertensives with any degree of ambulatory hypertension (one study suggested > 130/80 mmHg) should not be brushed aside, and should be actively treated [7]. White-coat hypertension may not be as common in type 2 patients as in non-diabetic patients.
- In suspected 'masked' hypertension, the converse of white-coat hypertension, there are normal clinic blood pressure measurements but elevated ambulatory measurements. This phenomenon seems to be common in type 2 diabetes, and is also prognostic. Masked nocturnal hypertension is also of interest, particularly in patients with nephropathy.
- In pre-hypertensive subjects.
- Where reaching target blood pressure values is prognostic, e.g. in diabetic nephropathy.
- In patients taking short-acting agents, especially to monitor overnight blood pressure control.
- In pregnancy complicated by hypertension.
- Where over-treatment is suspected (e.g. casual clinic measurements consistently < 120/80 mmHg) or symptoms suggesting postural hypotension. ABPM – usually every 30 min during the day, every hour during the night – are not frequent enough to detect transient or episodic falls in blood pressure, for example on getting out of bed in the morning.

---

lasted only 1.5–4 years. This legacy effect seems to be mediated in part through long-lasting reductions in sodium intake and awareness of dietary salt [10].

- *Dietary Approaches to Stop Hypertension (DASH).* Consider implementing the DASH diet, with increased consumption of fruit (but in moderation in diabetes), vegetables, legumes, beans, nuts, whole-grains and soy, and decreasing saturated and total fat. This can reduce SBP by 8–14 mmHg.

Table 11.2 Proposed reference values for ambulatory blood pressure monitoring relating to cardiovascular outcomes (2007)

Blood pressure category	24-hour average (mmHg)	Daytime average (mmHg)	Night-time average (mmHg)
Optimal	<115/75	<120/80	<100/65
Normal	<125/75	<130/85	<110/70
Ambulatory hypertension	≥130/80	≥140/85	≥120/70

- *Weight loss* of 8 kg can reduce blood pressure by 7/3 mmHg (Look AHEAD study; see Chapter 5). Sustained weight loss of this magnitude with diet alone is rare in practice, though studies with exenatide and a mean weight loss of about 3 kg, more easily achievable, show proportionate blood pressure reductions, i.e. 2/0.5 mmHg (see Chapter 6).
- *Exercise*: the standard recommendation of 30 min moderate exercise most days can reduce SBP by 4–9 mmHg.
- *Limit alcohol intake*: 21 units/week or less for men, 14 units/week or less for women can result in SBP reduction of 2–4 mmHg [11].
- Vitamin D supplements and high-dose ω-3 fatty acids (3 g daily) may reduce blood pressure slightly, but the evidence is not strong.

Pharmacological treatment: general features

The value of ranking antihypertensive agents

The near-universal adoption of treatment algorithms using strong recommendations for first-, second-and third-line treatments, habitual for the past 30 years or more, has been challenged by the European Society of Hypertension (ESH, 2007, 2009). The logic of their approach is that there are certain general agreements on blood pressure management.

- The major benefit of antihypertensive treatment is lowering of blood pressure itself, not the means by which it is achieved.
- Different classes of agents have only minor differences in cause-specific outcomes, and these are unlikely to be apparent in individual patients, as opposed to large RCT cohorts.
- When used at recommended doses, the various classes of agents have very similar blood pressure-lowering effects.
- The cardiovascular outcomes in an individual patient cannot yet be predicted.

- Relatively few combinations have formal hard-point outcome studies.
- Most patients will require two or more agents to achieve target blood pressure.
- All antihypertensive agents have benefits and side-effects.

Given these, in place of strict rankings, the European guidelines suggest preferred drugs in different specific conditions – not surprisingly, angiotensin blockade in diabetes – but then focus on strategies for combining agents. The contrasting approaches of NICE and ESH are shown in Fig. 11.4, with the high cardiovascular risk strategy, appropriate for many people with diabetes, selected for the ESH example. Most practitioners probably already use a combination of these approaches, but it is reassuring that a wide body of opinion supports a less hierarchical approach to the management of hypertension.

Aspirin

Still a controversial area in primary prevention, but there is no controversy over long-term low-dose aspirin use in secondary prevention patients with evidence of established atherosclerotic disease (myocardial infarction, stroke, coronary interventions, peripheral vascular disease, definite atheroma on coronary angiography, plaque on carotid Doppler scanning).

Primary prevention

No single clinical trial has given definitive results, and aspirin is no longer licensed in the UK for primary prevention (for details see www .mhra.gov.uk/drugsafetyupdate, October 2009). In meta-analyses, there are modest reductions in myocardial infarction and stroke, for example relative risk reductions of 9% for coronary heart disease, 15% for stroke. The effects are greater for coronary heart disease in men, and for stroke in women. Against this, there is a slightly increased risk of haemorrhagic (though not fatal) stroke, and around 50% increased risk of gastrointestinal bleeding in those without a history of ulcer disease. The more cardiovascular risk factors, the greater the increased bleeding risk. There is continuing concern about an increase in pharmacological aspirin resistance in people with diabetes, possibly through increased production of non-platelet-derived thromboxane A_2 (smoking, hypertension and hyperlipidaemia have similar, additional, effects). Recall, however, that apparent aspirin resistance may be caused simply by failure to take the medication: 40% of people with cardiovascular disease are reported not to take aspirin as prescribed.

The 2010 proposals, though based on a relatively weak level of evidence, are as follows.

- *Use a clinical risk calculator* (e.g. UKPDS risk engine, www.dtu.ox.ac/ riskengine/index/php). Suggest aspirin use in adults with a greater

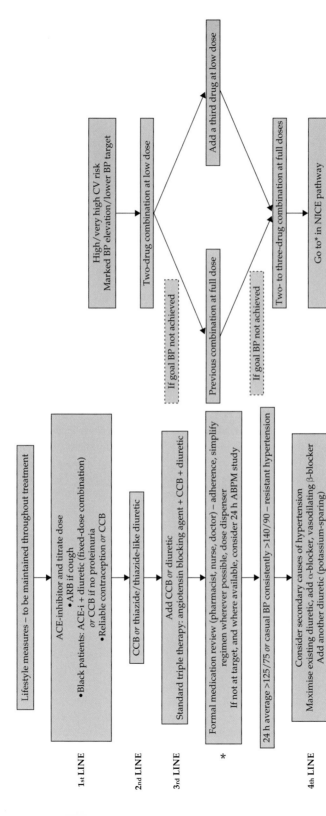

Fig. 11.4 Two approaches to the management of hypertension: (a) adaptation of NICE guideline (2009); (b) ESH guideline (2007). The two will frequently need integrating in treating hypertensive type 2 patients

than 10% 10-year cardiovascular disease event risk but who do not have increased risk of gastrointestinal bleeding (no previous bleed or peptic ulcer disease, no concurrent NSAID or warfarin use).

- *Use clinical approximation* (men over 50 and women over 60). The guideline suggests aspirin treatment if there is one or more additional cardiovascular risk factors (smoking, hypertension, dyslipidaemia, family history of premature cardiovascular disease, albuminuria), but as always these simple lists do not distinguish for example between current and past smokers, controlled or uncontrolled hypertension, statin-treated patients, and so on; most type 2 patients will have several of these factors.

- *Type 1 diabetes.* Very limited data. Patients with retinopathy or microalbuminuria or macroalbuminuria should probably take aspirin because of the significantly increased cardiovascular risk associated with these complications. There is no evidence for increased risk of retinal bleeding with aspirin, though dual antiplatelet therapy should probably not be used in retinopathy patients, especially if there is pre-proliferative or proliferative retinopathy. Patients with completely uncomplicated type 1 diabetes probably do not benefit, though after a very long duration (e.g. 20 years) there may be increased cardiovascular risk even if there is no microalbuminuria and strictly normal lipids. Discuss individually with patients; the decision may require specialist advice.

- *Hypertension.* The ADA (2004) recommends that hypertensive type 1 and 2 patients over 40 years old or with more than 10 years of known type 2 diabetes who achieve blood pressure below 150/90 mmHg should take low-dose aspirin, which reduces cardiovascular events by about 15% and myocardial infarction by 36%, in addition to the risk reduction of the antihypertensive medication itself.

Metabolic effects of thiazide or thiazide-like diuretics and beta-blockers

Concerns about the effects of thiazides and beta-blockers on glucose metabolism, lipid profiles and the risk of developing diabetes have been magnified to the point at which these valuable agents, especially the thiazides, are often considered forbidden in the management of diabetes. Hypertension in diabetes, especially resistant hypertension, cannot usually be managed without a thiazide or thiazide-like diuretic. It is therefore important to appreciate the magnitude of the effects.

1 Combined beta-blocker and thiazide treatment increases both mean fasting glucose and LDL by only about 0.1–0.3 mmol/L (glucose 2–5 mg/dL, LDL 4–12 mg/dL), triglycerides by about 0.2–0.5 mmol/L (18–44 mg/dL), and uric acid by 20%, values similar to those of the variability of the measurement.

2 Thiazide and beta-blocker treatment in most RCTs increases the risk of diagnosed diabetes; for example, in the ALLHAT study, the 4-year incidence of new-onset diabetes was 3.5% higher in the chlortalidone-treated group compared with the lisinopril-treated group (11.6% vs. 8.1%) [12].

3 Beta-blocker glucose effects are larger than those of thiazides. Non-selective beta-blockers, rarely used in long-term treatment now, reduce glucose uptake in muscle by blocking β_2-adrenergic stimulated blood flow, as well as first-phase insulin secretion. However, even selective beta-blockers such as metoprolol, widely used in ischaemic heart disease and heart failure, increase HbA_{1c}, though only by about 0.15%. In comparison with the metabolically neutral carvedilol, patients treated with metoprolol required more statin starts and up-titrations in clinical trials. In the individual patient, changes in glucose or lipid medication will be barely discernible. Nevertheless, these agents should be reserved as lower priority treatment in people whose diabetes management might require substantial shifts if they were to be used, especially in combination, for example:

(a) those with the dysglycaemia of the pre-existing metabolic syndrome, who may be precipitated into full-blown diabetes;

(b) those who are borderline for a change in diabetes treatment, for example from diet alone to oral hypoglycaemic agents or from oral hypoglycaemic agents to injectable treatment.

A more important consideration is whether conventional beta-blocker treatment is overall as effective in blood pressure lowering as other classes (see below).

Once-daily medication

Antihypertensive medication should nearly always be once daily. Most agents are intrinsically long-acting, and modified-release preparations of many short-acting agents are available.

Monotherapy versus combination therapy

Combination treatment with two different classes of agents is more effective than doubling the dose of one agent. This may be due in part to the problem that a proportion of patients will either not respond or have only a weak response to any single agent, but is made more attractive by the relatively low incidence of side-effects with most modern drugs. Initial therapy with two agents is likely to be useful in patients with high initial blood pressure or those with high cardiovascular risk: the blood pressure goal is likely to be achieved more quickly, there is a high risk of early events in these patients, and there is some evidence (e.g. from the VALUE study) that the event rate is reduced by prompt reduction in blood pressure. Fixed-dose combinations, now widely available, should

> **Box 11.5 Examples of fixed-dose antihypertensive drug combinations of value in high-risk or markedly hypertensive individuals**
>
> - ACE-i/CCB (amlodipine or verapamil)
> - ARB/amlodipine (reduces risk of peripheral oedema compared with amlodipine alone)
> - ACE-i/thiazide diuretic (usually hydrochlorothiazide 12.5 or 25 mg)
> - ARB/thiazide diuretic
> - ACE-i/thiazide-like diuretic (e.g. perindopril/indapamide)
> - Renin inhibitor (aliskiren)/hydrochlorothiazide (USA)
> - Thiazide or thiazide-like diuretic/potassium-sparing diuretic, e.g. co-amilozide (amiloride with hydrochlorothiazide, 2.5/25, 5/50)

be used whenever possible, and especially in moderate-risk (e.g. stage 2, SBP > 160 mmHg, DBP > 100 mmHg) or high-risk patients (see Fig. 11.3). Interestingly, in the very large ACCOMPLISH trial (2008) where 60% of the participants had diabetes, an ACE-i/calcium-channel blocker (CCB) combination (benazepril up to 40 mg daily plus amlodipine up to 10 mg daily) was better than an ACE-i/thiazide combination (hydrochlorothiazide up to 25 mg daily) in reducing major cardiovascular end points. (In addition, very low blood pressure levels were achieved in this study: mean blood pressure throughout was about 132/74 mmHg [13].) This study reinforces the European guidelines and should encourage increased use of fixed-dose combinations in high-risk patients, especially in the UK, where they are underused, possibly in part because prescriptions for people with diabetes are free of charge, but also because in the past academic teaching has frowned on them (Box 11.5).

Preferred treatment: angiotensin blockade

It is universally accepted that angiotensin blockade should be preferentially used in hypertensive diabetic patients. Although the evidence for greater cardiovascular risk reduction compared with other drug groups is not overwhelming, the renoprotective benefits in type 2 diabetes, and reduction in renal end points in both type 1 and type 2 diabetes, are so convincing that where possible any antihypertensive regimen should contain an angiotensin-blocking agent at maximum recommended dose. In practice, only severe hyperkalaemia, marked deterioration in renal function on starting treatment and angio-oedema should preclude use of one or other of these agents. Many uncontrolled studies have concluded that both ACE inhibitors and ARBs, especially ARBs, reduce the risk of developing AF.

In the GISSI-AF study (2009), valsartan did not reduce recurrent AF, though there is still hope that ARBs may reduce the risk of AF in high-risk primary prevention patients, for example those with LVH and hypertension, or left atrial enlargement. However, for the time being angiotensin blockade should not be used for either primary or secondary prevention of AF.

ACE-i or ARB?

Until recently a hotly contested question, with most systematic reviews and meta-analyses favouring ACE-i treatment over ARBs for cardiovascular event reduction in high cardiovascular risk subjects, but there are no comparative outcome studies in hypertension. HOPE (2000) established ramipril 10 mg daily as a default medication, in view of a significant reduction in cardiovascular events more than 2 years after the end of the active treatment phase of the study (HOPE-TOO, 2005). The combined results of HOPE and two further ACE-i studies in patients with high cardiovascular risk or previous cardiovascular events (EUROPA, 2003, perindopril; PEACE, 2004, trandolapril) confirmed the widespread cardiovascular benefit, but differences in achieved blood pressure, even though they are small, have continued to present difficulties in interpretation. Definitively, the prospective ONTARGET study (2008) of high-risk patients similar to the HOPE population found no benefit of telmisartan 80 mg daily over ramipril 10 mg daily in prevention of major cardiovascular outcomes [14]. The small additional blood pressure reduction with telmisartan carried no advantage, and was associated with a slightly increased risk of hypotension; ramipril, on the other hand, was slightly less well tolerated (cough and angio-oedema).

After the LIFE study (2002), the ARB losartan was favoured for diabetic patients with hypertension and LVH (though the comparator was atenolol with its weaker central antihypertensive effects). A detailed MRI substudy of the ONTARGET study found that ramipril and telmisartan improved left ventricular mass and volume to the same degree; since there was no difference in clinical outcomes between the two drugs, ACE-i and ARB treatment again seem to be equally valuable for this indication. Therefore, for hypertension and cardiovascular event reduction in high-risk patients, they are interchangeable.

ACE inhibitors (Table 11.3)

Captopril, the first ACE-i, was introduced nearly 30 years ago. We are still learning how to use them. Groups with low renin levels (older or black people) tend to have a weaker blood pressure response to an ACE-i (and to beta-blockers) than younger or white people (e.g. in ALLHAT mean SBP was 4 mmHg lower in black patients treated with chlortalidone compared with lisinopril). Low-sodium diets and diuretics help blood

Table 11.3 ACE inhibitors in current use (*British National Formulary*, section 2.5.5.1)

	Daily doses (number)	Starting dose (mg)	Maximum recommended daily dose (mg)	Comments
Benazepril	1	10	40	Used in ACCOMPLISH; not available in UK
Captopril	2–3	12.5 b.d. (or 6.25 b.d.)	~ 100	Prototype drug. Short-acting, twice or three times daily; occasionally of value in patients with daytime postural hypotension and nocturnal hypertension
Cilazapril	1	1	5	
Enalapril	1	5	40	Introduced shortly after captopril. Serviceable, and used in many clinical trials
Fosinopril	1	10	40	
Imidapril	1	5	20	
Lisinopril	1	5	40 (80 in *BNF*)	Intermediate-acting; high doses probably best given twice daily
Moexipril	1	7.5	30	
Quinapril	1–2	10	40 (80 has been used)	
Ramipril	1–2	2.5	10	Higher doses used in trials, e.g. DREAM (15 mg), and in other countries. Action < 24 hours; give at bedtime for improved overnight blood pressure control
Trandolapril	1	0.5	4	

pressure control by increasing renin levels. However, the evidence for worse clinical outcomes is not conclusive, especially in treat-to-target studies. For example, in the important AASK study (2002) African-Americans with established hypertensive renal disease (eGFR 20–65 mL/ min) had fewer hard renal end points with ramipril treatment than with either metoprolol or amlodipine, for a similar reduction in blood pressure [15]. ACE inhibitors should be priority treatment for all ethnic groups with hypertension associated with diabetes, renal impairment or proteinuria.

Cautions and side-effects
Increasing serum creatinine and falling eGFR
These powerful and beneficial drugs need careful use and diligent monitoring. However, continuing concern about precipitating acute kidney injury still prevents angiotensin blockade being started and, equally importantly, discourages titration of doses to maximum therapeutic levels, particularly in those with impaired renal function, the very patients who stand to gain the most benefit. Measure creatinine, electrolytes and eGFR about 1 week after starting treatment (see Box 11.4). For unknown reasons, serum creatinine often increases by up to 30% (this applies to ARBs as well). It is not associated with long-term harm; on the contrary, it markedly reduces renal end points, regardless of the stage of CKD. If the rise is greater than 30%, stop the medication and ask for advice. If there is no change in serum creatinine after the first dosage step, then it is unlikely with further increases. Those at risk of more rapid deterioration can be identified:

- widespread atherosclerotic disease, with an increased risk of bilateral renal artery stenosis;
- high-dose diuretics, often associated with hypotension, for example in heart failure;
- those taking NSAIDs or cyclooxygenase (COX)-2 inhibitors.

Once the need for angiotensin blockade is established, if there is concern about starting treatment, refer for further advice and careful monitoring.

Hyperkalaemia (serum $K^+ \geqslant 5.6$ mmol/L)
Hyperkalaemia is a major problem, more troublesome than changes in measurements of renal function, and a small proportion of patients, perhaps 5%, cannot have any angiotensin-blocking treatment because of severe hyperkalaemia ($K^+ > 6.0$ mmol/L) on even minimal doses. High serum potassium is common to begin with because of type 4 renal tubular acidosis (hyporeninaemic hypoaldosteronism). Angiotensin II stimulates adrenal aldosterone secretion, and both ACE inhibitors and ARBs therefore impair urinary potassium excretion; the risk of hyperkalaemia

> **Box 11.6 Management of hyperkalaemia when starting diabetic patients on angiotensin-blocking treatment**
>
> - Be alert to the possibility of hyperkalaemia when eGFR is < 90 mL/min in people with diabetes.
> - Discontinue drugs that may worsen hyperkalaemia (NSAIDs, COX-2 inhibitors, beta-blockers). Remember to ask about salt substitutes, herbal preparations and over-the-counter NSAIDs.
> - Always prescribe thiazide or loop diuretics, according to renal function.
> - If eGFR and serum potassium are normal, a single renal screen 1 week after starting angiotensin-blocking treatment is sufficient.
> - If baseline serum K^+ ≥ 5.0 mmol/L or eGFR < 90 mL/min, or both, measure renal screen 1 week after each dose increase.
> - If serum K^+ ≥ 5.6 mmol/L at any stage, discontinue or reduce the dose of medication. Renal physicians are often comfortable with stable serum K^+ up to 6.0 mmol/L, but at this level there is little room for manoeuvre in the non-dialysed patient if there is any acute deterioration in renal function (e.g. intercurrent infection, diarrhoea, vomiting).

in people with diabetes treated with angiotensin blockade is much higher than in non-diabetic renal disease (Box 11.6).

Cough and angio-oedema
ACE-i-induced cough is common, but the data from the literature varies. Most studies quote 5–20%. After stopping the medication, it usually lingers for about 1–4 weeks, occasionally up to 3 months. It seems to be more common in smokers. Rechallenging with another ACE-i is not worthwhile; move to an ARB. Angio-oedema is rare, occurring in about 1 in 500 starting ACE-i treatment. Most cases occur in the first 30 days, but at a constant low rate thereafter up to a year or longer. Smokers, black patients, and people with allergies are more susceptible.

Teratogenicity
ACE inhibitors and ARBs have been known for many years to be teratogenic when taken during later pregnancy. There is now evidence for increased risk after exposure during early pregnancy. Reliable contraception or alternative blood pressure medication must be used in women of childbearing age.

Angiotensin receptor blockers (Table 11.4)

Losartan was the first ARB, introduced in 1995. Its patent expired in 2009, and other compounds will shortly be available in generic form.

Table 11.4 Angiotensin receptor blockers in current use (*British National Formulary*, section 2.5.5.2)

	Starting dose (mg)	Maximum dose (mg)
Candesartan	4, 8	32
Eprosartan	600	800
Irbesartan	150	300*
Losartan	50	100
Olmesartan	10	40
Telmisartan	40	80
Valsartan	80	320*

*Increased antiproteinuric effects have been reported with very high doses of these drugs, but they are not licensed beyond the stated doses (see Chapter 8).

The accumulated evidence (see above and Chapter 8) is that ARBs and ACE inhibitors are entirely comparable in their cardiac and renal benefits, and adverse biochemical effects (hyperkalaemia and initial worsening of renal function) are also similar. However, they do not cause cough (though angio-oedema can occur rarely). They are all long-acting, and can be taken once daily.

Calcium-channel blockers

CCBs are the best 'broad-spectrum' antihypertensives. They have been around for many years – the prototype dihydropyridine CCB nifedipine was first used in the 1970s; amlodipine, currently the most widely used CCB, in the early 1990s – and their safety and benefits in diabetes have been underplayed (concerns were raised about their safety in the mid-1990s, though they were quickly allayed). The dihydropyridines do not have any antiproteinuric effects (see Chapter 8), but they seem to reduce the burden of carotid and coronary atherosclerosis, perhaps to a greater extent than ACE inhibitors. For example, in the CAMELOT study (2004), cardiac end points in normotensive type 2 patients were significantly reduced by amlodipine 10mg daily compared with enalapril 20mg daily, and ultrasound measurements of coronary atheroma tended to be lower [16].

Dihydropyridine CCBs are especially valuable in the following clinical settings:
- isolated systolic hypertension in elderly people and hypertension in black people;
- where there is associated angina;
- pregnancy;
- as initial treatment in patients with widespread atheroma while renal artery stenosis is being investigated;
- in suspected secondary causes of hypertension (e.g. Conn's syndrome, phaeochromocytoma) they are safe clinically and do not interfere with diagnostic endocrine chemical tests;
- where rapid reduction in SBP is required (acute or ambulatory setting), especially where there is impaired renal function.

They are metabolically neutral, with possibly a slightly increased risk of precipitating diabetes in the susceptible compared with angiotensin-blocking agents. They are potentiated by low-dose diuretics, and are particularly effective in combination with angiotensin-blocking agents. High-dose dihydropyridines frequently cause symptomatic peripheral oedema and headaches. Gum hypertrophy may occur in up to 40% of nifedipine-treated patients, but it also occurs occasionally with diltiazem, an important caution in diabetes, where gingival disease is already common. Dihydropyridines are safe in combination with beta-blockers, but diltiazem/verapamil and beta-blockade can cause profound bradycardia and heart block. Some guidelines suport the use of combination dihydropyridine and non-dihydropyridine CCBs in hypertension, but there is only one published report of the combination, and neither drug was used in maximum doses.

Antiproteinuric effects of diltiazem and verapamil

Dihydropyridines, though effective antihypertensive agents, do not reduce proteinuria, nor reduce progression to renal end points (IDNT; see Chapter 8). Verapamil/diltiazem are often stated to reduce proteinuria by up to 20%, but the data are inconsistent and there are no long-term studies of renal outcomes. Where there is residual proteinuria after maximum angiotensin blockade, starting diltiazem/verapamil and carefully monitoring proteinuria, or changing a dihydropyridine to diltiazem/verapamil might be of value, especially if there are dihydropyridine side-effects. However, the evidence for antiproteinuric effects of thiazide diuretics and some beta-blockers is more solid.

Prescribing CCBs (Table 11.5)

Apart from nifedipine and felodipine, the dihydropyridines have long half-lives, and are taken once daily. Nifedipine and diltiazem/verapamil

Table 11.5 Calcium-channel blockers (*British National Formulary*, section 2.6.2)

	Daily doses (number)	Starting dose (mg) (once daily unless otherwise stated)	Useful daily dose range (mg)	Comments
Dihydropyridine CCBs				
Amlodipine	1	5	5–10	
Felodipine	1	2.5 or 5	5–10	Modified-release preparations are available
Lacidipine	1	2	4–6	
Lercanidipine	1	10	10–20	
Nifedipine	1–2			Modified-release nifedipine preparations are twice daily, dose range 20–40 mg; longer-acting formulations (e.g. Adalat LA) are once daily, dose range 30–90 mg
*Non-dihydropyridine CCBs**				
Diltiazem	1–2			Modified-release diltiazem preparations are twice daily, dose range 90–120; longer-acting formulations (e.g. Tildiem LA) are once daily, usual maximum doses 300–360 mg
Verapamil	1–2			Modified-release verapamil (e.g. Securon SR), dose range 240–480 mg daily

*Because of their different clinical effects, the *BNF* suggests that these agents should be prescribed by brand name.

are short-acting agents, and must be prescribed as modified-release or long-acting preparations. The *British National Formulary* recommends prescribing by brand name not generically, because of variable bioavailability between brands. The difficulties are compounded by the wide dose range and multiple doses available, but these are valuable drugs and it is worthwhile taking care initiating and continuing prescriptions.

Beta-blockers (*British National Formulary, section 2.4*)

Non-selective beta-blockers (e.g. propranolol, timolol) are no longer used in hypertension. The β_1- selective agents (e.g. atenolol, bisoprolol, metoprolol) are still widely used as secondary prevention after myocardial infarction, but often at low doses compared with those recommended for hypertension. Recent clinical trial results have led to cooling of enthusiasm for beta-blockade in general, despite the similar outcomes compared with captopril in the intensive blood pressure arm of UKPDS. ALLHAT did not contain a beta-blocker arm, and the atenolol/bendroflumethiazide combination in ASCOT-BPLA was less effective in preventing stroke and cardiovascular events than the CCB/ACE-i arm, though there was no difference in the primary outcome, myocardial infarction. Atenolol in particular has weak effects on stroke prevention, but this may reflect the fact that beta-blockers, like angiotensin-blocking agents, are less effective in older people with their lower renin state, and because they have a weaker effect on central (aortic) pressures, a prominent problem in the systolic hypertension resulting from stiff arteries in older people and those with diabetes. They are still effective in younger, obese, hypertensive patients with high adrenergic drive. Although the side-effect profile is apparently poor (fatigue, depressive symptoms, sexual dysfunction), this is not reflected in clinical trials, where subjects were not more likely to discontinue treatment compared with placebo. Nevertheless, these symptoms may be disruptive in individual patients.

The newest ('third-generation') beta-blockers, in use since the mid-1990s, have a better metabolic profile than other agents in the class, and may be preferable in diabetes, though there are no long-term outcome studies.

- *Carvedilol*, a non-selective beta-blocker, also has vasodilating alpha-blocking effects. Carvedilol 6.25–25 mg b.d. was compared with metoprolol 50–200 mg b.d. in the GEMINI studies, which found that carvedilol improved insulin sensitivity. There was no change in HbA_{1c}, which increased only slightly, and not clinically significantly, by 0.15% with metoprolol [17]. Lipids were slightly better with carvedilol, and fewer patients progressed to microalbuminuria.

- *Nebivolol* is a highly selective β_1-adrenergic beta-blocker that also vaso-dilates, but through a direct endothelial effect mediated by nitric oxide. It is given as a fixed dose of 5 mg daily, though 10 mg daily has been used. It also improves measures of central blood pressure, while having similar effects to atenolol on brachial blood pressure.
- *Labetalol*, a combined beta- and alpha-blocking agent, is no longer used out of pregnancy.

Diuretics

Thiazide diuretics have been the mainstay of antihypertensive treatment since the first potent thiazide was introduced in 1957, and have often been the agents against which other drug classes have been compared in important clinical trials [18]. They are especially useful in low-renin (salt-sensitive) states, for example older people, and black or obese patients. Resistant hypertension (see below), common in these groups, is frequently due to inadequate diuretic therapy. Despite half a century of use, disagreement continues about their optimum dosing and whether blood pressure lowering effects and cardiovascular benefits are common to all agents in the class. There is continuing controversy about their potential metabolic disadvantages – concern about these, together with their low pharmaceutical profile, prevents their being used in many patients – but there is no evidence that these in any way blunt their cardiovascular benefits, even in people with diabetes (Box 11.7). They are as effective in

---

Box 11.7 Thiazides: metabolic problems and potential solutions

Hypokalaemia (K⁺ < 3.5 mmol/L)
Thiazide monotherapy reduces serum K⁺ by 0.3–0.4 mmol/L, and hypokalaemia occurs in 7–8%. There is a strong relationship between hypokalaemia and in-trial development of diabetes. Use angiotensin blockade or potassium-sparing diuretic, and restrict dietary salt. Target K⁺ > 4.0 mmol/L.

Hyperuricaemia
Thiazides cause dose-related rise in serum urate. Enquire about previous episodes of gout. If present, measure urate, and start allopurinol, or use alternative antihypertensive.

Hyponatraemia (Na⁺ < 135 mmol/L)
More common than hypokalaemia: up to 18% in those over 70. Can be insidious and symptomatic. Frequent monitoring of electrolytes, especially in elderly females. Remember the additional risk of hyponatraemia with SSRIs. Particularly common in hospitalized patients with other medical or surgical problems.

reducing coronary events as any other class of antihypertensive agents, but in ALLHAT were more effective in reducing heart failure and stroke than lisinopril or amlodipine.

Loop diuretics (furosemide, bumetanide, torsemide) have a shorter duration of action than the thiazides, and in patients with normal or moderately impaired renal function (eGFR > 30–40 mL/min), thiazides are more effective antihypertensives. In advanced renal impairment, where reduced eGFR limits the amount of sodium reaching the distal tubules, the site of action of the thiazides, loop diuretics are often needed for other indications (peripheral oedema, heart failure or nephrotic syndrome), but are more effective in blood pressure reduction.

Comparing the effectiveness of the thiazides is very difficult (Table 11.6). Chlortalidone (a thiazide-like agent) has been the drug used in most major clinical trials, but hydrochlorothiazide is almost universally used in fixed-dose combinations. Bendroflumethiazide is widely used in the UK, but is not available as monotherapy in the USA. Indapamide (another thiazide-like agent) is the only drug that is widely used in both monotherapy and fixed-dose combinations. There is reasonable evidence that the very long half-life of chlortalidone makes it a more effective 24-hour agent than the shorter-acting hydrochlorothiazide or bendroflumethiazide, and this may account for its remarkable cardiovascular benefits in large-scale studies; it may be effective if doses are occasionally missed, or even if taken on alternate days.

Potassium-sparing diuretics (*British National Formulary*, sections 2.2.3 and 2.2.4)

The potassium-sparing agents, weak diuretics that cause very little natriuresis on their own and which act on the collecting ducts of the renal tubule, should be more widely used, both in thiazide-treated patients and in resistant hypertension (see below). They also reduce urinary magnesium loss, often associated with hypokalaemia and difficulty in restoring normokalaemia. Amiloride is most often used in the UK, but triamterene and spironolactone are also suitable. Fixed-dose combinations of thiazides and potassium-sparing agents used to be widely promoted, but because of the potassium-retaining effects of the angiotensin-blocking agents and the recognition of type 4 renal tubular acidosis in diabetes with its associated tendency to hyperkalaemia, they are less used in diabetes. However, maintaining adequate serum potassium levels is important, because of the risk of symptoms and arrhythmias with hypokalaemia, but also because there is good epidemiological and clinical trial evidence that hypokalaemia is associated with increased risks of ischaemic events, and there is an association between hypokalaemia and hyperglycaemia. Co-amilozide (e.g. amiloride 2.5 mg and hydrochlorothiazide

Table 11.6 Thiazide and thiazide-like agents in use in the UK (*British National Formulary*, section 2.2.1)

	Elimination half-life (hours)	Dose range (mg)	Comments
Bendroflumethiazide	9	2.5–5	Widely used at the lower dose; evidence for increased antihypertensive effect at 5 mg daily (but prevalence of hypokalaemia increases from 8 to 18% at the higher dose)
Chlortalidone	40–60	25–50	One preparation available in the UK (25–50 mg). No fixed-dose combinations
Cyclopenthiazide	–	250–500 μg	
Hydrochlorothiazide	3–13	12.5–25	Used exclusively in fixed-dose combinations with ACE inhibitors or ARBs; not available separately. Choose the combinations containing 25 mg hydrochlorothiazide, probably the lowest effective dose (many combinations contain 12.5 mg)
Indapamide	14	2.5	Modified-release preparation (1.5 mg) available, as effective as hydrochlorothiazide 25 mg daily; also in fixed-dose with perindopril
Xipamide	–	20	

25 mg) is a typical example of the combination, but many others are available.

Other agents

Alpha-blocking agents (*British National Formulary*, section 2.5.4)

The alpha-blockers are overall metabolically neutral, with perhaps minor beneficial effects on the lipid profile. They are useful in men with symptomatic benign prostatic hypertrophy. The major drug in this class is doxazosin. Used in ALLHAT up to 4 mg daily, it was a less effective antihypertensive agent than chlortalidone, and was inferior to it in reducing cardiovascular events and episodes of heart failure. However, modified-release doxazosin up to 8 mg daily was a highly effective agent when added as a non-blinded third agent in ASCOT-BPLA (mean fall in blood pressure 12/7 mmHg). Dizziness, headache, fatigue and oedema were the commonest side-effects in ASCOT, resulting in withdrawal of 8% of patients. Use only the modified-release form, starting at 4 mg daily.

Centrally acting agents (*British National Formulary*, 2.5.2)

Prazosin and clonidine are obsolete, and methyldopa is used only in pregnancy. Moxonidine is the best tolerated of the centrally acting agents, but still has limiting central side-effects, especially dry mouth and headache. It may reduce microalbuminuria in type 1 diabetes through inhibition of afferent renal sympathetic nerves. Dose is 200–600 μg daily.

Resistant hypertension

Defined (in people with diabetes) as blood pressure above 130/80 mmHg, despite good adherence to treatment with three antihypertensive agents of different classes, including a diuretic. Given the difficulty of achieving this target in any hypertensive diabetic person, a more practical blood pressure definition might be that defining the goal in non-diabetic people (i.e. >140/90 mmHg). The definitions are arbitrary, but are important in drawing attention to a large group of people who require extra thought about the possibility of secondary or reversible causes of hypertension, and serious consideration of their therapeutic regimen (Box 11.8). The prevalence of resistant hypertension is not known, even in non-diabetic populations, but may be as high as 10–20%. Poor control of SBP is characteristic, and worsens with increasing age. Acknowledge the existence of true refractory hypertension – blood pressure that is never near target despite compliance with multiple medications – in patients often showing combinations of these characteristics.

Box 11.8 Characteristics of patients with resistant hypertension

- Older age (fourfold increased risk of poor control in those over 75 compared with those under 60)
- High starting blood pressure
- Systolic hypertension
- Nocturnal non-dippers on ABPM
- Obesity
- High dietary salt intake
- Chronic kidney disease
- Diabetes
- Left ventricular hypertrophy
- African/African-American/African-Caribbean ethnicity
- Female
- Obstructive sleep apnoea
- Patients intolerant of, or unsuitable for, treatment with one or more standard agents

Source: adapted from Calhoun *et al.* (2008)

Approach to patients with resistant hypertension
Assess drug adherence and drug-related causes

Although strictly a cause of 'pseudoresistance' rather than true treatment resistance, it is so common and so difficult to quantify that it qualifies as an important real-life factor. In clinical trials, almost 50% of participants stop taking their medication within the first year; of those continuing with treatment, another 50% had a 'drug holiday' lasting three or more days at least once a year [19]. Regular medication reviews, actively involving patients and their carers, are important. Make every attempt to simplify treatment, using once-daily fixed-dose combinations wherever possible, even if you were taught to despise them. Dose slippage or failure to increase doses to recommended levels is common, and results from many factors. Home monitoring of blood pressure improves adherence in resistant hypertension.

Although non-blood pressure medication is unlikely itself to be a cause of resistant hypertension, bear in mind the drugs that antagonize existing antihypertensives (e.g. NSAIDs) and those that worsen blood pressure (e.g. sympathomimetics, glucocorticoids).

Consider secondary causes of hypertension
Obstructive sleep apnoea

Strongly associated with all degrees of hypertension, but particularly when it is severe; up to 80% of treatment-resistant hypertensive subjects have objective evidence of sleep apnoea. It is particularly prevalent and severe in men. OSA and hypertension are probably linked through sympathetic nervous system activation, resulting in increased cardiac output, peripheral resistance, and salt and water retention. This link is supported by the finding that spironolactone may reduce OSA in people with resistant hypertension. Awareness of the link between OSA and poorly controlled hypertension is clearly important. Administering a simple questionnaire would be practical in the routine setting, for example the Epworth Sleepiness Score assesses the severity of daytime somnolence using eight simple questions (score $\geq$ 10: 'sleepy'; score $\geq$ 18: 'very sleepy') (sleepapnoeanz.org.nz/epworth_scale.html).

Renal disease
The presence of even a moderate degree of CKD (e.g. serum creatinine $>$ 130 μmol/L, 1.5 mg/dL) was associated with failure to achieve target blood pressure in ALLHAT. Seeking and stenting renal artery stenosis in severe or treatment-resistant hypertensive people used to be an important radiology sub-specialty, but medical treatment is probably now the best approach; it is not clear which agents are best in this situation.

Endocrine causes
Cushing's syndrome is usually listed as a cause of resistant hypertension, and it is, but the clinical diagnosis is likely to be evident in a severely hypertensive person, although poorly controlled diabetes rather than poorly controlled hypertension is more likely to be associated with clinically inapparent Cushing's syndrome. Phaeochromocytoma is associated with sustained rather than paroxysmal hypertension in about 50% of cases. Always think of this diagnosis in resistant hypertension. Plasma metanephrines are thought to be the best screening test, but they are not generally available, and triplicated 24-hour urinary free catecholamine measurements are the simplest initial tests.

Primary aldosteronism
The spectrum of hyperaldosteronism now extends from the uncommon aldosterone-secreting Conn adenoma of the adrenal, presenting with resistant hypertension and significant hypokalaemia, to normokalaemic hyperaldosteronism with no discrete adrenal lesion. There may be considerable overlap with the highly prevalent low-renin state. Depending on the diagnostic methods used, about 20% of patients with resistant hypertension may have underlying primary aldosteronism. Again, the link with obesity and sympathetic nervous system activation and its consequences is strong, but not yet confirmed causally. Until renin levels are routinely available, recognizing that hyperaldosteronism is common and

is likely to respond to specific agents should help achieve target blood pressure. Complex and time-consuming protocols are no longer needed for initial evaluation, and a random measurement of the aldosterone/renin ratio will be reliable in patients even on treatment, other than those taking potassium-sparing diuretics, especially spironolactone [20].

Assess diurnal blood pressure and white-coat effect
Patients with resistant hypertension should have ABPM. The white-coat effect is as frequent in treatment-resistant patients as it is in other groups, and is likely to carry the same increased risk of adverse cardiovascular events (in patients already at high risk) as has now been established in untreated people with the white-coat phenomenon. Consistently elevated clinic blood pressure readings should be factored into management unless ABPM measurements are strictly normal.

Management
Lifestyle intervention
The many lifestyle factors already described should be reinforced. In particular, resistant hypertension is often associated with high dietary salt intake. Aerobic exercise is important, and there may be substantial reductions in blood pressure with possibly some legacy effect after the exercise programme has finished in patients with very severe hypertension on triple therapy.

Pharmacological treatment
The greatest benefit in patients already taking three agents, including a diuretic, derives from optimizing the diuretic regimen, as many have inappropriate volume expansion. If there is poorly controlled hypertension without a diuretic, then initially introduce a diuretic and maximize its dose. In those already taking a thiazide, maximize the dose, or perhaps, in view of the strong evidence (see above), replace the existing thiazide with chlortalidone 25–50 mg daily. Ensure that any fixed-dose combination with an angiotensin blocker contains the 25-mg dose of hydrochlorothiazide, or consider increasing bendroflumethiazide to 5 mg daily. After stabilizing a patient on therapy in this way, an ABPM test would be wise. If still poorly controlled, then in view of the high prevalence of hyperaldosteronism in this group, consider adding the aldosterone antagonist spironolactone 25 mg daily, with careful monitoring of renal function and potassium levels (expect K^+ concentration to rise by about 0.5 mmol/L). Responses may be dramatic: for example, addition of this dose of spironolactone as a fourth agent in ASCOT-BPLA further reduced blood pressure by a mean of 22/10 mmHg. Because of its anti-androgenic action, spironolactone is absolutely contraindicated in women of childbearing age,

and breast tenderness with or without gynaecomastia is common in men. Amiloride, which acts as an indirect aldosterone antagonist, is better tolerated, and may be more effective in lowering blood pressure than spironolactone. Start at 5 mg daily, increasing gradually to 20 mg daily or more. Monitor renal function and serum potassium frequently; K^+ concentration will rise, possibly by up to 0.8 mmol/L.

References

1. Cushman WC, Evans GW, Byington RP *et al.* Effects of intensive blood-pressure control in type 2 diabetes mellitus. ACCORD Study Group. *N Engl J Med* 2010; 362:1575–85. PMID: 20228401.
2. Chew EY, Ambrosius WT, Davis MD *et al.* ACCORD Study Group and ACCORD Eye Study Group. Effects of medical therapies on retinopathy progression in type 2 diabetes. *N Engl J Med* 2010;363:233–44. PMID: 20587587.
3. Brown MJ. Renin: friend or foe? *Heart* 2007;93:1026–33. PMID: 17488768.
4. Rönnback M, Fagerudd J, Forsblum C, Pettersson-Fernholm K, Reunanen A, Groop PH. Altered age-related blood pressure pattern in type 1 diabetes. Finnish Diabetic Nephropathy (FinnDiane) Study Group. *Circulation* 2004;110:1076–82. PMID: 15326070.
5. Shimbo D, Pickering TG, Spruill TM, Abraham D, Schwartz JE, Gerin W. Relative utility of home, ambulatory, and office blood pressures in the prediction of end-organ damage. *Am J Hypertens* 2007;20:476–82. PMID: 17485006.
6. Verberk WJ, Kroon AA, Lenders JW *et al.* Self-measurement of blood pressure at home reduces the need for antihypertensive drugs: a randomized controlled trial. Home Versus Office Measurement, Reduction of Unnecessary Treatment Study Investigators. *Hypertension* 2007;50:1019–25. PMID: 17938383.
7. Spence JD. White-coat hypertension is hypertension. *Hypertension* 2008;51:1272. PMID: 18378857.
8. Kikuya M, Hansen TW, Thijs L *et al.* Diagnostic thresholds for ambulatory blood pressure monitoring based on 10-year cardiovascular risk. IDACO Investigators. *Blood Press Monit* 2007;12:393–5. PMID: 18277319.
9. Sacks FM, Campos H. Dietary therapy in hypertension. *N Engl J Med* 2010;362:2102–12. PMID: 20519681.
10. Cook NR, Cutler JA, Obarzanek E *et al.* Long term effects of dietary sodium reduction on cardiovascular disease outcomes: observational follow-up of the trials of hypertension prevention (TOHP). *Br Med J* 2007;334:885–8. PMID: 17449506.
11. Tejada T, Fornoni A, Lenz O, Materson BJ. Nonpharmacologic therapy for hypertension: does it really work? *Curr Cardiol Rep* 2006;8:418–24. PMID: 17059793.
12. Zillich AJ, Garg J, Basu S, Bakris GL, Carter BL. Thiazide diuretics, potassium, and the development of diabetes: a quantitative review. *Hypertension* 2006;48:219–24. PMID: 16801488.
13. Jamerson K, Weber MA, Bakris GL *et al.* Benazepril plus amlodipine or hydrochlorothiazide for hypertension in high-risk patients. ACCOMPLISH Trial Investigators. *N Engl J Med* 2008;359:2417–28. PMID: 19052124.
14. Yusuf S, Teo KK, Pogue J *et al.* Telmisartan, ramipril, or both in patients at high risk for vascular events. ONTARGET Investigators. *N Engl J Med* 2008;358:1547–59. PMID: 18378520.

15. Wright JT Jr, Bakris G, Greene T *et al*. Effect of blood pressure lowering and antihypertensive drug class on progression of hypertensive kidney disease: results from the AASK trial. African American Study of Kidney Disease and Hypertension Study Group. *JAMA* 2002;288:2421–31. PMID: 12435255.
16. Nissen SE, Tuzcu M, Libby P *et al*. Effect of antihypertensive agents on cardio-vascular events in patients with coronary disease and normal blood pressure: the CAMELOT study: a randomized controlled trial. *JAMA* 2004;292:2217–25. PMID: 15536108.
17. Bakris GL, Fonseca K, Katholi RE *et al*. Metabolic effects of carvedilol vs meto-prolol in patients with type 2 diabetes mellitus and hypertension: a random-ized controlled trial. *JAMA* 2004;292:2227–36. PMID: 15536109.
18. Ernst ME, Moser M. Use of diuretics in patients with hypertension. *N Engl J Med* 2009;361:2153–64. PMID: 19940300.
19. Vrijens B, Vincze G, Kristanto P, Urquhart J, Burnier M. Adherence to pre-scribed antihypertensive drug treatments: longitudinal study of electronically compiled dosing histories. *Br Med J* 2008;336:1114–17. PMID: 18480115.
20. Funder JW, Carey RM, Fardella C *et al*. Case detection, diagnosis, and treat-ment of patients with primary aldosteronism: an Endocrine Society clinical practice guideline. *J Clin Endocrinol Metab* 2008;93:3266–81. PMID: 18552288.

Further reading

Aspirin
Colwell JA. Aspirin therapy in diabetes. *Diabetes Care* 2004;27(Suppl. 1):S72–S73. PMID: 14693931.
Pignone M, Alberts MJ, Colwell JA *et al*. Aspirin for primary prevention of cardio-vascular events in people with diabetes: a position statement of the American Diabetes Association, a scientific statement of the American Heart Association, and an expert consensus document of the American College of Cardiology Foundation. *Diabetes Care* 2010;33:1395–402. PMID: 20508233.

European guidelines
Lurbe E, Cifkova R, Cruickshank JK *et al*. Management of high blood pressure in children and adolescents: recommendations of the European Society of Hypertension. *J Hypertens* 2009;27:1719–42. PMID: 19625970.
Mancia G, DeBacker G, Dominiczak A *et al*. Guidelines for the management of arte-rial hypertension: the Task Force for the Management of Arterial Hypertension of the European Society of Hypertension (ESH) and of the European Society of Cardiology (ESC). *J Hypertens* 2007;25:1105–87. PMID: 17563527.
Mancia G, Laurent S, Agabiti-Rosei E *et al*. Reappraisal of European guidelines on hypertension management: a European Society of Hypertension Task Force doc-ument. *J Hypertens* 2009;27:2121–58. PMID: 19838131.
Parati G, Stergiou GS, Asmar R *et al*. ESH Working Group on Blood Pressure Monitoring. European Society of Hypertension guidelines for blood pressure monitoring at home: a summary report of the Second International Consensus Conference on Home Blood Pressure Monitoring. *J Hypertens* 2008;26:1505–26. PMID: 18622223.

UK guidelines
National Institute for Health and Clinical Excellence. Hypertension: management of hypertension in adults in primary care (CG34). Available at www.nice.org.uk/CG034

Williams B, Poulter NR, Brown MJ *et al*. Guidelines for management of hypertension: report of the fourth working party of the British Hypertension Society, 2004: BHS IV. *J Hum Hypertens* 2004;18:139–85. PMID: 14973512.

Williams B, Poulter NR, Brown MJ *et al*. British Hypertension Society guidelines for hypertension management 2004 (BHS-IV): summary. *Br Med J* 2004;328: 634–40. PMID: 15016698.

USA guidelines

Urbina E, Alpert B, Flynn J *et al*. Ambulatory blood pressure monitoring in children and adolescents: recommendations for standard assessment. A scientific statement from the American Heart Association Atherosclerosis, Hypertension, and Obesity in Youth Committee of the Council on Cardiovascular Disease in the Young and the Council for High Blood Pressure Research. *Hypertension* 2008;52:433–51. PMID: 18678786.

Chobanian AV, Bakris GL, Black HR *et al*. Seventh report of the Joint National Committee on prevention, detection, evaluation, and treatment of high blood pressure. *Hypertension* 2003;42:1206–52. PMID: 14658957. Expected date of JNC 8, autumn 2011. Available at www.nhlbi.nih.gov/guidelines/hypertension/jnc8/index.htm

Calhoun DA, Jones D, Textor S *et al*. Resistant hypertension: diagnosis, evaluation, and treatment. A scientific statement from the American Heart Association Professional Education Committee of the Council for High Blood Pressure Research. *Hypertension* 2008;117:e510–e526. PMID: 18574054.

International

Shaw JE, Punjabi NM, Wilding JP, Alberti KG, Zimmet PZ. Sleep-disordered breathing and type 2 diabetes: a report from the International Diabetes Federation Taskforce on Epidemiology and Prevention. *Diabetes Res Clin Pract* 2008;81: 2–12. PMID: 18544448.

Websites

British Hypertension Society: www.bhsoc.org
Blood pressure measuring devices (supported by ESH): www.dableducational.org
Dietary Approaches to Stop Hypertension (DASH): www.nhlbi.nih.gov/health/public/heart/hbp/dash
Blood pressure levels in children and adolescents (age 1–17): www.nhlbi.nih.gov/guidelines/hypertension/child_tbl.htm

Lipids

CHAPTER 12

Key points

- Of the major cardiovascular risk factors, dyslipidaemia is often the easiest to control, even to the increasingly stringent target levels recommended especially for high-risk people.
- Type 2 diabetes is no longer considered a 'coronary risk equivalent' requiring secondary prevention/standard care in all patients. However, patients with known macrovascular disease remain at exceptionally high risk, and 'lower [LDL] is better' probably applies for cardiovascular outcomes in this group.
- Patients with uncomplicated type 1 diabetes generally have good lipid profiles and do not routinely require lipid-lowering treatment.
- Lipid profiles progressively deteriorate with increasing levels of proteinuria.
- LDL remains the primary treatment aim for type 2 patients, with target levels below 2.0 mmol/L (75 mg/dL) for all, and less than 1.7–1.8 mmol/L for those with previous cardiovascular events.
- Reduction of LDL to target still leaves high residual risk. Targeting the insulin-resistant dyslipidaemia features (low HDL-cholesterol, elevated triglycerides) with judicious combination treatment probably reduces risk further in secondary prevention patients and those with pronounced dyslipidaemia, but not in most primary prevention patients (FIELD, ACCORD studies).
- Lipid management is only one component of the multimodal management programme mandatory for patients with complications, especially microalbuminuria.

Practical Diabetes Care, 3rd edition. © David Levy.
Published 2011 by Blackwell Publishing Ltd.

Introduction

Dyslipidaemia in diabetes is usually the simplest cardiovascular risk factor to control. There are few patients whose lipid profile cannot be optimized, or at least markedly improved, with a combination of lifestyle interventions and single or combination drug therapy. The increasingly stringent targets recommended for high-risk patients, usually with pre-existing cardiovascular disease, proteinuria or both, are also attainable, but judicious combination therapy will be needed in some. There is persuasive evidence that low LDL levels maintained in the long term are associated with stabilization or even reversal of carotid and coronary atheroma, though we have yet to see the impressive intravascular ultrasound images correlate with event reduction in RCTs.

The difficulty lies not so much in achieving targets, but deciding which patients or groups of patients are likely to gain the most benefit from treatment. Statins do not consistently reduce total mortality, even in patients with diabetes, and although absolute event risk reductions in the early studies (e.g. 4S, 1994) were large (about 25–30%), in current trials they are much lower, about 3% over 5 years. Even with the most stringent LDL lowering, residual risk is still high; factors other than LDL must be important, and relatively modest lipid-lowering in the Steno type 2 study (2008) was associated with a very impressive absolute risk reduction, so long as it was accompanied by reasonable glycaemic and blood pressure control, lifestyle and aspirin treatment.

Lipids in type 1 diabetes

Type 1 patients without microvascular complications (especially microalbuminuria) and in good glycaemic control have a good lipid profile, similar to that of non-diabetic people of the same age. For example, baseline lipids in DCCT patients during the 1980s were as follows:
- total cholesterol 4.6 mmol/L (180 mg/dL)
- HDL-cholesterol 1.3 mmol/L (51 mg/dL)
- LDL-cholesterol 2.8 mmol/L (110 mg/dL)
- triglycerides 0.9 mmol/L (80 mg/dL).

Despite these impressive numbers, there are subtle lipoprotein abnormalities, for example slight increases in small atherogenic particles and minor differences in HDL subfractions, though total atherogenic particles are no different. Accordingly, the management of lipids in uncomplicated type 1 diabetes is quite different from that in type 2 diabetes, though the distinction is not sufficiently recognized in guidelines.

There is an intriguing association between exceedingly high HDL-cholesterol levels and long survival (50 years or more) in type 1 diabetes with a relatively low burden of vascular disease. In the UK and USA alike, these golden cohort patients have mean HDL-cholesterol levels of 1.7–1.9 mmol/L (66–74 mg/dL), with correspondingly low triglycerides (0.8–1.0 mmol/L, 70–90 mg/dL). Males comprised half the cohorts, which itself is remarkable, and hints at a causal link between lipid profiles and long survival. Contributing factors to the high HDL levels in these groups (mean age 70) might include current (and therefore probably long-standing) exercise and moderate alcohol intake, but other factors operate, for example familial longevity (see Chapter 4). Although the HDL in some people with numerically high levels may not be 'good', at least in this situation it appears to be benign.

Lipids in type 2 diabetes

Type 2 patients are usually considered to have similar or slightly higher total and LDL cholesterol levels compared with non-diabetic subjects, but contemporary studies, for example the Heart Protection Study (HPS), found slightly lower mean baseline total cholesterol levels (about 0.2 mmol/L, 8 mg/dL), possibly as a result of greater awareness of dyslipidaemia among people with type 2 diabetes. Even though LDL levels are not significantly elevated, at any LDL level coronary risk is higher than in non-diabetic subjects, though the studies from which these data come are now old (e.g. MRFIT, mid-1970s), and the current risk difference is likely to be considerably lower. Interestingly, there was also no difference in HDL-cholesterol levels in the HPS (mean 1.08 mmol/L, 42 mg/dL). However, whatever the mean levels, individual type 2 patients and those with the insulin resistance syndrome tend towards a characteristic profile, with increased triglycerides and depressed HDL-cholesterol.

Non-traditional lipid measurements that increase atherogenicity in type 2 diabetes include:
- increased apolipoprotein (apo)B, reflecting the total number of atherogenic particles, even though LDL may be normal;
- increased small, dense, atherogenic LDL particles that are prone to oxidation and glycation;
- possibly increased lipoprotein(a);
- altered HDL subfractions (HDL_2 is the most powerful anti-atherogenic fraction, and is reduced in diabetes; the antioxidant activity of the small dense HDL_3 fraction is reduced);
- increased non-HDL-cholesterol (easily calculated from the standard lipid profile).

Increased cardiac risk in type 2 diabetes, and a re-evaluation of the 'coronary equivalent' concept

These subtle differences together may account for some of the increased cardiovascular risk in type 2 diabetes. The level of increased risk is the subject of much academic discussion. In large diabetic populations studied in the past, coronary risks were often found to be approximately doubled compared with non-diabetic groups, and the concept of diabetes as a coronary risk equivalent is almost embedded – type 2 patients who have not yet suffered a coronary event have a similar coronary risk as non-diabetic patients who have already had an event. The therapeutic corollary of this view is that all patients require equally intensive secondary prevention treatment. More recent studies find a much lower coronary event rate in type 2 patients, and meta-analysis estimates the risk not as twofold increased but about half that of the non-diabetic population with a previous event. This may reflect the gradual but cumulatively important improvements in multimodal management resulting in better cardiovascular outcomes in type 2 diabetes. However, the statistic that is invariant across old and recent studies alike is the extremely high risk of type 2 patients who have had an event (e.g. 10% annual risk, compared with about 2% in those without an event) [1]. Guidelines do not yet reflect this revised view that implies we should individualize risk management with a strong emphasis on the highest risk patients.

Lipid profiles in poorly controlled diabetes and effects of intensive glycaemic treatment

In poorly controlled type 1 and 2 diabetes, insulin deficiency increases hepatic VLDL secretion leading to elevated serum triglycerides, sometimes massively so, resulting in lipaemic serum, difficulties in measuring many other serum components (including amylase), and an increased risk of acute pancreatitis. In large clinical studies improvement in glycaemic control from moderately poor levels primarily reduces triglycerides, with lesser falls in total and HDL cholesterol, but these would not usually be detectable in the individual patient (Table 12.1). Intensified glycaemic control in type 1 diabetes often causes weight gain, and intensively treated patients in the DCCT with the greatest weight gain (BMI 34 vs. 24) also showed a global deterioration in lipid profiles, with increased total and LDL cholesterol, increased triglycerides and lower HDL levels [2]. Systolic and diastolic blood pressure and high-sensitivity CRP all increased as well. There must be concern that worsening cardiovascular risk profiles in intensively treated type 2 diabetes may outweigh the limited advantages of tight glycaemic control as shown in the recent trials.

Table 12.1 Lipid profiles in well-controlled and poorly controlled diabetes			
	Total/LDL cholesterol	**Triglycerides**	**HDL-cholesterol**
Well controlled			
Type 1	Normal or ↓	Normal or ↓	Normal or ↑
Type 2	Normal or ↓	↑	↓
Poorly controlled			
Type 1	↑	↑	Normal
Type 2	↑	↑ or ↑↑	↓
Nephropathy	↑ or ↑↑	↑ or ↑↑	↓

There is little point in requesting lipid profiles in severely hyperglycaemic newly diagnosed or very poorly controlled patients; leave until control has been stabilized for at least a month (Box 12.1).

Familial hypercholesterolaemia may coexist with diabetes; suspect where there is high cholesterol (> 8.0 mmol/L, 310 mg/dL) and normal triglycerides. Clinical characteristics include:
- premature arcus senilis (in the 30–40 year age group);
- tendon xanthomata, xanthelasmata;
- family history of premature coronary artery disease (< 50 years of age) in non-diabetic first-degree relatives.

Familial combined hyperlipidaemia is an important, common (1 in 250) but complex polygenic disorder that shares many of the features of the insulin resistance syndrome, and is the most common familial form of hyperlipidaemia in young survivors of myocardial infarction. Definitions are not standardized but a typical lipid profile would show total cholesterol 7.0 mmol/L, HDL-cholesterol 0.9 mmol/L and triglycerides 3.0 mmol/L.

Screening for secondary causes of hyperlipidaemia

Simple screening tests will identify most secondary causes of hyperlipidaemia:
- liver function tests and gamma-glutamyltransferase;
- full blood count (mean corpuscular volume, alcohol);
- creatinine and electrolytes;

Box 12.1 Measuring lipids and lipid profiles

- LDL-cholesterol is the universal measurement of atherogenic lipoproteins in clinical trials and the primary goal of lipid management, though a better estimate of atherogenic (apoB-containing) particles is probably:

  non-HDL-cholesterol – [total cholesterol – HDL-cholesterol]

- LDL-cholesterol can be determined by:

  LDL-cholesterol = total cholesterol – (HDL-cholesterol + VLDL-cholesterol)

  VLDL particles ('triglyceride-rich particles') carry most of the plasma triglycerides, in a ratio of about 2.2 : 1 triglycerides to cholesterol (or 5 : 1 in non-SI units).

- Total cholesterol and HDL are measured directly in most laboratories, but LDL and VLDL cannot be routinely and cheaply measured. In the Friedewald equation used to calculate LDL, VLDL is therefore approximated by triglycerides/2.2 (or 5):

  LDL-cholesterol = total cholesterol – [HDL + triglycerides/2.18 (or 5)]

- When plasma triglycerides are high, the triglyceride/cholesterol ratio in VLDL particles is not maintained, so the equation is not valid in the postprandial state and when triglycerides are above 4.52 mmol/L (400 mg/dL).
- Because of the assumptions and approximations in the Friedewald equation, in addition to biological and laboratory variation and uncertainty about the quality and duration of fasting, take care not to over-interpret minor changes in LDL. This is of particular importance when discussing changes to drug therapy.
- 'Fasting' means 12 hours without calorie intake (water only). Do not underestimate the problems and anxiety caused by this duration of fasting in insulin-taking patients. Request fasting lipid profiles only when necessary.
- After ACS (and other acute medical or surgical illness), fasting lipid profiles are reliable within the first 24 hours, but not again until at least 6 weeks after the event.

- urate (associated metabolic syndrome, especially hypertriglyceridaemia);
- thyroid function.

Factors modifying lipid levels
Hypothyroidism
Overt hypothyroidism (TSH ≥ 10 mU/L) reduces hepatic LDL clearance, and profound hypothyroidism can be associated with very high

cholesterol levels, but in most cases even when total cholesterol is elevated (e.g. > 6.2 mmol/L, 240 mg/dL), expect only a modest reduction (~ 10%) after thyroxine treatment.

Subclinical hypothyroidism (TSH 5–10 mU/L) is not consistently associated with high cholesterol levels, though lipid profiles may improve with thyroxine treatment. There are no RCTs of thyroxine replacement and cardiovascular events in subclinical hypothyroidism, and treatment should be individualized [3]. Both hypothyroidism and statin treatment can give rise to muscle symptoms. Resistance to statin treatment may be caused by any degree of hypothyroidism (the upper limit of normal for TSH is now considered to be as low as 4.5 mU/L). Repeat thyroid function tests periodically in dyslipidaemic type 2 patients. There is still interest in thyromimetics in the treatment of dyslipidaemia; the hepatic-specific eprotirome improves the lipid profile of statin-treated patients, though it slightly reduces HDL.

Renal impairment
As proteinuria progresses, the lipid profile deteriorates, and is especially marked in nephrotic patients. High triglycerides and low HDL-cholesterol, partly related to decreased apoA1 synthesis, are characteristic. Surprisingly, patients with renal failure tend to have total and LDL cholesterol levels that are lower than patients without renal failure. Dyslipidaemia itself may impair renal function, for example abnormal LDL may increase angiotensin II and upregulate the AT_1 receptor, and increased chylomicron remnants may cause vasoconstriction. Naturally, angiotensin blockade and intensive lipid-lowering treatment are both required in patients with any degree of renal impairment or proteinuria, but lipid lowering does not reduce cardiovascular events once renal impairment has progressed to ESRD, presumably because advanced calcific coronary artery and valvular heart disease is not helped by statin treatment (see below).

Effects of drugs used in diabetes
Non-insulin agents
Only the glitazones have substantial effects on lipid profiles that may impact on cardiovascular outcomes. Pioglitazone has overall a beneficial effect. In particular HDL rises by about 9%, and triglycerides fall by 0.2–0.6 mmol/L (18–53 mg/dL), but LDL rises slightly. Other non-insulin agents are either lipid-neutral or have generally beneficial but minor effects that are not clinically significant compared with formal lipid-modifying treatment.

Antihypertensive agents
For information on beta-blockers and thiazide diuretics, see Chapter 11. Beta-blockers have occasionally been associated with severe hypertriglyceridaemia and acute pancreatitis.

Primary therapeutic target: LDL-cholesterol

Who should have statins for LDL lowering?

This list, derived from UK guidelines for diabetes, is largely uncontentious [4].

- Those with clinical evidence of macrovascular disease: angina, myocardial infarction, revascularization, peripheral vascular disease, cerebrovascular disease including transient ischaemic episodes.
- Concomitant familial hypercholesterolaemia or combined hyperlipidaemia.
- Treated hypertension.
- Microalbuminuria or macroalbuminuria (including those with previous microalbuminuria resolved by antiproteinuric and antihypertensive treatment).
- Impaired renal function (e.g. eGFR < 60 mL/min).
- Most diabetes patients over 50 years of age without additional cardiovascular risk factors.

There is insufficient evidence for universal statin treatment in the following groups, and judgement should be used in assessing individual risk:

- current smokers, irrespective of age (e.g. younger type 1 patients with no other cardiovascular risk factors);
- obesity (BMI > 30);
- metabolic syndrome.

Statin treatment in type 1 patients

Statin treatment should be individualized in type 1 patients under 50 years of age where there are no other cardiovascular risk factors and no microvascular complications. Uncomplicated patients under 40 probably do not require statin treatment. Microalbuminuric patients require statins, but there is nothing to guide us in the management of those with isolated retinopathy or neuropathy. These are rapidly expanding groups of patients, comprising possibly 5–10% of type 1 patients, for whom there is no evidence for the routine use of statin treatment. A meta-analysis of 1500 type 1 patients in RCTs between 1994 and 2005 found that the cardiovascular benefit of statins was similar to those with type 2 diabetes. However, nearly 40% had previous vascular events and hypertension, and their lipid profile was similar to that of the type 2 cohort (cholesterol 5.7 mmol/L, LDL 3.4 mmol/L, HDL 1.3 mmol/L, triglycerides 1.6 mmol/L), much more adverse than that of uncomplicated patients, for example those in the DCCT (see above) [5].

LDL targets for type 2 diabetes (Table 12.2)

The CARDS study (2005) established that maintaining LDL at about 2.0 mmol/L (80 mg/dL) reduced events in type 2 patients without known

Table 12.2 Progressive lowering of target LDL levels in type 2 diabetes since 1997

Target LDL (mmol/L, mg/dL)	Study/guideline and date published	Clinical features	Comments/drugs used
< 2.6 (100)	Post CABG Trial, 1997	CABG patients. LDL < 2.6 mmol/L reduced progression of atheroma and need for revascularization	Lovastatin 40–80 mg daily, cholestyramine 8 g daily added if necessary to achieve target
< 2.6 (100)	HPS, 2003	50% with, 50% without cardiovascular disease at baseline; small number of type 1 patients	Simvastatin 40 mg daily
< 2.6 (100)	NCEP ATP III, 2001, updated 2004	Target for all patients; supports LDL 1.7–1.8 mmol/L in patients with cardiovascular disease	Atorvastatin 10 mg daily
~ 2.0 (80)	CARDS, 2004	Type 2 patients with risk factors (retinopathy, albuminuria, current smoking, hypertension) but without overt cardiovascular disease	Atorvastatin 10 mg daily
2.0 (80)	TNT, 2005*	Secondary prevention: definite coronary artery disease	Atorvastatin 80 mg daily
2.1–2.2 (82–86)	ASCOT-LLA, 2005	Hypertensive type 2 patients	Atorvastatin 10 mg daily
< 1.8 (70)	PROVE-IT TIMI 22, 2005*	Post-ACS secondary prevention	Atorvastatin 80 mg or pravastatin 40 mg daily
1.6 (62)	ASTEROID, 2006*	Definite obstructive coronary disease in at least one artery. Decrease in intravascular ultrasound-measured atheroma volume (not clinical events)	Rosuvastatin 40 mg daily

*Studies not performed primarily in type 2 diabetes patients.

cardiovascular disease; this is an LDL level at which coronary and carotid atheroma probably stabilizes in those with established vascular disease (REVERSAL and ARBITER studies, respectively, using atorvastatin 80 mg daily). Coronary heart disease events fell within 6 months of starting treatment, and from 12 months until the end of the trial showed a consistent 37% relative risk reduction. Hypertensive patients in ASCOT-LLA also achieved an LDL of 2.1–2.2 mmol//L, with a substantial reduction in stroke; these and other RCTs support reducing LDL to 2.0 mmol/L in the general type 2 population. Unusually, epidemiological and clinical data agree on the log-linear relationship between LDL lowering and reduction in cardiovascular events, with no discernible plateau or J-shaped curve. Studies using angiographic measures of atheroma (e.g. ASTEROID, 2006) support LDL lowering to about 1.6 mmol/L (60 mg/dL), and to 1.7–1.8 mmol/L (66–70 mg/dL) in patients with ACS (PROVE-IT TIMI 22, 2004). Ultra-low LDL levels in the same trial (< 1.04 mmol/L and 1.04–1.55 mmol/L, 40–60 mg/dL) were associated with lower cardiac event rates than in other groups. There are no RCTs of these ultra-low LDL levels in either the general type 2 population or those with stable coronary disease, but they are attainable, do not seem to be associated with an increased risk of side-effects of the high doses of statins needed to achieve these levels (e.g. rosuvastatin 40 mg daily or atorvastatin 80 mg daily), and may well be justified in individuals at the very highest risk, for example people with stents or bypass grafts or who have evidence of extensive coronary artery disease or atheroma elsewhere [6].

Management

Diet therapy

Always considered the mainstay of dyslipidaemia management, significant reductions in LDL levels are difficult to achieve with diet except with long-term adherence to a regimen that most Western people would consider punitive. Changing the fatty acid constituents of diets to decrease ω-6 fatty acids while substantially increasing ω-3 fatty acids, for example through the Mediterranean diet (see Chapter 5), which is high in *cis*-monounsaturated fats and ω-3 fatty acids, may not substantially change the conventional lipid profile but may have important effects on cardiovascular and cancer outcomes, and is easier to incorporate long term into contemporary diets than the conventional advice on measures largely designed to reduce LDL levels by decreasing saturated fat intake (Box 12.2). Patients with very marked hypertriglyceridaemic syndromes, often genetic in origin (see below), should have primary diet therapy, as drug therapy may be relatively ineffective; modest reductions in weight and BMI, low alcohol intake and increased moderate exercise may have

---

Box 12.2 General advice about dietary fats

- Saturated fat < 7% of total energy intake
- Cholesterol intake < 200 mg/day
- *Cis*-monounsaturated fats (e.g. olive oil) can be up to 20% of total energy intake, with appropriate restriction of carbohydrate
- Restrict *trans*-fatty acids (e.g. solid vegetable oils and highly saturated fatty foods, contained especially in fast food)
- Dietary soluble fibre up to 10–25 g/day and plant sterols up to 2 g/day
- Lower ω-6/ω-3 dietary ratio: increase ω-3 fatty acids (e.g. oily fish); reduce ω-6 fatty acids (e.g. palm, soybean, sunflower oils and nuts)
- Increase sterol-enriched dairy products

---

significant effects on the underlying non-alcoholic fatty liver disease that seems to drive the excessive VLDL secretion.

Statins

Statins inhibit 3-hydroxy-3-methylglutaryl coenzyme A (HMG-CoA) reductase, which is rate-limiting in hepatic cholesterol synthesis. Lower intrahepatocyte cholesterol levels upregulate LDL receptors and enhance plasma clearance of LDL. Although the major effect of the statins is to lower LDL-cholesterol, the longer-acting, more powerful agents (atorvastatin and rosuvastatin) have a significant effect on triglyceride and HDL levels (Table 12.3). Whether these effects, or their powerful (but not always predictable) effects on lowering high-sensitivity CRP, contribute to their consistently beneficial effects on macrovascular events is less clear; statins are effective in reducing cardiovascular events in people with low HDL levels, and the clinical benefits of atorvastatin are seen at high doses, even though it is the only statin that tends to show an inverse relation between dose and HDL levels. The early secondary prevention statin studies (e.g. 4S, CARE and LIPID) recruited few diabetic subjects, and it was not clear initially whether they benefited to the same extent as non-diabetic subjects (the effectiveness of LDL lowering by statins in diabetes was not in question; the doubts included their lower initial LDL levels, the heterogeneity of the diabetes population and the relatively poor response of the lipid profile of the metabolic syndrome to statin treatment). However, from 2004, with the publication of the 'primary prevention' diabetes CARDS study, it became clear that statins reduced relative risks of cardiovascular events by a similar or even greater amount than in non-diabetes subjects, and also conferred higher absolute risk reductions. RCTs and guidelines are consistent in recommending a target LDL of 2 mmol/L (80 mg/dL) in all type 2 diabetic patients. The questions remaining

Table 12.3 Effects of different drug classes on lipid levels (typical mean percentage changes)

Drug/nutrient class	LDL	HDL	Triglycerides
Statins	↓20–50	↑4–10	↓10–20
Fibric acids	↓0–20	↑10–20 (inconsistent)	↓20–50
Niacin (nicotinic acid)	↓10–15	↑15–35	↓20–50
Ezetimibe	↓15–20	Minor ↑ (5)	Minor ↓ (10)
n-3 Fatty acids	Minor ↑	↔	↓15–35
Phytosterols/stanols	↓13–16	↔	↔

↑, increase; ↓, decrease; ↔, no change.

are whether attaining lower or even much lower LDL levels is of bene-fit in those with and without overt cardiovascular disease, what that LDL level should be, and whether combination treatment further improves the outlook (see below).

Dose–response relationships

Low starting doses of statins result in large reductions in LDL (10 mg of simvastatin, atorvastatin and rosuvastatin reduce LDL by about 25, 35 and 45% respectively). Thereafter doubling the dose further reduces LDL by only 4–6%, a small reduction that might not be apparent consider-ing the variability of routine clinical testing (see Box 12.1). Using doses intermediate between the tablet strengths available is therefore not log-ical. Since statin side-effects are dose-related, the highest doses carry an increased risk of side-effects while they may not be reliable in achiev-ing target LDL. However, when low- and high-dose atorvastatin (10 and 80 mg daily) were compared in the TNT study (2005), the (expected) 16% LDL difference between the two groups was associated with a 20% lower risk of cardiovascular events (absolute risk reduction 2%). The risk of per-sistent liver function test abnormalities was greater with the high dose, though the absolute risk was low; not all studies show a dose-related side-effect profile for atorvastatin. Southeast Asian and South Asian patients develop higher circulating statin levels than white subjects for a given drug and dose, and starting doses can be lower. This is reflected in clinical trials, where very low doses (e.g. simvastatin 10 mg daily) are often effective, and in clinical practice, where the most powerful statin, rosuvastatin, should be started at 5 mg daily, and the highest recommended dose is 20 mg in these ethnic groups (Table 12.4).

Analyses of many statin trials over a long period confirm the close relationship between achieved LDL and vascular events, whichever statin is used. Importantly, an analysis of TNT found that high dose atorvastatin (80 mg) not only reduced the risk of a first event, but also subsequent events up to the fifth. Using the standard measure in clinical trials – reducing the occurrence of first events – therefore substantially underestimates the total burden of cardiovascular events prevented [7]. In contrast to blood pressure studies, the majority of lipid trials are not treat-to-target, use fixed doses of specific statins, and retrospectively establish target LDL levels. The ideal approach would therefore be to match the statin to the required LDL reduction, and then rapidly change the dose to achieve target LDL. (As an example, simvastatin 40 mg will reduce LDL by about 40%; a patient with a baseline LDL above 3.2 mmol/L is unlikely to achieve the target LDL of 2.0 mmol/L). However, the significant cost difference between generic simvastatin and the other agents means that most guidelines suggest starting with simvastatin and only changing to other drugs if there are side-effects or an inadequate response. The situation will change as patents expire on other statins. In practice, because LDL will remain stable indefinitely on statin treatment as long as the medication is taken, it is worthwhile investing some time achieving target LDL.

Morning or evening dosing?

Cholesterol is mostly synthesized at night when dietary intake is low, and therefore the effect of statins is thought to be greater if they are taken in the evening. In small studies with simvastatin, LDL levels were about 10% lower with night-time dosing. However, drugs are generally taken more reliably in the morning, and since compliance is so important with statin treatment, reliable morning tablet-taking is preferable to intermittent evening dosing. The long-acting agents atorvastatin and rosuvastatin are equally effective whenever they are taken. Alternate day rosuvastatin 20 mg is nearly as effective as 10 mg daily.

Practical approach to statin treatment

Dose titration does not occur in practice, and most patients continue to take the dose on which they were started, but until we can routinely prescribe potent statins, active dose titration and changes of statin preparation are important in order to achieve target levels. After a change of statin or a dose, LDL will stabilize within 6 weeks, so it should be possible

Table 12.4 Currently available statins (*British National Formulary*, section 2.12)

Drug	Usual starting dose (mg)	Maximum clinically effective dose (mg)	Doses used in clinical trials	Comments
Atorvastatin	10	80	10 mg (CARDS, ASCOT-LLA); 80 mg (PROVE-IT, REVERSAL, TNT)	
Fluvastatin	20	80	Many smaller trials at 40–80 mg	Weak statin, but low risk of drug interactions; widely used in transplant patients
Simvastatin	20 or 40	40	40 mg (HPS, 4S)	The 80-mg dose, though recommended in NICE guidelines, carries a high rate of side-effects. Generics available
Pravastatin	40	40	40 mg (LIPID, ALLHAT-LLT, CARE)	Weak statin but effective at 40 mg where starting LDL is relatively low. Generics available. Low risk of drug interactions. Should be used more than it is
Rosuvastatin	5–10	40	40 mg (ASTEROID)	40-mg dose for hospital initiation only; maximum 20 mg in Asian patients (start at 5 mg). Low risk of drug interactions

to establish a well-tolerated effective regimen in most patients within a few months. UK clinical guidelines do not specify in detail the practical place of statins other than simvastatin. The following is a possible strategy for secondary prevention.

1 Trial of simvastatin up to 40 mg or maximum tolerated dose (since most of the effect is seen with 10 or 20 mg, it is worthwhile starting with these lower doses, especially in patients anxious about statins and in those with pre-existing musculoskeletal symptoms).
2 If target LDL is not reached, trial of atorvastatin up to 40 mg (80 mg with caution).
3 If still not at target, trial of rosuvastatin up to 40 mg daily (20 mg in South Asian and Southeast Asian patients).
4 If still not at target, add ezetimibe 10 mg daily.
5 If titration of a statin is limited by side-effects, use ezetimibe as monotherapy or add-on to maximum tolerated statin.

Adverse effects

Statins are worldwide the most widely prescribed drugs. More than 20 years of clinical experience confirms them also as some of the safest, but their massive usage has highlighted the burden of adverse effects. However, they are often carelessly prescribed with medications known to interact with them, some combinations resulting in increased plasma levels that increase the risk of adverse effects [8].

Muscle side-effects
The spectrum of muscle side-effects is wide, and their mechanism not known. Fulminating rhabdomyolysis, associated with gross elevations of CK ($>10\,000\,U/L$) is usually idiosyncratic and occurs within 3 months of starting statin treatment. Drug–drug interactions account for about half of cases, and renal impairment and hypothyroidism are also suspected contributory factors. Rhabdomyolysis can present with muscle weakness, and not always muscle pain and tenderness. Much feared, and undoubtedly 30–40 times more common in statin-treated patients compared with the general population, it is still extremely rare. Much more common and variable is myopathy or myalgia, neither reliably associated with increased CK levels. Myopathy with elevated CK levels is probably dose-related, for example there is a fourfold increased risk in patients taking simvastatin 80 mg daily compared with those taking 20–40 mg daily; also uncommon, its incidence is between 0.1 and 0.2%. Minor myalgia is common; for example, in the HPS, almost one-third of patients in the placebo and simvastatin-treated groups reported minor muscle aches and pains. These and other 'minor' symptoms commonly reported with statins (gastrointestinal symptoms, headache, functional impairment and

flu-like symptoms) are apt to be dismissed as having a doubtful causal link to statin treatment, but they are lifelong treatments and should not be discounted so lightly. Review drug interactions; if there are none, stop the statin and suggest a rechallenge. The patient's view is paramount. Trying another agent is worthwhile, though there is scant data on the value of this manoeuvre. Stereotyped symptoms on taking more than one agent should be a signal to discontinue further attempts at instituting long-term treatment, though dogged persistence with multiple agents, with a misplaced emphasis on the life-saving as opposed to the risk-reducing properties of statins, is depressingly common. Try other strategies (see below). CK levels are often measured for various reasons in asymptomatic patients and statins consequently not prescribed. It is safe to use statins in patients with asymptomatic elevations in CK up to five times the upper limit of the reference range.

Liver side-effects
Significant elevations in transaminases (more than three times upper limit of normal on two occasions separated by days or a few weeks) are about 10 times more common at the highest doses of statins than at the lowest. They usually occur within the first 3 months of treatment, in about 0.6 per 1000 clinical trial participants, and nearly always resolve after discontinuing the statin. Liver failure is very rare, and occurs at a rate no higher than that in the general population. Baseline checks of liver function, repeated 2–3 months after starting treatment, are still recommended, and caution required in patients with more than threefold elevation of alanine aminotransferase/aspartate aminotransferase. The background rate of liver function abnormalities in type 2 patients is high, and careful selective monitoring is needed. However, there is increasing evidence for the safety of statins in patients in non-alcoholic fatty liver disease, and expert opinion is that cardiovascular benefits outweigh hepatic risks in patients with stable chronic liver disease.

Drug interactions (Table 12.5)
The importance of drug interactions with statins is not fully appreciated in routine practice. All statins undergo extensive first-pass metabolism by liver cytochrome (P450/CYP) systems, and therefore circulating levels are markedly influenced by concomitant drug therapy that also relies on this system for metabolism. Enzyme-inducing drugs will reduce statin levels, enzyme-inhibiting drugs will increase statin levels. Increased levels are associated with a greater risk of muscle side-effects. Unfortunately, it is not known whether 'minor' side-effects are increased when statins are prescribed with CYP inhibitors. In patients taking complex antiretroviral or immunosuppressive drug regimens, consider using pravastatin,

Table 12.5 Clinically significant drug interactions with statins

Statin and CYP substrates	Drugs reducing statin levels (CYP inducers)	Drugs increasing statin levels (CYP inhibitors)
Atorvastatin, simvastatin (CYP3A4)	Carbamazepine Dexamethasone Omeprazole Phenytoin Rifampicin	Amiodarone Clarithromycin, erythromycin Diltiazem, verapamil Fluoxetine, sertraline, venlafaxine, tricyclics Glucorticoids Grapefruit juice Ketoconazole, fluconazole Protease inhibitors St John's Wort Tacrolimus, ciclosporin Tamoxifen Telmisartan Warfarin
Rosuvastatin, fluvastatin (CYP2C9; minor interaction)	Phenytoin Rifampicin	Ketoconazole, fluconazole
Pravastatin (largely eliminated by other routes)	–	–

fluvastatin or rosuvastatin rather than simvastatin; careful discussion with pharmacist colleagues is needed.

There is a striking increase in muscle side-effects in patients taking statin–fibrate combinations. Gemfibrozil appears to be the chief culprit, but it was little used in the UK in any case. It should be considered obsolete. Myopathy/myositis is not increased when fenofibrate is combined with a statin, but the clinical indications for using the combination are now much less compelling, and other drug combinations are probably more clinically effective in patients with mixed or insulin-resistant dyslipidaemias (see below). There is much interest in the interaction between statins and grapefruit juice. Grapefruit juice inhibits CYP3A4 and increases systemic exposure to statins. Taking a glass of standard grapefruit juice every day modestly increases plasma simvastatin and atorvastatin levels, but pravastatin has no effect, as it is not metabolized by the CYP3A4 pathway. Large quantities of grapefruit juice should not be part of the dietary portfolio of people with diabetes in any case (one suggestion is that more than 1 L a day could be clinically significant), but a regular small intake is of no clinical consequence. The non-dihydropyridine CCBs diltiazem and verapamil are mild-to-moderate CYP3A4 inhibitors. Clinically, statin side-effects do not seem to be more common when atorvastatin or simvastatin are combined with these agents, but bear in mind the possibility.

Statins in renal disease
See Chapter 8.

Ezetimibe
Ezetimibe is the first cholesterol absorption inhibitor, acting at a gastro-intestinal cholesterol target now known to be Niemann–Pick C1-like protein, which is involved in the accumulation of free cholesterol. It lowers LDL-cholesterol, with minor effects on other lipids (see Table 12.3). Its mode of action is quite different from that of other lipid-lowering agents acting on the gut, for example the bile-acid sequestrants and the plant sterols/stanols.

The indications for ezetimibe are as follows.
- As add-on therapy to high-dose (or maximum-tolerated dose) statin where target LDL has not been reached.
- Where there is a poor response to statins: type 1 patients have high intestinal cholesterol absorption, and respond well to ezetimibe.
- As monotherapy when statins are not tolerated.
- In CKD (including pre-dialysis and dialysis patients), combined with low-dose simvastatin [9].

Ezetimibe acts synergistically with statins and, importantly, its LDL-lowering effect is constant and independent of baseline LDL. Individual responses to ezetimibe vary widely, but most studies show a mean LDL fall of about 15–18%. This drop is equivalent to the effect of three statin dosage steps (e.g. an eightfold increase in dose of simvastatin, from 10 to 80 mg), and therefore avoids the need for intensive statin dose titration, as it is well tolerated and does not add to the side-effect rate of statins. Concern about increased risks of cancer with ezetimibe has been allayed by careful analysis.

Enthusiasm for ezetimibe has been tempered by the results of three contentious RCTs, and the absence of hard end-point studies.
- There was no reduction in CIMT in familial hypercholesterolaemia over 2 years in the ENHANCE trial (2008), despite the expected additional 17% LDL lowering when added to existing maximum statin therapy. However, this result was not unexpected given the clinical circumstances.

- Ezetimibe with simvastatin also had no effect on echocardiographic measurements or operative intervention in aortic stenosis (SEAS, 2008), but again the outcome was not unexpected – even potent statins are ineffective in this condition.
- In the ARBITER-6 HALTS study (2009), niacin added to statin treatment reduced CIMT while ezetimibe had no effect, but the trial was stopped early, and this probably biased the outcome.

A more conventional study, IMPROVE-IT, due to finish in 2011, is using simvastatin 40 mg with or without ezetimibe in post-ACS patients [10].

In contrast to this controversy, studies dating back many years have shown consistent benefits from LDL lowering, whatever the method used. In clinical practice, ezetimibe remains valuable in secondary prevention and very high risk primary prevention patients. There is a single dose, 10 mg daily. No significant drug interactions are known. In small studies it is safe and effective when combined with fibrates or niacin, though these combinations are not licensed.

Fibric acid drugs

The fibrates (gemfibrozil, ciprofibrate, bezafibrate and fenofibrate) are PPAR-α agonist drugs with a broad spectrum of lipid actions, though their major clinical effects are to:

- increase HDL and decrease triglycerides;
- reduce fasting and postprandial levels of triglyceride-rich lipoproteins;
- shift LDL from the small dense pattern, thought to be atherogenic, to a larger more buoyant fraction.

Other than reducing triglycerides, the fibrates do not have effects that can be measured on a simple lipid profile, and in long-term studies they do not significantly reduce LDL (see Table 12.3).

The indications for the fibrates are:

- Hypertriglyceridaemia, particularly where there is a risk or history of acute triglyceride-induced pancreatitis (e.g. triglycerides > 10 mmol/L, 890 mg/dL).
- After myocardial infarction in cautious combination with a statin where there is an insulin-resistant dyslipidaemia.
- In patients with cardiovascular risk factors when there is a severe insulin-resistant dyslipidaemia (e.g. HDL < 0.75 mmol/L, 30 mg/dL; triglycerides > 3.2 mmol/L, 284 mg/dL; ACCORD).
- Patients with retinopathy.

Fibrates were widely used as monotherapy until the introduction of the statins in the late 1980s, and a further series of clinical trials reported from the late 1990s onwards. The most unequivocally positive was the secondary prevention VA-HIT (1999), in which gemfibrozil reduced events in a group of post-myocardial infarction patients with low-normal LDL (mean 2.9 mmol/L, 113 mg/dL), mildly raised triglycerides (1.8 mmol/L, 160 mg/dL) and low HDL (0.8 mmol/L, 31 mg/dL). Greatest benefit was seen in subjects with diabetes or the insulin resistance syndrome. However, implementing the findings of this study in practice was difficult: gemfibrozil could not be safely combined with a statin in routine practice, and the results of studies of intensive post-myocardial infarction statin therapy were uniformly impressive.

Angiographic progression of atheroma was reduced by fenofibrate in the DAIS (2001). There have been two large recent primary prevention studies in diabetes, both using fenofibrate. FIELD (2005) was negative for its primary major cardiovascular end points, and several reasons have been cited. The baseline lipid profile was remarkably normal, and the effects of fenofibrate were limited to a 30% fall in triglycerides from a high-normal level of 1.7 mmol/L (150 mg/dL). The placebo group had a high rate of 'drop in' statin treatment. It may simply be that fenofibrate, in contrast to the other fibrates, is relatively ineffective, though safe, both as monotherapy and in combination with a statin. Much has been made of other benefits of fenofibrate seen in FIELD (e.g. significant reductions in laser-treated retinopathy and of below-ankle amputations) for which there are no mechanistic explanations, but may be related to the many non-lipid effects of fibrates, for example improvement in procoagulant and inflammatory states [11]. Of great interest, and confirming this unexpected outcome, ACCORD Eye also found that patients with some retinopathy at baseline had a lower risk of significant retinopathy progression if treated with fenofibrate (in addition to simvastatin).

The ACCORD lipid study (2010) was the first completed primary prevention study using combination simvastatin and fenofibrate treatment. The baseline lipid profile was again unremarkable and, apart from a lower HDL, was similar to VA-HIT (LDL 2.56 mmol/L, 100 mg/dL; HDL 0.97 mmol/L, 38 mg/dL; triglycerides 1.8 mmol/L, 162 mg/dL). By the end of the study (mean follow-up 4.7 years) only triglycerides were significantly different in the fenofibrate group. There was no reduction in cardiovascular end points when compared with a group treated with simvastatin alone, but patients with the most severe insulin-resistant dyslipidaemia (e.g. HDL < 0.75 mmol/L, 30 mg/dL; triglycerides > 3.2 mmol/L, 284 mg/dL) benefited, with a significant 10–13% risk reduction in major cardiovascular and coronary events [12]. This finding, that patients with the most atherogenic dyslipidaemia, gain real benefit with fibrate treatment has now been replicated across several major studies, but most analyses have been post hoc, and it is difficult to draw firm messages for primary care teams.

In the light of the failure of these two definitive end-point studies, fibrates can no longer be considered to have a routine place in primary prevention or in high-risk patients. In post-myocardial infarction patients, combination therapy with a statin plus niacin has a stronger overall evidence base (see below). However, where dramatic triglyceride lowering to a safe level (i.e. < 5 mmol/L, 445 mg/dL) is required for reducing the risk of acute pancreatitis, the fibrates are more effective than either the potent statins or niacin (see below), neither of which should be used as initial treatment in patients with predominant hypertriglyceridaemia. Patients with retinopathy that is progressing or not regressing could be considered for fibric acid treatment, especially if their lipid profile approximated that of the high-risk ACCORD subjects.

Gemfibrozil has the strongest evidence base of all the fibrates in clinical trials, but in practice modified-release bezafibrate (400 mg daily) is probably the fibrate of first choice where it is available, followed by fenofibrate (micronized, 160, 200 and 267 mg daily). Fibrates are renally excreted, and doses should be reduced according to eGFR (see *British National Formulary*, section 2.1.2); do not use fibrates where eGFR is below 15 mL/min.

Because of the general move away from fibric acid drugs, there is often no clear plan how to manage the many patients still taking them. Patients with a clear history of triglyceride-induced pancreatitis should not change therapy, but in others withdrawing the fibrate is safe and has little effect on the lipid profile so long as the statin is maintained. However, always carefully review the history for the initial indication(s).

Adverse effects
Non-specific side-effects are common, as with statins, but the risk of muscle side-effects is lower. Statistically significant increases in CK levels have been reported with fenofibrate. Serum creatinine can reversibly increase by up to 15% resulting from increased creatinine synthesis; if a fibrate is coprescribed with an angiotensin-blocking agent, the cumulative effect on serum creatinine can be quite dramatic. Trial withdrawal of one or both agents can be reassuring. Combination statin–fibrate treatment must not be used in renal impairment.

Phytosterols/phytostanols

Plant sterols, hydrogenated to stanols, reduce cholesterol absorption. At the recommended intake of 2 g/day they can lower total cholesterol by 12–14% and LDL by 13–16% (e.g. 0.3 mmol/L, 12 mg/dL) in both type 1 and 2 patients. Like ezetimibe, they have no effect on HDL or triglycerides (see Table 12.3) or on inflammatory markers such as high-sensitivity CRP.

The indication for these agents is as a nutraceutical at a fixed dose of 2 g/day in mild hypercholesterolaemia.

Though there is the expected variability in clinical response, at its maximum it is a clinically useful effect, though only about one-third as potent as a statin, and is additive to that of other LDL-lowering agents (including ezetimibe). The difficulty and paradox is that at present they are mostly incorporated into dairy products, as they are fat-soluble (though a soy-based drink is available in the UK). They therefore have to be taken daily as a food (nutraceutical), for example 1.5 tablespoons of margarine, or more conveniently as a small yoghurt drink. The products are expensive and compliance is a problem. In the UK, Benecol and Flora pro.activ brands are available; the former is lower in carbohydrate calories.

The ω-3 polyunsaturated fatty acids

The ω-3 (also known as *n*-3) polyunsaturated fatty acids are 'essential' in that they cannot be endogenously synthesized and must be obtained from food. The major long-chain fatty acids EPA and DHA are found in greatest concentrations in the flesh of oily fish, and the livers of both oily and non-oily fish.

The indications for the ω-3 polyunsaturated fatty acids are:
- post-myocardial infarction prophylaxis starting within 3 months of an event;
- in combination with a statin in mild–moderate mixed hyperlipidaemia;
- in patients with macrovascular disease (stroke and heart failure);
- in vitamin D insufficiency.

Low dose (EPA + DHA 1 g daily)

There is no effect on the conventional lipid profile, but there is significant reduction in:
- sudden death in post-myocardial infarction patients (GISSI-Prevenzione, 1999);
- secondary stroke events in Japanese (JELIS, 2008; EPA 600 mg t.d.s.);
- hospitalization for heart failure (GISSI-HF, 2008).

High dose (EPA + DHA 2–8 g daily)

Hepatic VLDL synthesis is lowered, and hepatic β-oxidation and peripheral VLDL clearance is increased, resulting in dose-dependent triglyceride lowering (~10% at 2 g, ~40% at 8 g) (see Table 12.3). LDL and HDL levels both increase by about 6%, depending on the baseline triglyceride level. Although effective and well tolerated, very large doses of fish oils are needed to achieve the same degree of triglyceride lowering as more convenient doses of fibrates or niacin (see below). Prescription preparations (e.g. Omacor, UK; Lovaza, USA) contain 1 g EPA + DHA per capsule, compared with standard high-strength fish oil capsules which contain about 300 mg each, while 10 mL of high-strength liquid fish oil contains about 1.9 g, usually in an EPA/DHA ratio of 3 : 2. Though fish consumption is important, oily fish provides only 1 g per serving of 56–84 g (2–3 ounces), and it is therefore difficult to achieve adequate intakes for triglyceride lowering through fish intake alone. Dietary intake in Americans with diabetes is very low indeed, with a mean of 160 mg/day in the Look AHEAD study (though intake still correlated well with triglyceride level and more weakly with HDL-cholesterol) [13]. Flax (linseed) and other plant seeds contain long-chain fatty acids, for example linolenic acid, and these can be substituted for fish oils in vegetarians. However, it is generally thought that conversion to the ω-3 series is low.

Up to 4 g daily of ω-3 fatty acids (Omacor) are safe in combination with statins in combined hyperlipidaemias; other combinations, for example with niacin or fibrates, would be logical in patients with severe hypertriglyceridaemia, but there are no formal studies and the combinations are unlicensed. There have been concerns about worsening glycaemic control with ω-3 fatty acid treatment, but the effect is small and not clinically relevant. Proprietary preparations of fish oils may contain small amounts of vitamin D, for example 5 μg (200 units) per 10 mL.

Niacin (nicotinic acid)

Niacin (nicotinic acid, vitamin B_3) has a long history of use in lipid disorders. While it only modestly reduces total cholesterol by about 10%, the effect on LDL-cholesterol may be as much as 30% because of its powerful effects on metabolic syndrome-related lipid abnormalities of elevated triglycerides and depressed HDL-cholesterol, improving each by 20–30%. It can therefore be considered a broad-spectrum antidyslipidaemic agent.

The indications for niacin are:
- secondary myocardial infarction prevention combined with a statin, especially in insulin-resistant dyslipidaemia (elevated triglycerides, depressed HDL);
- after CABG.

Secondary prevention studies combining niacin with either a statin or bile-acid resin in patients with established coronary artery disease have shown decreased progression of atherosclerosis (quantitative coronary angiography and CIMT) and, allowing for the small numbers of patients recruited into trials of this vintage (1970s to 1990s), reduced recurrent clinical events. Patients with the metabolic syndrome appear to benefit even more [14].

Niacin has been less used of late because the high doses required to produce these benefits (1–2 g daily) frequently cause flushing and itching which can be severe, although the intensity and frequency of the attacks decreases with use. Nevertheless, in clinical practice persistence with niacin treatment is poor. There have also been concerns about increased insulin resistance and blood glucose levels in both diabetic and non-diabetic patients. In diabetic patients, mean fasting glucose levels rise by a median of only 0.2 mmol/L (4 mg/dL) and HbA_{1c} by 0.2% (2 mmol/mol), undetectable on routine testing, and clinically not relevant compared with the benefit of niacin treatment.

An extended-release preparation (Niaspan) has been joined by a fixed-dose combination (Tredaptive), containing laropiprant, a selective blocker of the receptor for the prostaglandin PGD_2 responsible for the cutaneous flushing. Still, 60% of patients will experience mild flushing or worse in the first week of treatment, compared with 80% taking other forms of nicotinic acid; in maintenance treatment, 55% will have some flushing, though 40% are classified as mild. This important treatment still requires detailed explanation and support in the early phases of treatment if adherence is to be maximized. Medication is taken at night, increasing from 1 g nicotinic acid/20 mg laropiprant to 2 g/40 mg after a month (there is likely to be increased flushing for about 3 weeks when the dose is increased). The triple combination of niacin, ezetimibe and simvastatin is effective and safe in patients with mixed hyperlipidaemias treated for over a year [15].

Bile-acid sequestrants

The first agents to be effective in LDL lowering, but usually difficult to use in practice because of limiting gastrointestinal side-effects and the inconvenience of taking unpalatable and insoluble powders several times a day. They rapidly fell out of use after the introduction of statins.

The indications for the bile-acid sequestrants are as follows:
- LDL lowering in patients intolerant of statins;
- in combination with statins where further LDL lowering is required to reach target.

Colesevelam, more potent than the earlier agents, better tolerated and presented as tablets rather than resin, was introduced in 2000. LDL can fall a further 10–16% when added to a statin and although the mechanisms are not known, HbA_{1c} may fall by up to 0.8% (this is a consistent effect in RCTs, and in the USA it is licensed for its blood glucose-lowering effect). Gastrointestinal side-effects are still quite frequent, for example constipation in 20%, and high doses are required for the full LDL-lowering effect (six 625-mg tablets daily). It is effective, safe and well tolerated in patients with familial hypercholesterolaemia already taking a statin and ezetimibe. While potentially valuable in some patients, it is currently very expensive in the UK.

Severe hypertriglyceridaemia (Box 12.3)

Syndromes with very high triglycerides (> 20 mmol/L, 2000 mg/dL) are uncommon (e.g. 1 in 1000 in the population), but are over-represented in diabetes and alcoholism (presumably especially so where the two are combined). The underlying genetic conditions are uncommon but there are several of them, contributing to a common phenotype in clinical practice, including:

- lipoprotein lipase gene mutations;
- associated apoC2 abnormalities (Fredrickson hyperlipoproteinaemia type I), exacerbated by insulin deficiency;
- Fredrickson hyperlipoproteinaemia types IIb, III (dysbetalipoprotein-aemia) and V;
- chylomicronaemia syndrome.

Poorly controlled type 2 diabetes, at diagnosis or beyond, is a common cause of severe mixed hyperlipidaemia, often remitting completely when the diabetes comes under control. Lipid-lowering treatment is not needed under these circumstances, unless there is residual hypertriglyceridaemia once the diabetes is treated. Fatty liver, a common accompaniment,

---

Box 12.3 Management of severe hypertriglyceridaemia

Consider underlying conditions
- Poorly controlled or undiagnosed diabetes
- Alcohol (possibly not very large quantities)
- Non-alcoholic fatty liver disease
- Medication (uncommon: high-dose thiazides, oestrogens)
- High-carbohydrate diets (high intake of fruit juice or non-diet soft drinks)

Investigations
- Liver ultrasound
- Repeated fasting lipid profile, including apoB measurement where available (discuss with chemical pathology or lipid clinic)

Lifestyle management
- Restrict alcohol to one drink a day
- Reduce fat intake as much as possible, to less than 10% if feasible
- Reduce weight, increase activity
- Frequent follow-up

Medication
- Optimize diabetes control (especially with metformin and insulin)
- Fibric acid drugs, high-dose fish oil (up to 8 g EPA + DHA daily), niacin; combination treatment often needed

exacerbates the problem. Triglycerides above 10 mmol/L predispose to acute pancreatitis, and the National Cholesterol Education Program guidelines in the USA recommend triglycerides should be the primary therapeutic target when above 5 mmol/L.

References

1. Bulugahapitiya U, Siyambalapitiya S, Sithole J, Idris I. Is diabetes a coronary risk equivalent? Systematic review and meta-analysis. *Diabetic Med* 2009;26:142–8. PMID: 19236616.
2. Purnell JQ, Hokanson JE, Marcovina SM, Steffes MW, Cleary PA, Brunzell JD. Effect of excessive weight gain with intensive therapy of type 1 diabetes on lipid levels and blood pressure: results from the DCCT. *JAMA* 1998;280:140–6. PMID: 9669786.
3. Duntas LH, Wartofsky L. Cardiovascular risks and subclinical hypothyroidism: focus on lipids and new emerging risk factors. What is the evidence? *Thyroid* 2007;17:1075–84. PMID: 17900236.
4. Feher MD, Winocour PH, on behalf of the Association of British Clinical Diabetologists. ABCD position statement on lipid modifying drug therapy in diabetes. *Practical Diabetes International* 2007;24:458–62.
5. Cholesterol Treatment Trialists' (CTT) Collaborators. Efficacy of cholesterol-lowering therapy in 18,686 people with diabetes in 14 randomised trials of statins: a meta-analysis. *Lancet* 2008;371:117–25. PMID: 18191683.
6. Wiviott SD, Cannon CP, Morrow DA, Ray KK, Pfeffer MA, Braunwald E. Can low-density lipoprotein be too low? The safety and efficacy of achieving very low low-density lipoprotein with intensive statin therapy: a PROVE-IT TIMI 22 substudy. *J Am Coll Cardiol* 2005;46:1411–16. PMID: 16226163.
7. LaRosa JC, Deedwania PC, Shepherd J et al. Comparison of 80 versus 10 mg of atorvastatin on occurrence of cardiovascular events after the first event (from the Treating to New Targets [TNT] trial). *Am J Cardiol* 2010;105:283–7. PMID: 20102935.
8. Bellosta S, Paoletti R, Corsini A. Safety of statins: focus on clinical pharmacokinetics and drug interactions. *Circulation* 2004;109(23 Suppl. 1):III50–III57. PMID: 15198967.
9. Landray M, Baigent C, Leaper C et al. The second United Kingdom Heart and Renal Protection (UK-HARP-II) Study: a randomized controlled study of the biochemical safety and efficacy of adding ezetimibe to simvastatin as initial therapy among patients with CKD. *Am J Kidney Dis* 2006;47:385–95. PMID: 16490616.
10. Cannon CP, Giugliano RP, Blazing MA et al. Rationale and design of IMPROVE-IT (IMProved Reduction of Outcomes: Vytorin Efficacy International Trial): comparison of ezetimibe/simvastatin versus simvastatin monotherapy on cardiovascular outcomes in patients with acute coronary syndromes. *Am Heart J* 2008;156:826–32. PMID: 19061694.
11. Rajamani K, Colman PG, Li LP et al. Effect of fenofibrate on amputation events in people with type 2 diabetes mellitus (FIELD study): a prespecified analysis of a randomised controlled trial. *Lancet* 2009;373:1780–8. PMID: 19465233.

12. Ginsberg HN, Elam MB, Lovato LC *et al.* Effects of combination lipid therapy in type 2 diabetes mellitus. ACCORD Study Group. *N Engl J Med* 2010;362:1563–74. PMID: 20228404.
13. Belalcazar LM, Reboussin DM, Haffner SM *et al.* Marine omega-3 fatty acid intake: associations with cardiometabolic risk and response to weight loss intervention in the Look AHEAD (Action for Health in Diabetes) study. *Diabetes Care* 2010;33:197–9. PMID: 19841042.
14. Zhao XQ, Krasuski RA, Baer J *et al.* Effects of combination lipid therapy on coronary stenosis progression and clinical cardiovascular events in coronary disease patients with metabolic syndrome: a combined analysis of the Familial Atherosclerosis Treatment Study (FATS), the HDL-Atherosclerosis Treatment Study (HATS), and the Armed Forces Regression Study (AFREGS). *Am J Cardiol* 2009;104:1457–64. PMID: 19932775.
15. Fazio S, Guyton JR, Polis AB *et al.* Long-term safety and efficacy of triple combination ezetimibe/simvastatin plus extended-release niacin in patients with hyperlipidemia. *Am J Cardiol* 2010;105:487–94. PMID: 20152243.

Further reading

Betteridge DJ (ed.) *Case Studies in Lipid Management*. London: Informa Healthcare, 2006.

British Cardiac Society; British Hypertension Society; Diabetes UK; HEART UK; Primary Care Cardiovascular Society; Stroke Association. JBS 2: Joint British Societies' guidelines on prevention of cardiovascular disease in clinical practice. *Heart* 2005;91(Suppl. 5):v1–v52. PMID: 16365341.

Brunzell JD, Davidson M, Furberg CD *et al.* Lipoprotein management in patients with cardiometabolic risk: consensus statement from the American Diabetes Asdociation and the American College of Cardiology Foundation. *Diabetes Care* 2008;31:811–22. PMID:18375431.

Haffner SM. American Diabetes Association. Dyslipidemia management in adults with diabetes. *Diabetes Care* 2004;27(Suppl. 1):S68–S71. PMID: 14693930.

Levy D, Galton D. Diabetes, lipids, and atherosclerosis. In: DeGroot LJ, Jameson JL (eds) *Endocrinology*, 5th edn, chapter 135. Philadelphia: Elsevier Saunders, 2005.

National Institute for Health and Clinical Excellence. Statins for the prevention of cardiovascular events. NICE Technology Appraisal Guidance 94, January 2006. Available at www.nice.org.uk/TA94

National Institute for Health and Clinical Excellence. Lipid modification. NICE Clinical Guideline 67 (2008, expected revision May 2011). Available at www.nice.org.uk/CG67

Websites

National Cholesterol Education Program Adult Treatment Panel (NCEP ATP) III (2001, updated 2004) (NCEP ATP IV expected autumn 2011): www.nhlbi.nih.gov/guidelines/cholesterol/

Management of severe hypertriglyceridemia: www.emedicine.medscape.com/article/126568-overview

Psychological aspects of diabetes

CHAPTER 13

Key points

Type 1

- Disordered eating, insulin omission and hypoglycaemia avoidance are common in young people, especially girls, with type 1 diabetes.
- Formally diagnosed eating disorders are infrequent, but have a poor prognosis.
- Psychosocial factors, especially parental well-being, are closely associated with metabolic control in young people.
- The number of insulin injections a day does not impact on quality of life, but high total daily doses of insulin and BMI do.
- About one-third of young adults do not access specialist diabetes services. This group is in poor glycaemic control and has a higher rate of significant psychiatric problems.

Type 2

- Depression is a risk factor for developing type 2 diabetes, may contribute to and accelerate complications, and is associated with worse glycaemic control; when severe, it is associated with increased all-cause mortality.
- Only about one-quarter of patients with high anxiety and depression scores are recognized in primary care or by diabetes specialist nurses, and most patients go untreated. These are likely to be patients with more chronic complications, who in turn may benefit most from active intervention.

(Continued)

Practical Diabetes Care, 3rd edition. © David Levy.
Published 2011 by Blackwell Publishing Ltd.

- Screening for depression does not improve management, increase antidepressant prescription rates, or improve outcomes, and has a high false-positive rate.
- Flexible management of depression with antidepressants, psychological treatments or both is no less successful than in non-diabetic individuals.

Introduction

That there is a close link between long-term conditions and psychological functioning is to state the obvious. But the complexity of the relationship, especially in a condition that spans a lifetime, such as diabetes, has only relatively recently been explored. In addition, the therapeutic options, once the often very subtle problems have been identified, are only just emerging. Finally, the literature is full of studies describing cross-sectional associations, many of them expected or unsurprising, but only longitudinal studies can uncover causality; fortunately, detailed and validated measures of psychological function are now routinely included in many current large-scale RCTs, and the next few years should give us a much clearer understanding of the dynamics of psychological aspects of diabetes and, more importantly, an insight into therapies. Because the fundamental processes at work in type 1 and type 2 diabetes are different, it is worthwhile discussing them separately, especially in relation to the intimate association between family functioning and type 1 diabetes in young people.

Type 1 diabetes

The literature on the effect of psychological and psychosocial stresses on people with type 1 diabetes has rapidly increased since DCCT published, and there is a view that family stresses, particularly over the imperative for 'good' glycaemic control, established by the DCCT, have increased since then, especially in relation to questions of blood glucose testing, disordered eating and the closely linked problem of omitting insulin doses.

Events around the time of diagnosis

About one-third of children develop a clinically significant adjustment disorder in the 3–12 months following the diagnosis of type 1 diabetes; although this usually resolves, if it persists it is associated with later psychological difficulties. Although less common, major depression and generalized anxiety disorder are at their peak in the year following diagnosis; parents also respond to the diagnosis with a form of post-traumatic stress disorder, twice as commonly in mothers than fathers. The theme of increased psychological problems in mothers, usually the main carers in young people with diabetes, is recurrent. There is little evidence from retrospective studies that psychological events are more frequent in the run-up to clinical diagnosis, but hospital admission or serious illness, unrelated to diabetes, is much more common, a finding that ties in with clinical experience and also with the concept of a physical stressor precipitating the final autoimmune insult to residual β-cell function.

Eating disorders in type 1 diabetes (Box 13.1)

These are difficult to diagnose (standard questionnaires are too complicated for routine use), but repeated sensitive questioning based on the clues in the box may help. Formally diagnosed eating disorders are rare in type 1 diabetes, but they carry a high mortality and are frequently associated with characteristic advanced complications, especially retinopathy, peripheral neuropathy (though rarely with foot ulceration) and visceral

---

Box 13.1 Clinical features of eating disorders in type 1 diabetes

Anorexia and bulimia

'Classical' eating disorders (anorexia and bulimia) are rare, but when anorexia occurs it carries a high mortality (e.g. one-third at 12 years).

Disordered eating

Most eating disorders in type 1 diabetes should be considered 'disordered eating', with the following features:
- Dieting and strenuous exercise for weight control
- Insulin omission for weight loss
- Self-induced vomiting and laxative use are uncommon
- HbA_{1c} usually 1–2% higher in those with disordered eating

Binge eating disorder

Binge eating disorder, short of bulimia, is common. Clues include:
- Excessive concerns about body shape and weight
- Extreme exercising
- Recurrent DKA
- Amenorrhoea
- Unusually elevated HbA_{1c} levels
- Increased levels of depression, diminished self-worth over physical appearance and increasing body weight may predict disturbed eating behaviour

Source: after Goebbel-Fabbri *et al.* [1,2]

autonomic neuropathy, especially gastroparesis. Because of the very poor control often associated with gastroparesis (see Chapter 10) this is likely to be a factor accelerating the progression of other microvascular complications. Disordered eating behaviour is much more common than formal eating disorders.

Insulin omission

Missing insulin is an early learned method for weight control and loss, and repeated sensitive questioning is required to assess it in individuals. Nearly 40% of patients between 15 and 30 years old report intentional insulin omission. Overall, up to age 60, one-third omit insulin, and it is surprisingly common even in older women aged between 45 and 60. More extreme omission, effectively stopping insulin treatment entirely for up to 2 weeks at a time, is common during adolescence and early adulthood. Taking more daily injections is associated with insulin omission – again no surprise – so there is no point suggesting more injections for people in poor control if the current injections are not being taken. Try to fix the underlying problem first.

'Brittle' diabetes

A controversial and fortunately uncommon disorder, described especially in the UK and USA, usually occurring in young women, with onset at puberty, and defined as a patient whose life is 'constantly disrupted by episodes of hypo- or hyperglycaemia, whatever their cause' [3]. Its characteristics are unstable glycaemic control not responding to intensive management, recurrent hospital admissions (predominantly either hypoglycaemia or DKA), high insulin requirements, overweight, long-term oligomenorrhoea/amenorrhoea, major psychiatric problems and severe family disruption. Eating disorders and gastroparesis add to the distressing and difficult mix [4]. Variants are described in males, though much less frequently, and also in the elderly, where psychosocial factors are not nearly as conspicuous. Where implantable pumps have been used, insulin requirements appear to be unexceptional, and insulin manipulation is often suspected and documented. Severe microvascular complications, poor pregnancy outcomes and possibly an increased risk of death are associated with this most taxing and stressful clinical situation. Fortunately, the syndrome usually seems to remit by the early thirties. Intensive medical, educational and psychological support is required during the long interim period.

Quality of life in adolescence and young adults

Overall measures of quality of life are reduced in adolescents, though specific domains (e.g. formation of close personal relationships) show great variability. Girls, single-parent families and ethnic minorities have depressed quality-of-life measures (and worse HbA_{1c}), and it has been suggested that targeting these groups with repeated quality-of-life questionnaires and subsequent discussion of the results may be helpful, though no change in HbA_{1c} should be expected [5].

The intensive commitment required to participate in the DCCT (1993) was associated with lower quality of life, despite improved HbA_{1c} levels, but studies in situations without such intensively enforced adherence have consistently shown an association between higher quality of life and better glycaemic control and lower HbA_{1c}, though the causal direction is not clear. In general, as expected, well-functioning family units, with high cohesion, good organization and an affective environment, are beneficial and, conversely, poorer psychosocial environments (e.g. single parenthood, lower income, ethnic minority status, family dysfunction) are associated with poor glycaemic control and recurrent DKA (Box 13.2). In the 12 years after the onset of type 1 diabetes, young people (average age 21) were 20% more likely to have needed mental health referrals and not to have completed school than non-diabetic people. Mental health care usage was particularly high in the one-third no longer in specialist diabetes care, and not surprisingly glycaemic control was worse. Returning these youngsters to diabetes care services is therefore very important, and primary care teams can play an important part in achieving this [6].

Within a few years of diagnosis, one in five adolescents is probably not attending a hospital clinic. These young people are often not engaging

---

Box 13.2 Aspects of family dynamics impacting on diabetes

- Conflict over specific areas of diabetes management, including insulin administration, but especially blood glucose monitoring, is frequently a focus of disagreement about responsibility.
- Decreasing parental involvement and increasing general disagreements between the person with diabetes and their parents may predict worse glycaemic control.
- Poor parental psychological well-being, especially maternal.
- Having two parents at home is associated with better glycaemic control, but family structure is not related to quality of life.
- Difficulty in establishing a balance between *laissez-faire* and 'helicopter' parenting.
- Obsessive tendencies in parents and/or the young person. This may lead to 'good' HbA_{1c} measurements, but at the cost of anxiety and low mood.

Source: after Cameron *et al.* [7]

with their primary care team either; contributory factors include reluctance to discuss medical matters with professionals much older than they are, and organizational disorder associated with disrupted families and high divorce rates. Transition care from paediatric to adult clinics is often weak, and innovative approaches, for example employing a 'health navigator' in the team, very likely improve outcomes. However, much more is required, and recognition that the adult clinic is a relatively unfriendly place for a young person compared with the paediatric clinic could be a useful starting point for service redesign [8]. The importance of psychological support during the transition phase is universally recognized, but few centres in the UK provide comprehensive services, despite good evidence that they lead to less stress, fewer symptoms and improved glycaemic control.

Interventions

Cognitive behaviour therapy is the most commonly used intervention in young people and their families. Systematic review of this approach showed a modest effect on both glycaemia (HbA_{1c} improved by about 0.5%, 5 mmol/mol) and distress levels; nevertheless these are better outcomes than in adults. Motivational interviewing is relatively new, and seems promising; it is based on counselling that emphasizes facilitating behavioural change. Depression in young people is common, much more prevalent in females, and about two to three times more frequent than in the general population. It runs a more prolonged course, and is prone to recur.

Psychological problems in adults with type 1 diabetes

Relatively little has been written on psychological problems in adults with type 1 diabetes. Depression is common, but predates the onset of late complications. It may share some of the somatic features of poorly controlled diabetes (e.g. fatigue, daytime somnolence, weight loss and waking at night), but enquiring about affective symptoms (low mood, anhedonism, anxiety, shame and fear) should help make the distinction – these factors are more likely to be associated with depression. Patients with complications, for example visual failure, erectile dysfunction and cheiroarthropathy, are likely to be in a self-reinforcing cycle of poor self-care, impelled by depression. Relatively simple interventions may be of value, and have been demonstrated for improved blood pressure control in patients with successfully treated erectile dysfunction. Not surprisingly, once microvascular complications are established, the depression rate further increases twofold to threefold. Nearly one-third of a group of type 1 and 2 patients presenting with a first foot ulcer were considered to have major depression. In this same group, depression was associated with a threefold increased mortality over 18 months compared with those who were not depressed [9]. This dramatic finding hints that there are problems beyond those of self-management, poor adherence and even serious events such as amputation, and changes in the hypothalamic–pituitary–adrenal axis, autonomic neuropathy (itself associated with increased mortality) and cytokine responses may be contributory or even causal. Other studies come to the same conclusion, that hyperglycaemia and depression are linked in type 1 diabetes, but the mediator(s) of the interaction are factors other than poor diabetes self-care behaviours.

Type 2 diabetes

Much of the literature concerns the important problem of type 2 diabetes and depression and, in comparison with type 1 diabetes, little about the psychological disturbances associated with specific phases of type 2 diabetes. However, we are entering an important phase of research in which detailed and validated measures of psychological function are being incorporated into large-scale longitudinal studies investigating earlier phases of diabetes (e.g. Look AHEAD, Diabetes Prevention Program) with much more reliable quantitative outcome data.

Causal link between depression and type 2 diabetes

There has been much debate over whether type 2 diabetes causes depression or, more intriguingly, whether the reverse applies. Until recently the bidirectionality was appreciated but there was no strong evidence to support one model over the other (Table 13.1). Several meta-analyses of longitudinal studies have now concluded that there is a stronger link between baseline depression and incident type 2 diabetes than vice versa (about 40–60% increased risk in the former direction compared with about 15–20% in the latter) [10]. In the period leading up to the diagnosis of type 2 diabetes, patients were twice as likely to be taking antidepressants as control subjects. This finding, that depression itself is a risk factor for the development of type 2 diabetes, is partly, but only partly, supported by the Diabetes Prevention Program (see Chapter 1), in which the diagnosis of diabetes was precisely defined. Elevated depression scores at study entry were not associated with the progression of IGT to diabetes, but in the intensive lifestyle and placebo metformin groups, baseline antidepressant use and continuous antidepressant use during the study was associated with a marked (2–3.5-fold) increased risk of developing diabetes, independent of other risk factors. This suggests that antidepressants themselves may contribute to the development of diabetes, and that metformin treatment prevents it. However, it may be that more severe depression, for which antidepressant use is a marker, is associated with

---

Table 13.1 Factors in the link between depression and type 2 diabetes

Depression predisposing to type 2 diabetes
Decreased physical activity

Increased calorie intake

Central obesity and dysglycaemia

Neuroendocrine changes, e.g. increased sympathetic activity, increased hypothalamic–pituitary–adrenal axis activity, increased levels of proinflammatory
cytokines

Type 2 diabetes predisposing to depression
At diagnosis: increased threat, anxiety and loss

Increasing emphasis on implementing lifestyle changes leads to disruption

---

developing diabetes, as found in the meta-analysis [11]. Details apart, the
message for clinicians is that diagnosed and treated depression are strong
risk factors for diabetes. The diagnosis of type 2 diabetes does not appear
to have a severe psychological impact, other than short-lived anxiety, and
a transient rise in the use of antidepressant medication in the year after
diagnosis.

Other emotional problems in type 2 diabetes

Emerging after diagnosis, generalized anxiety disorder is common
in type 2 (and type 1) diabetes, estimated at about 40% in both conditions, significantly more frequent in women. The relationship between
anxiety and poor glycaemic control is statistically significant. Diabetes-
specific emotional problems are common (notably worry about the
future, the possibility of serious complications, guilt or anxiety when
straying from recommendations about management, and concern that
mood or feelings are related to blood glucose levels). These concerns, particularly perception of disease severity and worry about the burden of
self-care, are more common among insulin-treated patients than in non-
insulin-treated patients, but there are no differences between tablet- and
diet-treated patients. It will be interesting to see what impact the concerns
about insulin treatment itself have in comparison with the new injected
GLP-1 analogues. The prevalence of diabetes-specific distress increases
with severity of depression.

There is a disconnection between the frequently reported improvement in quality of life seen with insulin treatment in type 2 diabetes and
the finding that patients report greater distress with insulin treatment

than with either diet alone or oral hypoglycaemic agents. The difference is explained by the *improvement* in symptoms with initiating insulin treatment compared with the long-term distress of insulin-treated patients. However, much of the difference is explained by more advanced disease associated with insulin treatment and greater expected burden of self-care. Nevertheless, other treatment modalities carry their own sources of distress, especially acceptance of the condition in those treated with diet and oral hypoglycaemic agents; diet-treated patients are distressed by unclear management goals [12].

Associations with depression in type 2 diabetes

In the Look AHEAD study, about 15% had symptoms of mild–moderate depression, about 17% were current users of antidepressant medication, and about 4% both [13]. Other studies in the USA have described higher rates, up to 25%, of more severe depression, with all ethnic groups (white, African-American, Latinos and others) recording similar rates. Not surprisingly, depression in diabetes is associated with non-adherence to diabetes self-care (this applies to type 1 as well); although a wide variety of behaviours has been studied (including diet, medication and glucose monitoring), the most consistent association is with missed medical appointments, and impaired interpersonal functioning in depressed people may be an important mediator of this behaviour. Once again, there is difficulty in ascribing a causal association (though it might seem self-evident) between depression and impaired diabetes self-care, never mind a direction of causality, but a longitudinal study found that worsening levels of self-care and depression were associated with baseline depression in type 2 diabetes.

In Look AHEAD, depression scores and use of antidepressant medication were independently associated with:
• hypertension and use of antihypertensive medication;
• current smoking;
• obesity;
• lower peak exercise activity.
Again, the management corollary of these unspectacular findings is important: identification of clusters of these factors should be an alert to the presence of depression. In established neuropathy, neurological disability predicts increased depressive symptoms; slightly more counterintuitively, depression was most strongly linked with the symptom of unsteadiness, an important factor limiting a wide spectrum of activities and resulting in diminished self-worth.

There are clearly barriers to identifying depression in those who are most likely to suffer it, namely those with more chronic complications. Biomedical priorities and targets steer the time-limited agenda of a medical consultation, and in primary care (and possibly even more likely in secondary care) the greater the number of medical comorbidities, the less likely depression will be recognized.

Interventions in depression in type 2 diabetes

Many psychological interventions have been described (especially group cognitive behaviour therapy, but also stress management, relaxation therapy and individual cognitive behaviour therapy). A meta-analysis of 12 trials that measured HbA_{1c} over a period of usually up to 6 months found that intervention was associated with a significant fall in HbA_{1c} of 0.76%, but it was not possible to determine which intervention method was most successful nor how the various treatments exerted their effect. Psychological treatments seem to be of real value, and about twice as effective as antidepressants in inducing remission in a major depressive illness, though long-term effects are not known [14]. Inevitably, not all studies have found that glycaemic control improved with even enhanced antidepressant therapy (psychological or pharmacological), but improved glucose control cannot reasonably be required to be a primary outcome of a therapy intended to alleviate a psychological problem. There is a hint that interventions designed to manage depressive symptoms may be more effective in improving self-care than those that reduce distress. Patients report a high degree of satisfaction (60–80%) with all modalities of treatment (antidepressants, mental health provider, alternative healers) [15].

In the short-term, antidepressant treatment (e.g. tricyclics, SSRIs and SNRIs) is reasonably effective, but increases the likelihood of recovery from the index episode of depression by only 20–30%; sertraline has no effect beyond placebo in those over 55 years old, and those with higher pain scores had a particularly poor response. The long-term outlook is poor. Fewer than 50% of patients remained well in the year after treatment, about 15% develop chronic depression resistant to current treatments, a high proportion relapse as often as once a year, and very few remain free of depression in the following 5 years. Depression treated with antidepressants seems to correspond reasonably well with glycaemia, improving with treatment and deteriorating with relapse, and maintenance antidepressant treatment is more effective than placebo in deferring relapse.

The important Pathway study (2006) found that patients (nearly all type 2) with two or more chronic complications of diabetes benefited over a year with a comprehensive depression care pathway compared with usual care. The intervention was intensive, involving primary care physicians, nurse specialists in depression management, and an initial strategy (according to patients' wishes) of either antidepressant therapy or sessions of problem-solving therapy. Routine and intensive input were equally effective in those with fewer complications, but patients with one or more macrovascular complications seemed to do especially well [16]. The forthcoming TEAMcare study will further explore a comprehensive biopsychosocial intervention programme in patients with depression, and poor diabetes control with or without coronary heart disease.

References

1. Goebbel-Fabbri AE, Fikkan J, Connell A, Vangsness L, Anderson BJ. Identification and treatment of eating disorders in women with type 1 diabetes mellitus. *Treat Endocrinol* 2002;1:155–62. PMID: 15799208.
2. Goebbel-Fabbri AE, Fikkan J, Franko DL, Pearson K, Anderson BJ, Weinger K. Insulin restriction and associated morbidity and mortality in women with type 1 diabetes. *Diabetes Care* 2008;31:415–19. PMID: 18070998.
3. Tattersall RB. Brittle diabetes revisited: the Third Arnold Bloom Memorial Lecture. *Diabetic Med* 1997;14:99–110. PMID: 9047086.
4. Saunders SA, Williams G. Difficult diabetes. In: DeFronzo R, Ferrannini E, Keen H, Zimmet P (eds) *International Textbook of Diabetes Mellitus*, 3rd edn, chapter 87. Oxford: Wiley-Blackwell, 2004.
5. deWit M, Delemaare-van de Waal HA, Bokma JA *et al.* Monitoring and discussing health-related quality of life in adolescents with type 1 diabetes improve psychological well-being: a randomized controlled trial. *Diabetes Care* 2008;31:1521–6. PMID: 1850924.
6. Northam EA, Lin A, Finch S, Werther GA, Cameron FJ. Psychosocial well-being and functional outcomes in youth with type 1 diabetes 12 years after disease onset. *Diabetes Care* 2010;33:1430–7. PMID: 20357379.
7. Cameron FJ, Northam EA, Ambler GR, Daneman D. Routine psychological screening in youth with type 1 diabetes and their parents: a notion whose time has come? *Diabetes Care* 2007;30:2716–24. PMID: 17644619.
8. Weissberg-Benchell J, Wolpert H, Anderson BJ. Transitioning from pediatric to adult care: a new approach to the post-adolescent young person with type 1 diabetes. *Diabetes Care* 2007;30:2441–6. PMID: 17666466.
9. Ismail K, Winkley K, Stahil D, Chalder T, Edmonds M. A cohort study of people with diabetes and their first foot ulcer: the role of depression on mortality. *Diabetes Care* 2007;30:1473–9. PMID: 17363754.
10. Mezuk B, Eaton WW, Albrecht S, Golden SH. Depression and type 2 diabetes over the lifespan: a meta-analysis. *Diabetes Care* 2008;31:2383–90. PMID: 19033418.
11. Rubin RR, Ma Y, Marrero DG *et al.* Elevated depression symptoms, antidepressant medicine use, and risk of developing diabetes during the Diabetes Prevention Program. *Diabetes Care* 2008;31:420–6. PMID: 18071002.
12. Delahanty LM, Grant RW, Wittenberg E *et al.* Association of diabetes-related emotional distress with diabetes treatment in primary care patients with type 2 diabetes. *Diabetic Med* 2007;24:48–54. PMID: 17227324.
13. Rubin RR, Gaussoin SA, Peyrot M *et al.* Cardiovascular disease risk factors, depression symptoms and antidepressant medicine use in the Look AHEAD (Action for Health in Diabetes) clinical trial of weight loss in diabetes. *Diabetologia* 2010;53:1581–9. PMID: 20422396.
14. Jenkins DJ. Psychological, physiological, and drug interventions for type 2 diabetes. *Lancet* 2004;363:1569–70. PMID: 15145627.

15. De Groot M, Pinkerman B, Wagner J, Hockman E. Depression treatment and satisfaction in a multicultural sample of type 1 and type 2 diabetic patients. *Diabetes Care* 2006;29:549–53. PMID: 16505504.
16. Kinder LS, Katon WJ, Ludman E *et al.* Improving depression care in patients with diabetes and multiple complications. *J Gen Intern Med* 2006;21:1036–41. PMID: 16836628.

Further reading

Anderson BJ, Rubin RR (eds) *Practical Psychology for Diabetes Clinicians*, 2nd revised edn. Alexandria, VA: American Diabetes Association, 2002.

Lustman PJ, Penckofer SM, Clouse RE. Recent advances in understanding depression in adults with diabetes. *Curr Psychiatry Rep* 2008;10:495–502. PMID: 18980733.

Petrak F, Herpertz S. Treatment of depression in diabetes: an update. *Curr Opin Psychiatry* 2009;22:211–17. PMID: 19553878.

Pouwer F. Should we screen for emotional distress in type 2 diabetes mellitus? *Nat Rev Endocrinol* 2009;5:665–71. PMID: 19884900.

Young-Hyman DL, Davis CL. Disordered eating behaviour in individuals with diabetes: importance of context, evaluation, and classification. *Diabetes Care* 2010;33:683–9. PMID: 20190297.

Index

Abbott, 27, 31, 78
abdominal infections, 146
abdominal pain, in hyperglycaemic
    emergencies, 28
acarbose, 17, 93, 117
ACCORD, 40, 204, 219, 228, 231, 233
ACCORD Eye, 188, 189, 190, 281
ACE-i and ARB treatment, 173, 244
ACE-i/calcium-channel blocker (CCB)
    combination, 243
ACE inhibitors, 17, 38, 54, 172, 219,
    244–7
ACE-i/thiazide combination, 241, 242,
    243, 249, 252, 254, 268
acetoacetate, 26–7
acetone, 26, 27
Actrapid, 31, 70
acute coronary syndromes (ACS), 48
    CABG, 51–2
    diabetes prevalence, 49
    diabetes status identification, 49
    glycaemic control, 49–51
    PCI in, 51
    post-coronary interventions, 52–4
acute diabetic foot, 44–5, 210
acute pancreatitis, 28, 121, 268
Addison's disease, 6, 37, 77
adult-onset diabetes mellitus, *see* type 2
    diabetes
ADVANCE trial, 95, 98
advanced diabetic eye disease, 192–3
albiglutide, 124
albumin excretion, *see* urinary albumin
    excretion
albuminuria, 167
    definitions of, 164
alcohol, 26, 41, 199, 286
    intake limit, 238, 239
aliskiren, 173
alpha-blocking agents, 255

α-glucosidase inhibitors, 117, 135
alprostadil, 223
ambulatory blood pressure monitoring
    (ABPM), 227, 236, 237, 238
amiloride, 243, 253, 259
amiodarone, 278
amitriptyline, 214, 215
amlodipine, 172, 243, 246, 248, 250, 253
amoxicillin, 143, 149
AMP-activated protein kinase (AMPK),
    104
ampicillin, 149
anaemia, 115, 170, 177–8
anaerobes, 147, 152
anaerobic streptococci, 147
angiotensin blockade, 156, 165, 166,
    169, 171, 243
    ACE inhibitors, 244–7
    ACE-i versus ARB, 244
    angiotensin receptor blockers,
        247–8
angiotensin blocker treatment, 189, 231
    and blood pressure, 189
angiotensin receptor blockers (ARBs), 17,
    243, 247–8
ankle–brachial pressure index, 207
anorexia, 211, 218, 291
antiepileptic drugs, 215
antihypertensive agents, 92, 172, 220,
    249, 253, 255, 268
    ranking, value of, 238–9
anti-obesity agents, 88–9
apolipoprotein B, 158, 264
aspirin, 38, 54, 166, 189–90, 239, 241
asymptomatic bacteriuria, 142–3
atenolol, 244, 251
atorvastatin, 54, 175, 190, 193, 272, 273,
    274, 275, 276, 278, 279
atrial fibrillation, 54
autoimmune hepatitis, 6